VITILIGO

This monograph on vitiligo is dedicated to
Dr Taeha Woo, a pioneer for Korean dermatology,
who encouraged, motivated and supported the editors
in the preparation of this book.

VITILIGO

A MONOGRAPH ON THE BASIC AND CLINICAL SCIENCE

EDITED BY

SEUNG-KYUNG HANN MD
Department of Dermatology
Yonsei University College of Medicine
Seoul, Korea

AND

JAMES J. NORDLUND MD
Department of Dermatology
University of Cincinnati College of Medicine
Cincinnati, Ohio, USA

FOREWORD BY

AARON B. LERNER
Professor, Department of Dermatology
Yale University College of Medicine
New Haven, Connecticut, USA

Blackwell
Science

Editorial Offices:
Osney Mead, Oxford OX2 0EL
25 John Street, London WC1N 2BL
23 Ainslie Place, Edinburgh EH3 6AJ
350 Main Street, Malden
MA 02148-5018, USA
54 University Street, Carlton
Victoria 3053, Australia
10, rue Casimir Delavigne
75006 Paris, France

Other Editorial Offices:
Blackwell Wissenschafts-Verlag GmbH
Kurfürstendamm 57
10707 Berlin, Germany

Blackwell Science KK
MG Kodenmacho Building
7–10 Kodenmacho Nihombashi
Chuo-ku, Tokyo 104, Japan

First published 2000

Set by Excel Typesetters Co.,
Hong Kong
Printed and bound in France
by Imprimerie Pollina, Luçon

A catalogue record for this title
is available from the British Library

ISBN 0-632-05071-3

Library of Congress
Cataloging-in-publication Data

Vitiligo / edited by Seung-kyung
Hann, James Nordlund.
p.; cm.
Includes bibliographical references.
ISBN 0-632-05071-3
1. Vitiligo.
I. Hann, Seung-kyung.
II. Nordlund, James J.
[DNLM: 1. Vitiligo—diagnosis.
2. Vitiligo—etiology.
3. Vitiligo—therapy. WR 265
V844 2000]
RL790. V55 2000
616.5′5—dc21

99-046475

DISTRIBUTORS

Marston Book Services Ltd
PO Box 269
Abingdon, Oxon OX14 4YN
(*Orders*: Tel: 01235 465500
Fax: 01235 465555)

USA
Blackwell Science, Inc.
Commerce Place
350 Main Street
Malden, MA 02148-5018
(*Orders*: Tel: 800 759 6102
781 388 8250
Fax: 781 388 8255)

Canada
Login Brothers Book Company
324 Saulteaux Crescent
Winnipeg, Manitoba R3J 3T2
(*Orders*: Tel: 204 837 2987)

Australia
Blackwell Science Pty Ltd
54 University Street
Carlton, Victoria 3053
(*Orders*: Tel: 3 9347 0300
Fax: 3 9347 5001)

For further information on
Blackwell Science, visit our website:
www.blackwell-science.com

Contents

List of Contributors

DANIEL M. ALBERT, MD *Department of Ophthalmology and Visual Science, University of Wisconsin*

WAYNE D. BEAZLEY, BSc *Clinical and Experimental Dermatology, Department of Biomedical Sciences, University of Bradford, Bradford, BD7 1DP*

MAVIS BILLIPS, MD *Suite 617, 321 North Larchmont Blvd, Los Angeles, CA 90020*

RAYMOND E. BOISSY, PhD *Department of Dermatology, University of Cincinnati College of Medicine, 231, Bethesda Avenue, ML-0592, Cincinnati, OH 45267-0592*

JEAN-CLAUDE BYSTRYN, MD *The Ronald O. Perelman Department of Dermatology, New York University School of Medicine, 560, First Avenue, New York, NY 10016*

WOO-HYUNG CHUN, MD *Department of Dermatology, Yonsei University College of Medicine, CPO Box 8044, Seoul, Korea*

JIAN CUI, MD, PhD *Ronald O. Perelman Department of Dermatology, New York University School of Medicine, 560, First Avenue, New York, NY 10016*

RAFAEL FALABELLA, MD *Universidad del Valle, Facultad de Salud, Departmento de Dermatologia, Apartado Aereo 253600, Cali, Colombia*

PEARL E. GRIMES, MD *Suite 617, 321, North Larchmont Blvd, Los Angeles, CA 90020*

REBAT M. HALDER, MD *Department of Dermatology, Howard University College of Medicine, 2041 Georgia Avenue, NW Washington, DC 20060*

SEUNG-KYUNG HANN, MD *Department of Dermatology, Yonsei University College of Medicine, CPO Box 8044, Seoul, Korea*

SUNGBIN IM, MD *Department of Dermatology, Ajou University School of Medicine, 5 Wonchon-dong, Paldal-ku, Suwon, 442-721, Korea*

DAISY KOPERA, MD *Department of Dermatology, University of Graz, Auenbruggerplatz 8, A-8036 Graz, Austria*

LYNN LAMOREUX, PhD *Department of Vetrinary Pathobiology, Texas A&M University, College Station, TX 77843-4463*

PARTHA P. MAJUMDER *Anthropology and Human Genetics Unit, Indian Statistical Institute, 203 B. T. Road, Calcutta 700 035, India*

MONTE D. MILLS, MD *Department of Ophthalmology and Visual Science, University of Wisconsin Medical School*

LEIGH MIYAMOTO, MD *Department of Dermatology, Cleveland Clinic Foundation, 9500 Euclid Avenue, Cleveland, OH 44195–5032*

JEREMY MOORE, PhD *Clinical and Experimental Dermatology, Department of Biomedical Sciences, University of Bradford, Bradford, BD7 1DP*

WARWICK L. MORISON, MD *Department of Dermatology, John Hopkins University, Baltimore, MD*

JAMES J. NORDLUND, MD *Department of Dermatology, University of Cincinnati, Cincinnati, OH 45267-0592*

GIOVANNI E. ORECCHIA, MD *Clinica Dermatologica, IRCCS S. Matteo, P.le Golgi 2, 27100 Pavia, Italy*

JEAN-PAUL ORTONNE, MD *Hôpital L'Archet 2, Department of Dermatology, BP79, Nice Cedex 3, France 06202*

JUDITH PORTER, *Department of Sociology, Bryn Mawr College, Bryn Mawr, Pennsylvania*

KARIN U. SCHALLREUTER, MD *Clinical and Experimental Dermatology, Department of Biomedical Sciences, University of Bradford, UK and Institute for Plymentary Disorders in association with E.M. Arndt, University of Greifswald, 17489 Greifswald, Germany*

PRANAV B. SHETH, MD *Department of Dermatology, University of Cincinnati, PO Box 670592, Cincinnati, OH 45267-0592*

JAMES S. TAYLOR, MD *Section of Industrial Dermatology, Department of Dermatology, Cleveland Clinic Foundation, 9500 Euclid Avenue, Cleveland, OH 44195*

JOHN M. WOOD, PhD *Clinical and Experimental Dermatology, Department of Biomedical Sciences, University of Bradford, Bradford, BD7 1DP*

Foreword

Knowing how most victims of vitiligo feel about their disfigurement, and knowing the relationship between vitiligo and disorders of immunity and melanoma, my major goal has been to make vitiligo a 'real disease'. That is, to make it a disorder important to both patients and physicians. Vitiligo is always of major significance to patients who have it, in contrast to the indifference of many physicians. This timely and comprehensive monograph by Drs Hann and Nordlund is of great help. Many aspects of the basic biology of pigment cells, as they relate to vitiligo, are reviewed by 27 authors. The history of vitiligo, the hypotheses of melanocyte destruction, the treatment of patients and many other topics are well covered in this book. For those interested in vitiligo, it is essential to have this book.

More than 20 years ago, I wrote a review article entitled *Vitiligo: What is it? Is it important?* The answer is yes. Vitiligo is important. Knowing more about the processes involved in the destruction of pigment cells as they occur in vitiligo will not only provide us with a method to stop the spread of vitiligo, but also help us to know more about autoimmunity and ways to control melanomas. Vitiligo is a real disease.

Aaaron B. Lerner

Preface

Vitiligo is an enigmatic disorder and thus fascinating to dermatologists, pigment cell biologists and to others who love biology. That the disorder can destroy melanocytes in the interfollicular epidermis, in the eyes, and possibly the ears but spare those melanocytes in the hair follicle is a remarkable phenomenon. Equally bizarre is the observation that vitiligo can be spreading in one area of the integument while melanocytes are proliferating in other areas and repigmenting the skin. How the pathogenic mechanisms can be active in one site while inactive in other sites is puzzling indeed.

Depigmentation is common in the animal kingdom, especially notable in the mammalian species. There are many types of pigment loss, many of which resemble vitiligo and from which we all can learn much about the pigmentary system. It is especially mystifying that melanomas, an uncontrolled proliferation of melanocytes, can be associated with destruction of melanocytes in skin surrounding the cancer or at distal sites, although this type of pigmentary loss might be different from classical vitiligo. And that depigmented halos occur around naevi, angiomata and other cutaneous structures is well known but a phenomenon for which there is no explanation.

This monograph is intended to bring these and related topics into a single repository for dermatologists and other biologists. In addition it is the hope that a review of the pathogenic mechanisms might be a stimulus to others to become interested in and investigate this disorder so prevalent world wide. The chapters on therapy are intended to assist the practitioner in gaining sufficient expertise to care for those with vitiligo but the principles of treating vitiligo should be applicable to many other types of skin disorders as well.

Finally, it is the hope of the editors that this volume can be revised and updated every five years because of the profusion of new information that becomes available from scientists and clinicians from around the world as an indicator that the dermatological world is closer to solving the problem of vitiligo and its treatment.

The editors wish to acknowledge the critical role of their teachers and thank them for being a stimulus for their interest in studying vitiligo and in preparing a monograph on vitiligo. There were special teachers who motivated us to study this disorder, its treatment and other issues related to pigmentation. Drs Taeha Woo and Yoon-Kee Park introduced Dr Hann to the fascination of this mysterious disorder of pigmentation. Dr Aaron Lerner was the inspiration for Dr Nordlund to begin his interest in pigmentation and vitiligo.

We thank all the contributors for their assistance in making this a comprehensive treatise on the basic and clinical science related to vitiligo and other forms of depigmentation.

Acknowledgements

The editors and authors wish to thank Ms Joan Griggs, Mrs Mary Brocker, Mrs Isook Kim, and Mrs Bobbie Lambert without whose help this volume could not have been completed. Their cheerfulness, dedication and efforts made preparation of this monograph a joy.

PART 1
GENERAL TOPICS ABOUT VITILIGO

1: Definition of Vitiligo

SEUNG-KYUNG HANN AND JAMES J. NORDLUND

The definition of vitiligo

Vitiligo is a specific type of leukoderma manifested characteristically by depigmentation of the epidermis. Occasionally the loss of melanin is partial, i.e. hypopigmentation. Vitiligo is best defined as an acquired, progressive disorder that selectively destroys (or that results in the selective disappearance) of some or all melanocytes residing in the interfollicular epidermis and occasionally in the hair follicles as well. The mechanism(s) by which the melanocytes are lost (or by which melanocytes are made to disappear) may be multiple but is not yet identified unequivocally.

Clinically vitiligo is characterized by white macules on the skin that can be few or many in number. The depigmentation can be localized, moderate in extent or wide spread, even resulting in a complete loss of all interfollicular melanocytes. Very rarely all melanocytes in both the interfollicular and follicular epidermis are destroyed. Such individuals will have entirely white skin and hair.

There are several clinical types of vitiligo. The unilateral (segmental) form usually does not cross the midline and does not have a classical dermatomal distribution but affects one segment of the integument. The segment might be composed of several or parts of several adjacent dermatomes or have no relationship to dermatomes at all. The progression is usually limited to months or a few years (Barona *et al.* 1995; Hann & Lee 1996).

The bilateral (non-segmental) form is characterized by bilateral, usually symmetrical, depigmented macules. It is further subdivided into a localized form (type), limited to small areas of the integument, and into the generalized type. The latter is characterized by widespread extensive depigmentation that most commonly spreads throughout the life of the individual. In addition there is a very rare variety of generalized vitiligo that seems to be a manifestation of a systemic autoimmune disease. This disorder is manifested by vitiligo, as well as multiple endocrine failures such as diabetes mellitus, adrenal insufficiency, thyroid dysfunction and gonadal dysfunction. All of the latter endocrine abnormalities seem to be caused by autoantibodies but the cause of the loss of melanocytes remains unidentified.

Persisting enigmas about vitiligo

Much clinical and basic research on vitiligo has been done and new concepts have been developed. Therefore, a new definition of vitiligo should be made in accordance with the new concepts. In order to make a new definition, some controversies concerning the definition or nomenclature of vitiligo should be discussed.

One very important question is whether vitiligo is only a cutaneous pigmentary disorder or a systemic disorder of the pigmentary system. The pigmentary system of the ears and eyes shows degenerative changes in some patients with vitiligo. Discrete areas of depigmentation, with associated pigment hyperplasia involving the choroid and retinal pigment epithelium as well as active uveitis, have been observed in as many as 40% of patients with vitiligo (Albert *et al.* 1979, 1983). Vitiligo patients exhibit some audiologic abnormalities such as sensorineural hypoacusis, which may be related to involvement of the inner ear melanocytes (Tosti *et al.* 1987). Because most patients with vitiligo who have audiological and ophthalmological changes are usually free of symptoms or have vague complaints, involvement of melanocytes in the extracutaneous parts of the body is easily overlooked. Vogt–Koyanagi–Harada and the Alezzandrini syndromes might be the most severe examples of vitiligo of the skin and the pigment system of the eyes. Most investigators consider the Vogt–Koyanagi–Harada and Alezzandrini syndromes to be different diseases to vitiligo.

A second question is whether chemical depigmentation or occupational depigmentation, which occurs following contact with a phenolic compound or monobenzyl ether of hydroquinone, is in fact vitiligo with a known precipitating cause or some other depigmenting disorder. In our opinion, they are different disorders because chemical and occupational depigmentation tend to be limited to sites of exposure to the melanocytotoxic material. In addition, the clinical course of depigmentation differs. Vitiligo tends to be progressive throughout the life of affected individuals. In contrast, chemical depigmentation usually stops spreading after the offending agent is removed. We propose separating vitiligo vulgaris from chemical and occupational leukoderma until there is definitive data to show the two disorders have a common pathogenesis.

A third question that must be addressed is whether halo naevi are a form of vitiligo. The answer is unknown. Both halo naevi and vitiligo vulgaris are common in children and teenagers. However, there are striking differences between vitiligo and halo naevi. Halo naevi tend to have spontaneous repigmentation. They do not tend to enlarge by centrifugal spread without limit nor do they progress over the whole body. It is our opinion that halo naevi associated with vitiligo are an example of common abnormalities occurring together.

A fourth question that must be addressed is whether grey hair or white hair are a form of vitiligo. Grey hair is the ageing of melanocytes of hair follicles, a process that is associated with interruption of melanogenesis. In contrast, white hair usually means a complete absence of melanocytes from the papilla of the hair follicle. White hair is classified into two types. One is genetic or familial and is a rather common cause of total loss of pigment of the scalp hair in younger adults in the third and fourth decade of life. It is our opinion that this type of depigmentation of the hair is not the same disorder as vitiligo vulgaris and the two forms of depigmentation should be distinguished. The other type of complete white hair of the scalp is uncommon but is associated with vitiligo. White hair is often accompanied by interfollicular depigmentation especially when it is associated with vitiligo. It seems likely that loss of melanocytes in the follicles of those with vitiligo represents the same destructive process active within the hair bulb.

A fifth issue is the association of depigmentation with other disorders. Depigmentation can occur on normal skin or on lesions of patients with malignant melanoma (Koh *et al.* 1983; Nordlund *et al.* 1983). Depigmentation in patients with metastatic melanoma is a surprisingly common and striking phenomenon. It has been suggested that it might represent a good prognostic sign for those with metastatic melanoma (Nordlund *et al.* 1983). The distribution of depigmentation associated with melanoma is different from that of vitiligo. Depigmentation begins as small, round macules which are most prominent on the chest and upper back. It is our opinion that depigmentation associated with melanoma should be distinguished from vitiligo.

In conclusion, vitiligo is a type of leukoderma that should be defined as an acquired, progressive depigmentation with unpredictable course. It classically involves integument and probably affects the pigmentary system of other organs. Other forms of leukoderma should be distinguished from vitiligo until more information is available about their pathogenesis, and these disorders labelled as specific forms of depigmentation such as chemical or occupational depigmentation or depigmentation associated with melanoma.

References

Albert, D.M., Nordlund, J.J. & Lerner, A.B. (1979) Ocular abnormalities occurring with vitiligo. *Ophthalmology* **86**, 1145–1160.

Albert, D.M., Wagoner, M.D., Pruett, R.C., Nordlund, J.J. & Lerner, A.B. (1983) Vitiligo and disorders of retinal pigment epithelium. *British Journal of Dermatology* **67**, 153–156.

Barona, M.I., Arrunategui, A., Falabella, R. & Alzate, A. (1995) An epidemiological case-control study in a population with vitiligo. *Journal of the American Academy of Dermatology* **33**, 621–625.

Hann, S.K. & Lee, H.J. (1996) Segmental vitiligo: clinical findings in 208 patients. *Journal of the American Academy of Dermatology* **35**, 671–674.

Koh, H.K., Sober, A.J. *et al.* (1983) Malignant melanoma and vitiligo-like leukoderma: an electron microscopic study. *Journal of the American Academy of Dermatology* **9**, 696–708.

Nordlund, J.J., Kirkwood, J.M., Forget, B.M., Milton, G., Albert, D.M. & Lerner, A.B.

(1983) Vitiligo associated with melanoma: a good prognostic sign. *Journal of the American Academy of Dermatology* **9**, 689–696.

Tosti, A., Bardazzi, F., Tosti, G. & Monti, L. (1987) Audiologic abnormalities in cases of vitiligo. *Journal of the American Academy of Dermatology* **17**, 230–233.

2: The Loss of Melanocytes from the Epidermis: the Mechanism for Depigmentation of Vitiligo Vulgaris

JAMES J. NORDLUND

Patients with vitiligo note the loss of colour from their skin when the disorder first begins or spreads. Melanin is synthesized within the melanocytes and later transferred to surrounding keratinocytes. The colour of the skin is determined to a large extent by the amount and type of melanin within the epidermis (Nordlund *et al.* 1998). There are two mechanisms by which the melanin might disappear from the skin and the skin turn white. The first is dysfunction of the melanocytes, the second is loss of the melanocytes themselves. There are many examples of both types of mechanism being involved in various abnormalities of skin colour (Nordlund *et al.* 1998).

Albinism is a disorder characterized by genetic defects that partially or completely impede the synthesis of melanin. The number of melanocytes in the epidermis of an albino is the same as that in a normally pigmented person, only the machinery for the production of melanin is defective. The skin of an albino can have varying amounts of colour, from virtually no melanin (the classical tyrosinase negative albino) to moderate amounts of melanin in all three forms of oculocutaneous albinism (King 1998). Other disorders of hypopigmentation that are caused by a defect in melanin production or transfer include the Chediak–Higashi syndrome, Hermansky–Pudlak syndrome, the Angelman and Prader–Willi syndrome (reviewed in Nordlund *et al.* 1998).

The other mechanism for absence of melanin from the epidermis is a deficiency of melanocytes. Melanocytes can be absent from the epidermis at the time of birth or can be lost later in life. Absence of melanocytes from the epidermis at birth is called piebaldism, a term that means white striped. Such individuals usually have a family history of white macules present from birth. During embryogenesis melanocytes fail to complete their migration from the neural crest to the epidermis (Spritz 1998). As a result there are no melanocytes in the interfollicular or follicular epidermis and the skin and hair are completely white.

In contrast, some individuals acquire white macules on the skin after birth from the condition vitiligo vulgaris. In general most investigators have concluded that the white macules characteristic of vitiligo are a manifestation of loss of melanocytes. There are numerous data upon which this conclusion is based. However, it is not easily proven beyond doubt that melanocytes are absent from the epidermis. A few investigators have recently proposed that melanocytes remain in the skin but become dysfunctional due to biochemical defects (Schallreuter *et al.* 1994a, b, c).We present here the data which make us conclude that the depigmentation observed in patients with vitiligo is a result of loss of melanocytes from the epidermis.

Histological studies

There have been a number of studies reported in which investigators examined the skin of vitiligo lesions for persistence of melanocytes. Some melanocytes can be found in epidermis of early lesions (Galadari *et al.* 1993) that are only partially depigmented and in which some colour persists. In late lesions that were totally depigmented, there was complete absence of melanocytes by light or electron microscopy (Bleehen 1976; Morohashi *et al.* 1977; Ortonne *et al.* 1979, 1980; Moellmann *et al.* 1982; Galadari *et al.* 1993; Arrunategui *et al.* 1994). These studies have been confirmed by more recent studies in which the investigator utilized a series of fluorescent tagged antibodies directed against a battery of antigens on the surface molecules on melanocytes (Le Poole *et al.* 1993). The antibodies failed to identify mature or immature melanocytes in the depigmented skin from patients with vitiligo. The results of these studies confirm those of prior studies (see Chapter 5).

Melanocyte cultures

Several investigators have noted that the melanocytes from an individual with vitiligo exhibit abnormal behaviour in culture, an indication that the cells are intrinsically abnormal (Puri *et al.* 1987, 1989; Ramaiah *et al.* 1989; Boissy *et al.* 1991a, b). The unidentified abnormality makes the culture of melanocytes from individuals with vitiligo difficult. This problem recently has been solved (Medrano & Nordlund 1990). Using the techniques described by the latter investigators, others have attempted to culture melanocytes from the depigmented patches of vitiligo. The attempts were unsuccessful (R. Boissy, personal communication), a result that supports the absence of melanocytes rather than dedifferentiation or dysfunction of melanocytes.

Response to therapy

Possibly the strongest evidence that melanocytes are, in fact, truly absent from the epidermis in the depigmented skin of vitiligo is the response to medical and surgical therapies. Medical therapies like psoralen with long wavelength ultraviolet light (PUVA) or topically applied steroids presumably rely on pre-existing melanocytes in the follicular apparatus to repigment the skin. The reservoir for melanocytes seems to reside in the hair follicle (reviewed in Nordlund & Ortonne 1998 and Dourmishev *et al.* 1982; Cui *et al.* 1991; Arrunategui *et al.* 1994, see Chapter 20). Glabrous skin which is, by definition, devoid of hair follicles is found on the palms, soles, tips of the fingers and toes, the genitalia and the lips. It is well known that depigmented patches of vitiligo on glabrous skin do not respond to medical therapies for vitiligo. There should be no difference in response to therapy between the glabrous and nonglabrous skin if melanocytes persisted in the vitiligo patches and the melanocyte reservoir were unnecessary.

It also has been observed that hair-bearing skin in which the hair is white (not grey) also does not respond to medical therapies like PUVA or topically applied steroids. This response is in contrast to skin with pigmented hairs that commonly, although not always, responds to treatments like PUVA (Nordlund & Ortonne 1998) (see Chapter 21). It is common to observe white hairs in segmental vitiligo (personal observation), possibly the reason why segmental vitiligo often is resistant to medical therapies (Koga 1977; Falabella 1983; Behl 1985; Koga & Tango 1988; Ando *et al.* 1993). In addition, results of several studies have demonstrated that when skin does respond to therapy with PUVA or topical steroids, the melanocytes migrate from the hair follicle (Ortonne *et al.* 1979, 1980; Cui *et al.* 1991). That pigmented hairs are required for vitiligo skin to repigment strongly supports the conclusion that melanocytes are absent from the depigmented skin.

Finally, vitiligo patches that do not respond to medical therapies can be repigmented surgically (see Chapter 24). The successful use of autografts of various types to repigment depigmented skin indicates that the epidermis is capable of supporting a population of visible, identifiable and functioning melanocytes. There are numerous successful techniques to transplant autologous melanocytes from one site on the integument to another (Behl & Bhatia 1973; Bonafe *et al.* 1983; Suvanprakorn *et al.* 1985; Beck & Schmidt 1986; Falabella 1983, 1986, 1988; Koga 1988; Brysk *et al.* 1989; Gilhar *et al.* 1989; Plott *et al.* 1989; Chitale 1991; Gauthier & Surleve-Bazeille 1992; Zachariae 1994; Agrawal & Agrawal 1995; Boersma *et al.* 1995; Hann *et al.* 1995; Kahn & Cohen 1995). That surgical techniques repigment skin when medical therapies are unsuccessful can be interpreted to indicate that there is no factor produced by the keratinocytes that is responsible for dedifferentiating melanocytes. If the keratinocytes were masking (without killing) melanocytes, then surgical therapies should be no more successful than medical therapies. Surgical therapies are a simple but neat method to replace a missing reservoir.

The data presented in this chapter all support only one conclusion, i.e. that the white skin of vitiligo is characterized by the loss of melanocytes from the epidermis. In this monograph, this conclusion will be the basis for many comments and recommendations.

References

Agrawal, K. & Agrawal, A. (1995) Vitiligo: repigmentation with dermabrasion and thin split-thickness skin graft. *Dermatologic Surgery* **21**, 295–300.

Ando, I., Chi, H.I., Nakagawa, H. & Otsuka, F. (1993) Difference in clinical features and HLA antigens between familial and non-familial vitiligo of non-segmental type. *British Journal of Dermatology* **129**, 408–410.

Arrunategui, A., Arroyo, C., Garcia, L., Covelli, C., Escobar, C., Carrascal, E. & Falabella, R. (1994) Melanocyte reservoir in vitiligo. *International Journal of Dermatology* **33**, 484–487.

Beck, H.I. & Schmidt, H. (1986) Graft exchange in vitiligo. Studies on the outcome of exchanging biopsies from vitiliginous skin to normal, pigmented skin and vice versa. *Acta Dermato-Venereologica (Stockholm)* **66**, 311–315.

Behl, P.N. (1985) Repigmentation of segmental vitiligo by autologous minigrafting (letter). *Journal of the American Academy of Dermatology* **12**, 118–119.

Behl, P.N. & Bhatia, R.K. (1973) Treatment of vitiligo with autologous thin Thiersch's grafts. *International Journal of Dermatology* **12**, 329–331.

Bleehen, S.S. (1976) The treatment of vitiligo with topical corticosteroids. Light and electronmicroscopic studies. *British Journal of Dermatology* **94**, 43–50.

Boersma, B.R., Westerhof, W. & Bos, J.D. (1995) Repigmentation in vitiligo vulgaris by autologous minigrafting: results in nineteen patients. *Journal of the American Academy of Dermatology* **33**, 990–995.

Boissy, R.E., Beato, K.E. & Nordlund, J.J. (1991a) Dilated rough endoplasmic reticulum and premature death in melanocytes cultured from the vitiligo mouse. *American Journal of Pathology* **138**, 1511–1525.

Boissy, R.E., Liu, Y.Y., Medrano, E.E. & Nordlund, J.J. (1991b) Structural aberration of the rough endoplasmic reticulum and melanosome compartmentalization in long-term cultures of melanocytes from vitiligo patients. *Journal of Investigative Dermatology* **97**, 395–404.

Bonafe, J.L., Lassere, J., Chavoin, J.P., Baro, J.P. & Jeune, R. (1983) Pigmentation induced in vitiligo by normal skin grafts and PUVA stimulation: a preliminary study. *Dermatologica* **166**, 113–116.

Brysk, M.M., Newton, R.C., Rajaraman, S., Plott, T., Barlow, E., Bell, T., Penn, P. & Smith, E.B. (1989) Repigmentation of vitiliginous skin by cultured cells. *Pigment Cell Research* **2**, 202–207.

Chitale, V.R. (1991) Overgrafting for leukoderma of the lower lip: a new application of an already established method. *Annals of Plastic Surgery* **26**, 289–290.

Cui, J., Shen, L.Y. & Wang, G.C. (1991) Role of hair follicles in the repigmentation of vitiligo. *Journal of Investigative Dermatology* **97**, 410–416.

Dourmishev, A.L., Aleksandrov, I.I., Zlatkov, N.B. & Trifonov, S.D. (1982) On the mechanism of perifollicular repigmentation in vitiligo. *Doklady Bolgarskoi Academii Navk* **35**, 789–791.

Falabella, R. (1983) Repigmentation of segmental vitiligo by autologous minigrafting. *Journal of the American Academy of Dermatology* **9**, 514–521.

Falabella, R. (1986) Repigmentation of stable leukoderma by autologous minigrafting. *Journal of Dermatologic Surgery and Oncology* **12**, 172–179.

Falabella, R. (1988) Treatment of localized vitiligo by autologous minigrafting. *Archives of Dermatology* **124**, 1649–1655.

Galadari, E., Mehregan, A.H. & Hashimoto, K. (1993) Ultrastructural study of vitiligo. *International Journal of Dermatology* **32**, 269–271.

Gauthier, Y. & Surleve-Bazeille, J.E. (1992) Autologous grafting with noncultured melanocytes: a simplified method for treatment of depigmented lesions. *Journal of the American Academy of Dermatology* **26**, 191–194.

Gilhar, A., Pillar, T., Eidelman, S. & Etzioni, A. (1989) Vitiligo and idiopathic guttate hypomelanosis. Repigmentation of skin following engraftment onto nude mice. *Archives of Dermatology* **125**, 1363–1366.

Hann, S.K., Im, S., Bong, H.W. & Park, Y.K. (1995) Treatment of stable vitiligo with autologous epidermal grafting and PUVA. *Journal of the American Academy of Dermatology* **32**, 943–948.

Kahn, A.M. & Cohen, M.J. (1995) Vitiligo: treatment by dermabrasion and epithelial sheet grafting. *Journal of the American Academy of Dermatology* **33**, 646–648.

King, R. (1998) Albinism. In: *The Pigmentary System: Physiology and Pathophysiology* (eds J.J.Nordlund, R.E.Boissy, V.J.Hearing, R.A.King & J.-P.Ortonne), pp. 553–575. Oxford University Press, New York.

Koga, M. (1977) Vitiligo: a new classification and therapy. *British Journal of Dermatology* **97**, 255–261.

Koga, M. (1988) Epidermal grafting using the tops of suction blisters in the treatment of vitiligo. *Archives of Dermatology* **124**, 1656–1658.

Koga, M. & Tango, T. (1988) Clinical features and course of type A and type B vitiligo. *British Journal of Dermatology* **118**, 223–228.

Le Poole, I.C., van den Wijngaard, R.M., Westerhof, W., Dutrieux, R.P. & Das, P.K. (1993) Presence or absence of melanocytes in vitiligo lesions: an immunohistochemical investigation. *Journal of Investigative Dermatology* **100**, 816–822.

Medrano, E.E. & Nordlund, J.J. (1990) Successful culture of adult human melanocytes obtained from normal and vitiligo donors. *Journal of Investigative Dermatology* **95**, 441–445.

Moellmann, G., Klein-Angerer, S., Scollay, D.A., Nordlund, J.J. & Lerner, A.B. (1982) Extracellular granular material and degeneration of keratinocytes in the normally pigmented epidermis of patients with vitiligo. *Journal of Investigative Dermatology* **79**, 321–330.

Morohashi, M., Hashimoto, K., Goodman, T.F. Jr, Newton, D.E. & Rist, T. (1977) Ultrastructural studies of vitiligo, Vogt–Koyanagi syndrome, and incontinentia pigmenti achromians. *Archives of Dermatology* **113**, 755–766.

Nordlund, J.J. & Ortonne, J.P. (1998) Vitiligo vulgaris. In: *The Pigmentary System: Physiology and Pathophysiology* (eds J.J.Nordlund, R.E.Boissy, V.J.Hearing, R.A.King & J.-P.Ortonne), pp. 513–551. Oxford University Press, New York.

Nordlund, J.J., Boissy, R.E., Hearing, V.J., King, R.A. & Ortonne, J.-P., eds. (1998). *The Pigmentary System: Physiology and Pathophysiology*. Oxford University Press, New York.

Ortonne, J.P., MacDonald, D.M., Micoud, A. & Thivolet, J. (1979) PUVA-induced repigmentation of vitiligo: a histochemical (split-DOPA) and ultrastructural study. *British Journal of Dermatology* **101**, 1–12.

Ortonne, J.P., Schmitt, D. & Thivolet, J. (1980) PUVA-induced repigmentation of vitiligo: scanning electron microscopy of hair follicles. *Journal of Investigative Dermatology* **74**, 40–42.

Plott, R.T., Brysk, M.M., Newton, R.C., Raimer, S.S. & Rajaraman, S. (1989) A surgical treatment for vitiligo: autologous cultured-epithelial grafts. *Journal of Dermatologic Surgery and Oncology* **15**, 1161–1166.

Puri, N., Mojamdar, M. & Ramaiah, A. (1987) *In vitro* growth characteristics of melanocytes obtained from adult normal and vitiligo subjects. *Journal of Investigative Dermatology* **88**, 434–438.

Puri, N., Mojamdar, M. & Ramaiah, A. (1989) Growth defects of melanocytes in culture from vitiligo subjects are spontaneously corrected *in vivo* in repigmenting subjects and can be partially corrected by the addition of fibroblast-derived growth factors *in vitro*. *Archives of Dermatological Research* **281**, 178–184.

Ramaiah, A., Puri, N. & Mojamdar, M. (1989) Etiology of vitiligo. A new hypothesis. *Acta Dermato-Venereologica (Stockholm)* **69**, 323–326.

Schallreuter, K.U., Buttner, G., Pittelkow, M.R., Wood, J.M., Swanson, N.N. & Korner, C. (1994a) Cytotoxicity of 6-biopterin to human melanocytes. *Biochemical and Biophysical Research Communications* **204**, 43–48.

Schallreuter, K.U., Wood, J.M., Pittelkow, M.R., Gutlich, M., Lemke, K.R., Rodl, W., Swanson, N.N., Hitzemann, K. & Ziegler, I. (1994b) Regulation of melanin biosynthesis in the human epidermis by tetrahydrobiopterin. *Science* **263**, 1444–1446.

Schallreuter, K.U., Wood, J.M., Ziegler, I., Lemke, K.R., Pittelkow, M.R., Lindsey, N.J. &

Gutlich, M. (1994c) Defective tetrahydrobiopterin and catecholamine biosynthesis in the depigmentation disorder vitiligo. *Biochimica et Biophysica Acta* **1226**, 181–192.

Spritz, R.A. (1998) Piebaldism, Waardenburg syndrome and related genetic disorders. In: *The Pigmentary System: Physiology and Pathophysiology* (eds J.J.Nordlund, R.Boissy, V.Hearing, R.A. King & J.P.Ortonne), pp. 505–510. Oxford University Press, New York.

Suvanprakorn, P., Dee-Ananlap, S., Pongsomboon, C. & Klaus, S.N. (1985) Melanocyte autologous grafting for treatment of leukoderma. *Journal of the American Academy of Dermatology* **13**, 968–974.

Zachariae, H. (1994) Autotransplantation in vitiligo: treatment with epithelial sheet grafting or cultured melanocytes. *Journal of the American Academy of Dermatology* **30**, 1044.

3: History and Cultural Aspects of Vitiligo

DAISY KOPERA

Historical references about vitiligo

Several authors have noted interesting ancient, historical references to vitiligo (Brocq 1892; Sutton 1965; Goldman *et al.* 1966; Nair 1978; Lee 1982; Ortonne *et al.* 1983; Koranne & Sachdeva 1988; Hann & Chung 1997). However these commentaries may be contested by historians as references to vitiligo because of semantic difficulties and possible errors in the translation and interpretation of ancient writings. Therefore, the following review has to be seen more as a chapter reviewing historical writings on 'patchy skin lesions', some of which might be vitiligo but not necessarily all.

Vitiligo in writings from dates before Christ (BC)

The earliest reports on patchy skin diseases that may be interpreted as today's vitiligo date back to approximately 1500BC. The *Ebers Papyrus* mentions two types of skin diseases characterized by changes in the colour of the skin. One disorder could be interpreted as leprosy as 'thou shalt not do anything to it'. The other seems to be characterized only by a lack of pigmentation and is likely to be vitiligo (Nair 1978).

References of the same age can also be found in the ancient vedic scripture of India, *Atharva Veda* (Koranne & Sachdeva 1988). It reports on the disease 'Kilas'. The term 'kilas' derives from the sanskrit word 'kil' meaning 'white' in the sense of 'casting away'. In a translation of the *Atharva Veda* in 1905 'kilas' was equated with the term 'vitiligo'. A collection of Shinto prayers from the Far East known as *Makatominoharai* (1200BC) report on 'shira bitu' meaning 'white man', and in some incidences it may also be interpreted as vitiligo. *Charak Samhita* (800BC), another medical compilation found in the Indian literature, mentions a disease called 'svitra', a sanskrit word meaning 'spreading whiteness'. The *Ashtangahidaya* (600BC) tries to explain prognostic factors of these eruptions (Nair 1978). For the management of white spots, in ancient Egypt or India, the active ingredient of *Psoralea corylifolia* or *Ammi majus* was applied on depigmented spots and exposed to sunlight.

Much emphasis on 'white spots' can be found in the Greek literature. Herodotus (484–425BC), a Greek historian, wrote in his book *Clio* that foreigners who suffered from such lesions, must have 'sinned against the sun' and had to leave the country immediately (Goldman *et al.* 1966). The Indian *Manu Smirti* (200BC) describes 'Sweta Kushtha', meaning 'white disease', skin lesions which probably were vitiligo (Koranne & Sachdeva 1988).

Biblical references to vitiligo

The Bible refers to certain skin conditions using the Hebrew word 'Zara'at' in Leviticus XIII in the Old Testament. This term in actuality alludes to many different cutaneous afflictions. Some of them have been interpreted as the sign of a sin, which in Hebrew theology symbolizes a punishment sent by God. The term 'Zara'at' in the Bible denotes 'white spots' but this does not necessarily indicate vitiligo (Goldman *et al.* 1966). The roots of this controversy about the different interpretations of 'Zara'at' can be found from the events occurring around 250BC when Ptolemy II demanded the translation of the Bible into Greek in order to make it understandable to a larger population. For all statements where a human being is declared unclean by reason of 'Zara'at', the scholars of the Septuagint retained the term 'leprosy' without regard to modern dermatological terminology (Leviticus XIV, 34). The confusion arising from this definition is an important cause for the social stigma attached to 'white spots on the skin' as they may either denote leprosy or vitiligo or many other cutaneous lesions (Table 3.1). Since then theologians also proposed the term 'psoriasis' to be used synonymously for these afflictions. They reasoned that to change the biblical concept of leprosy, the substitution of the term 'psoriasis' seemed useful because it does not denote the idea of an associated 'moral sin'. The term psoriasis in the Bible should be understood to mean any 'affection of the skin'.

For many years dermatologists have been interested in the true nature of 'biblical white spots'. Most dermatologists have concluded that the medical terms used in the Bible are not related to leprosy in many instances. Rather, the terms probably represent a variety of skin conditions and sometimes also mean vitiligo (Table 3.1) (Goldman *et al.* 1966).

Table 3.1 Classification of the meaning of 'White spots' in the Bible (see also Goldman *et al.* 1966).

Description of the Lesion	Interpretation
White spots per se	Vitiligo
White spots associated with inflammation	Postinflammatory leucoderma Leprosy (?)
White spots associated with scaling	Psoriasis Leprosy (?)
White spots associated with atrophy	Morphea Leprosy (?)
White spots associated with the regrowth of hairs which turn white	Alopecia areata

Vitiligo references from writings Anno Domino (AD)

It is said that in the Chinese literature skin disorders were mentioned much earlier than in western literature but their descriptions were rather vague. Around 600AD Dohi wrote clear descriptions of 'Pin-yüan-hon-lun' which was probably today's lepra (Goldman *et al.* 1966). In ancient Arabic books 'white skin' was expressed as 'baras' and with terms like 'bahak' or 'bohak' (Koranne & Sachdeva 1988). From the Koran the story has been transmitted that Jesus was able to cure patients with 'baras' (Ortonne *et al.* 1983). Patchy skin lesions, likely to be of a leprous nature, were the most important cutaneous diseases that were mentioned in the writings of the early European medical schools up to the 15th Century. At the end of that century leucoderma syphiliticum became a new, important differential diagnosis as the number of lepers decreased and the 'new' lues venera, later known as syphilis, spread far and wide over Europe.

In Korea, hypopigmentary disorders, such as vitiligo, tinea versicolor, naevus depigmentosus, naevus anaemicus and albinism, as well as their treatment, were written about in an old Korean Oriental medical book published in the early 17th Century, the *Doney Bogam*. As a method of treatment sulphur or specially formulated arsenic or mercury ointment was applied on vitiligo lesions and primitive phototherapy was used (Hann & Chung 1997). An example of vitiligo was drawn on the portrait of Chang-Myeong Song (1689–1767), a high ranking official of the Yi dynasty of Korea (1392–1910) (Fig. 3.1) (Lee 1982). There was obviously no misconception about vitiligo in Korea. Otherwise a portrait of a member of the noble class showing vitiliginous skin would not have been published.

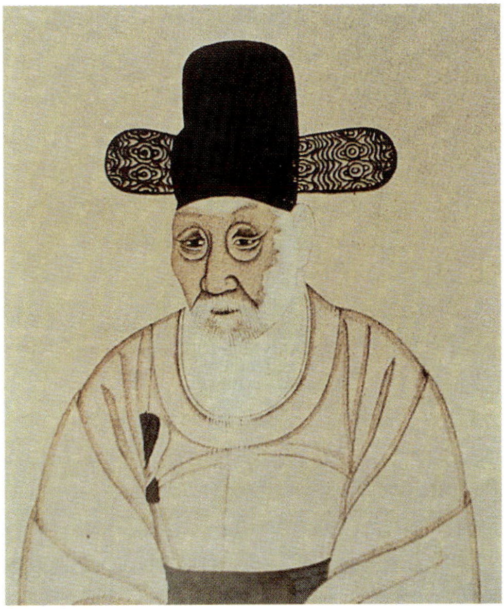

Fig. 3.1 Portrait of Chang-Myeong Song (1689–1767), a high ranking official of the Yi dynasty of Korea (1392–1910), showing vitiligo. (See also Lee 1982).

The origin of the word vitiligo

The word 'vitiligo' itself is said to have been first used by Celsus in his Latin medical classic *De Medicina* in the 1st Century AD. Regarding the roots of the term 'vitiligo' there seems to be some difference of opinion between lexicographers and dermatologists. Some suggest that the word vitiligo comes from the Latin word for veal because the white skin has an appearance resembling the white glistening of the flesh of calves ('vituli'). Others suggest that it may be derived from 'vitelius', the Latin word for 'calf' itself because of the white patches in a calf's fur. Some early writers, like Hieronymus Mercurialis who wrote in the 16th Century, believed that the word vitiligo represents a blemish or fault which in Latin is called 'vitium'. The addition of the 'l' in the word 'vitiligo' is uncertain. It may just have been introduced for reasons of euphony (Nair 1978; Ortonne *et al.* 1983). Finally, the *Lexicon of the Latin Language* published by Facciolati and Forcellini in Boston 1841, did not clarify the origin of the terminology. Instead of settling the confusion this lexicon aggravated the issue by its statement, 'Vitiligo (vitium): a kind of leprosy or cutaneous eruption consisting of spots, sometimes black (?), sometimes white, called morphea, alphus, melas, leuce; also in general a cutaneous eruption. Celsus & Pliny' (2nd Century AD) (Sutton 1965).

Vitiligo in the 19th Century

Near the end of the 19th Century, when skin diseases were still presented in alphabetical order in many textbooks of dermatology, vitiligo was defined as a pigmentary dystrophy. Moreover, Louis Brocq (1856–1928) noted the lack of pigmentation (achromy) in vitiliginous lesions combined with an increase of pigmentation (hyperchromy) in the lesion's periphery which he called 'dyschromy' (Brocq 1892). Moritz Kaposi (1837–1902) was one of the first to describe the histopathological features of vitiligo. He stated that the only anatomical change in vitiliginous skin is the lack of pigment granules in deep rete cells. In the periphery of the lesion there is an increase of pigmentation. Sparse pigment laden cells in the corium are unable to add much to the clinical aspect of the skin's pigmentation (Fig.3.2) (Kaposi 1879).

Obscure aetiological mechanisms like emotional stress or other traumatic factors triggering the eruption of vitiligo have been discussed by our dermatological forefathers. For them, a connection with the nervous system seemed to be evident (Neumann 1880; Brocq 1892).

At the turn of the century different approaches were made in the treatment of vitiligo. Systemic administration of bromides, iodides or valerianates, of mercury, antimony, and arsenic did not show much effect. Ernest Besnier (1831–1909) recommended subcutaneous injection of pilocarpine, and saline or bromoiodic baths. Different mixtures with croton oil, iodine, sublimate, and naphtol have been used topically without convincing therapeutic results (Neumann 1880; Brocq 1892).

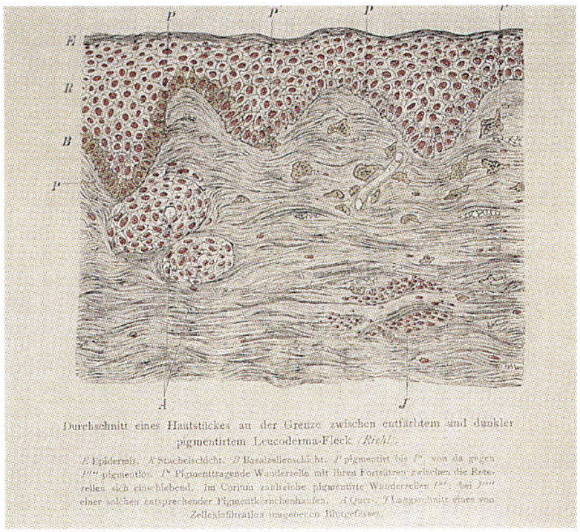

Fig. 3.2 Vitiligo/Leucoderma. Illustration from Kaposi's textbook: *Pathologie und Therapie der Hautkrankheiten*. (1st edn 1879) 5th edn 1899, p. 624 (see also Kaposi 1879).

Acknowledgements

We gratefully mention Professor Sungnack Lee for providing the historic portrait of Chang-Myeong showing vitiligo (Lee 1982).

References

Brocq, L., ed. (1892) *Traitement des Maladies de la Peau*, pp. 853–855. Doin, Paris.

Goldman, L., Moraites, R.S. & Kitzmiller, K.W. (1966) White spots in biblical times. *Archives of Dermatology* **93**, 744–753.

Hann, S.K. & Chung, H.S. (1997) Historic view of vitiligo in Korea. *International Journal of Dermatology* **36**, 313–315.

Kaposi, M., ed. (1899) *Pathologie und Therapie der Hautkrankheiten*. 5th edn, pp. 703–707, Urban und Schwarzenberg, Berlin/Wien. (1st edn 1879).

Koranne, R.V. & Sachdeva, K.G. (1988) Vitiligo. *International Journal of Dermatology* **27**, 676–681.

Lee, S. (1982) Vitiligo auf einem historischen Portrait. *Hautarzt* **33**, 335–336.

Nair, B.K.H. (1978) Vitiligo—A retrospect. *International Journal of Dermatology* **17**, 755–757.

Neumann, I., ed. (1880) *Lehrbuch der Hautkrankheiten*, p. 438, Braumüller, Wien.

Ortonne, J.P., Mosher, D.B. & Fitzpatrick, D.B., eds. (1983). *Vitiligo and Other Hypomelanoses of Hair and Skin*, pp. 129–132. Plenum Publishing Co., New York/London.

Sutton, R.L. (1965) On definition of vitiligo (letter). *Archives of Dermatology* **91**, 288.

4: Genetics and Prevalence of Vitiligo Vulgaris

PARTHA P. MAJUMDER

Familial aggregation of vitiligo was noted as early as 1933 by Cockayne (Cockayne 1933). In the early 1950s, both members of monozygotic twin pairs were reported to be afflicted with vitiligo (Lerner 1959). Vitiligo has been reported in several children of one family (Halder *et al.* 1987). Many subsequent studies have noted high degrees of positive family history and familial aggregation (Hafez *et al.* 1983; Das *et al.* 1985; Nath *et al.* 1994). These observations support a genetic involvement in the aetiology of vitiligo (Hafez *et al.* 1983; Majumder *et al.* 1988; Nath *et al.* 1994; Lacour & Ortonne 1995).

Early studies on determination of the mode of inheritance of vitiligo yielded equivocal results. While all these studies concluded that the genetic factor controlling vitiligo was autosomal, all plausible modes of inheritance were proposed (El-Mofty 1968). These included single locus autosomal dominant with incomplete penetrance, autosomal recessive and multifactorial with a high ($\approx$ 70%) heritability. One of the major problems with these early studies on genetics of vitiligo was that they did not take into account the variable age at onset of vitiligo. It is known that when this variability is ignored while analysing family data, inferences about the mode of inheritance are likely to be incorrect.

The prevalence and mean age at onset of vitiligo varies considerably among different geographical regions and ethnic groups. Based primarily on clinical records of hospitals and dermatology clinics, the prevalence is estimated to be about 2% of the population in Japan, 1% in the USA and Egypt, 0.24% in the UK and 0.14% in Russia. These estimates are probably upwardly biased. From epidemiological surveys conducted in Denmark and India, the estimated prevalence is about 0.5% (Hafez *et al.* 1983). Prevalence of vitiligo increases significantly with age. The trend of increase with age differs among geographical regions. The prevalence has also been consistently reported to be higher, although not always significantly, among females than among males. The mean or modal age at onset varies among geographical regions and by gender. Epidemiological data from India have shown that the mean ages at onset among males and females are, respectively, about 25 years and 20 years (Das *et al.* 1985). In Denmark, these ages are reported to be about 39 years and 37 years, respectively. A recent study on Caucasian families resident in the USA showed that there was no significant difference in mean ages at onset between males and females. This age was estimated to be about 22 years (Nath *et al.* 1994; Nordlund & Majumder 1997).

About 20% of vitiligo patients have at least one first-degree relative with vitiligo. The relative risk of vitiligo for first-degree relatives (parents, children, siblings) is elevated by 7- to 10-fold (Nath *et al.* 1994). Second-degree relatives also have significantly elevated relative risks. The patterns of inheritance and recurrence risks among relatives of patients with vitiligo do not conform to those expected for an autosomal, single gene trait. Results of recent family studies that have taken variability of the age at onset into account indicate that vitiligo is controlled by recessive genes at three or four autosomal loci (Majumder *et al.* 1988; Nath *et al.* 1994; Nordlund & Majumder 1997). Of the various models of inheritance proposed and investigated, the most parsimonious model is that, for manifestation of vitiligo, an individual should be homozygous for the recessive genes at all the loci controlling the disease. This implies that in the vast majority of families there will be only one member afflicted with vitiligo. In a small number of families, there will be multiple affected members. Recurrence risks will usually be small.

Vitiligo has been considered an autoimmune disorder because of its positive association with other disorders such as thyroiditis, diabetes mellitus and alopecia areata, all of which are thought possibly to have an immune-mediated aetiology (Lerner & Nordlund 1978; Nordlund 1987). However, it remains unclear whether this association is due to chance alone. Case control studies on human leucocyte antigens (HLA) have consistently shown positive association of HLA DR4 with vitiligo and negative association of DR3. Other HLA associations that have been reported are with Dw7, DR7, DR1, B13, A2, B21, Cw6, DR53, A19 and DR52 (Foley *et al.* 1983). No consistent association of inherited deficiencies of components of the human complement system has been found (Venneker *et al.* 1992). While such association studies shed little light on genetics of vitiligo, it has recently been reported that missense mutations in guanosine triphosphate (GTP)-cyclohydrolase I gene may cause vitiligo (Fuente-Fernendez 1997). It may be noted that GTP-cyclohydrolase I is the initial and rate-limiting enzyme in tetrahydrobiopterin synthesis. Tetrahydrobiopterin might be essential for synthesis of melanin. However, it remains unclear whether mutations in this gene are the only causes of vitiligo. It is more likely that mutations in multiple genes may precipitate the disease. It is also important to point out that several environmental factors, including stress, extreme exposures to pesticides, sunlight, etc., have been implicated in the aetiology of vitiligo (Slominski *et al.* 1989). However, no consistent environmental risk factor has so far been found. It is possible that an environmental trigger is essential to precipitate the disease in genetically predisposed individuals.

References

Cockayne, E.A. (1933) *Inherited Abnormalities of the Skin and its Appendages*. Oxford University Press, London.

Das, S.K., Majumder, P.P., Chakraborty, R., Majumder, T.K. & Halder, B. (1985) Studies on vitiligo. I. Epidemiological profile in Calcutta, India. *Genetic Epidemiology* **2**, 71–78.

El-Mofty, A.M. (1968) *Vitiligo and Psoralens*. Pergamon Press, New York.

Foley, N.R., Lowe, N.J., Misheloff, E. & Tiwari, J.L. (1983) Association of HLA-DR4 with vitiligo. *Journal of the American Academy of Dermatology* **8**, 39–40.

Fuente-Fernendez, R. de la (1997) Mutations in GTP-cyclohydrolase I gene and vitiligo. *The Lancet* **350**, 640.

Hafez, M., Sharaf, L. & El-Nabi, S.M.A. (1983) The genetics of vitiligo. *Acta Dermato-venereologica (Stockholm)* **63**, 249–251.

Halder, R.M., Grimes, P.E. & Cowan, J. (1987) Childhood vitiligo. *Journal of the American Academy of Dermatology* **16**, 948–954.

Lacour, J.P. & Ortonne, J.P. (1995) The genetics of vitiligo. *Annales de Dermatologie et de Venereologie* **124**, 167–171.

Lerner, A.B. (1959) Vitiligo. *Journal of Investigative Dermatology* **32**, 285–310.

Lerner, A.B. & Nordlund, J.J. (1978) Vitiligo: What is it? Is it important? *Journal of the American Medical Association* **239**, 1183–1187.

Majumder, P.P., Das, S.K. & Li, C.C. (1988) A genetical model for vitiligo. *American Journal of Human Genetics* **43**, 119–125.

Nath, S.K., Majumder, P.P. & Nordlund, J.J. (1994) Genetic epidemiology of vitiligo: Multilocus recessivity cross-validated. *American Journal of Human Genetics* **55**, 981–990.

Nordlund, J.J. (1987) Hypopigmentation, vitiligo and melanoma: New data, more enigmas. *Archives of Dermatology* **123**, 1005–1011.

Nordlund, J.J. & Majumder, P.P. (1997) Recent investigations on vitiligo vulgaris: advances in clinical research. *Dermatologic Clinics* **15**, 69–78.

Slominski, A. Paul, R. & Bomirski, A. (1989) Hypothesis: possible role of melatonin receptors in vitiligo. *Journal of the Royal Society of Medicine* **82**, 539–541.

Venneker, G.T., Westerhof, W., de Vries, I.J., Drayer, N.M., Wolthers, B.G., de Waal, L.P., Bos, J.D. & Asghar, S.S. (1992) Molecular heterogeneity of the fourth component of complement (C4) and its genes in vitiligo. *Journal of Investigative Dermatology* **99**, 853–858.

PART 2
CLINICAL PRESENTATION OF VITILIGO

5: Histology of Vitiliginous Skin

RAYMOND E. BOISSY

Histological evaluation of skin from patients with vitiligo has been performed in order to obtain insights about the pathophysiology of the disease. Specifically, the amelanotic lesion, the pigmented skin and the border or interface between the two have been examined by routine histology, histochemistry, immunocytochemistry and electron microscopy. The clinical presentation of this disease can be quite variable and complex. Likewise the histological profile of vitiliginous skin is not necessarily uniform in all specimens from various patients. However, the current consensus on the histological presentation in vitiligo is that the amelanotic lesion is devoid of melanocytes, the border exhibits melanocytic as well as keratinocyte damage plus occasional mononuclear leucocyte infiltrates. The pigmented skin may exhibit minimal aberrations of the melanocyte and the keratinocyte. A compilation of the literature on the histological profile in vitiligo is presented in this chapter.

The histology of the amelanotic vitiligo lesion

Melanin stains

Histological evaluation of skin from patients with vitiligo was originally performed to determine whether the amelanotic lesions were devoid of melanocytes or, alternatively, contained melanocytes defective in their ability to make melanin. Results of histological studies on epidermal sheets derived from vitiliginous skin were first reported in the late 1950s (Jarrett & Szabo 1956; Hu *et al.* 1959). These initial publications demonstrated that melanin was absent or dramatically reduced in the white lesions. To augment the visualization of melanin synthesis and deposition in the epidermis, the Masson–Fontana silver reduction staining technique (Masson 1948) was performed on split skin obtained from depigmented lesions (Hu *et al.* 1959). Most specimens remained unreactive throughout the lesional area, an observation that confirms the absence of melanin. The investigators did observe occasional, weakly silver-positive cells within the intermediate zone between the depigmented lesion and the surrounding normally pigmented skin.

DOPA staining

Histochemical procedures specific for the identification of melanocytes have been developed to detect and/or highlight quiescent or inactive melanocytes, i.e. amelanotic and/or hypomelanotic cells, respectively, in tissue (Bloch 1917; Okun *et al.* 1969). For these histochemical procedures, tissue or cells are fixed and incubated in a buffer solution containing either tyrosine or l-dihydroxyphenylalanine (DOPA), the substrates for melanin. During the incubation period, the exogenously supplied substrate penetrates through the tissue/cells and is enzymatically converted to a melanin reaction product at sites where functional tyrosinase exists, i.e. within the melanosomes located in the cytoplasm of melanocytes. Tyrosine or DOPA histochemistry has been used very effectively to distinguish between tyrosinase-related forms of oculocutaneous albinism, i.e. OCA1 that results from mutations inhibiting the function of tyrosinase, and tyrosinase-positive forms of OCA (Kugelman & Van Scott 1961; King *et al.* 1994) caused by mutations in other genes that are involved in synthesis of melanin. Hu *et al.* (1959) performed DOPA histochemistry on their specimens in the study described in the preceding paragraph and demonstrated that most vitiligo lesions were DOPA negative. On occasion, islands of DOPA-positive cells were observed in the vitiliginous lesions. These DOPA-positive cells were smaller and less dendritic than normal melanocytes. The cytoplasmic staining of the reaction product was more diffuse and less granular than in normal melanocytes. The authors suggested that these cells probably represented 'inactive' melanocytes. However, one could interpret these observations to be consistent with the presence of unhealthy or moribund melanocytes. In their conclusion, these authors suggested that the melanocytes were generally not present in the amelanotic vitiligo lesions. Subsequent DOPA histochemistry studies on split vitiligo skin also demonstrated the absence or the presence of a few abnormal melanocytes in the depigmented lesions (Bleehen 1979; Koh *et al.* 1983). However, it remained to be definitively determined whether the melanocyte in vitiligo underwent dedifferentiation resulting in a cell that was undetectable by the histological and histochemical techniques used in these initial studies.

Routine histology

Other histological studies of the amelanotic lesions continued to focus on determining whether melanocytes were absent or nonfunctional in the white lesions. By routine paraffin or plastic embedding and counterstaining, melanocytes in the basal layer of normally pigmented epidermis appear as clear cells (Quevedo & Holstein 1998). The transparent appearance of the cytoplasm is due to a retraction artefact from the fixation of the tissue with formalin. Investigators have used this phenomenon to search for melanocytes in various types of hypopigmenting disorders. In vitiliginous skin from patients with vitiligo, several investigators demonstrated independently the absence of clear dendritic cells in the basal layer of the epidermis (Birbeck *et al.* 1961; Moellmann *et al.* 1982; Le Poole *et al.* 1997). These results contrasted with the histological profile of skin from patients with various forms of albinism (Fig. 5.1). Albinism is a form of cutaneous hypopigmentation caused by mutations of one of a series of genes that necessarily participate in the synthesis of melanin by the melanocytes. Amelanotic, nonfunctioning albino melanocytes such as those found in OCA-1 can be detected in their normal position in the basal epithelium where they appear as clear cells (Becker *et al.* 1952). Therefore, the absence of clear cells in the basal layer of vitiliginous epidermis is consistent with the conclusion that nonfunctional melanocytes were not present in the depigmented epidermis and that the melanocytes had disappeared from these sites.

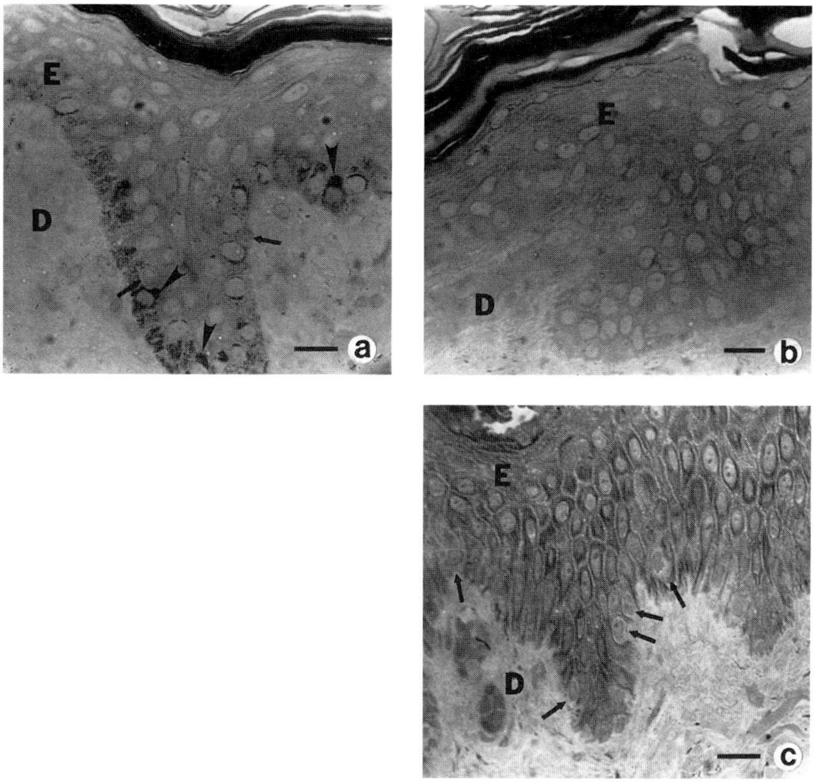

Fig. 5.1 Histological thin sections of skin derived from (a) a normally pigmented African-American individual, (b) a patient with vitiligo and (c) a patient with tyrosinase-related oculocutaneous albinism (OCA1) that were embedded in EPON resin, sectioned at one micron thickness, and stained with 1% toluidine blue. Melanocytes in the stratum basalum of the epidermis appear as roundish cells with relatively clear cytoplasm (arrows) in the African-American individual (a) and the OCA1 patient (c) but are absent from the lesional skin of the patient with vitiligo (b). Also note the presence of melanosomes transferred to keratinocytes that form a prominent apical aggregate over the nucleus (arrowheads) in the African-American individual and the complete absence of melanin in both patients with vitiligo and OCA1. E = epidermis; D = dermis. Bars = 20 microns.

Other histochemical stains

In contrast, atypical clear cells have been reported to exist in the stratum basale of vitiliginous lesions. Birbeck *et al.* (Birbeck *et al.* 1961) initially reported the presence of DOPA-negative, gold chloride-positive dendritic cells in the basal layer of vitiliginous epidermis. These unique cells existed in numbers similar to that of the basal melanocytes of normal epidermis. Langerhans cells, described as high level clear cells with these specific tinctorial properties, appeared more numerous in vitiliginous lesions (Birbeck *et al.* 1961). The authors noted that these two populations of cells, i.e. basal clear dendritic cells and suprabasal Langerhans cells, were ultrastructurally indistinguishable from each other. Both cells exhibited indented nuclei, characteristic granules that differ from premelanosomes, and an absence of both keratin fibrils and desmosomes. This would suggest that the basal clear dendritic cells in reality were Langerhans cells migrating into the vitiliginous epidermis. The presence of basal Langerhans cells in vitiliginous skin was demonstrated in subsequent publications (Breathnach *et al.* 1966; Mishima *et al.* 1972; Breathnach 1975) (Fig. 5.2). However, a recent study evaluating Langerhans cell distribution in vitiliginous epidermis by immunocytochemistry demonstrated that there were no topographical differences in the presence of Langerhans cells in lesions, at the border or in pigmented skin of patients with the inflammatory form of vitiligo (Le Poole *et al.* 1996).

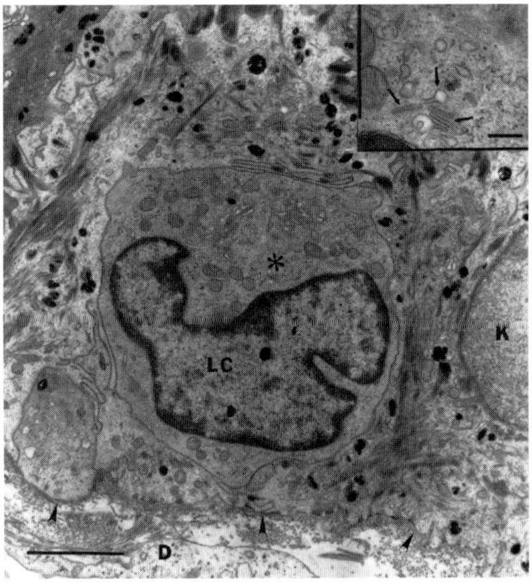

Fig. 5.2 Electron micrograph of a Langerhans cell (LC) residing in the Stratum basalum of the epidermis at the pigmented border of a lesion in a patient with vitiligo. The perinuclear cytoplasmic area (*) is magnified in the inset of the upper right hand corner to demonstrate the presence of Birbeck granules (arrows). K = keratinocyte; D = dermis; arrowheads = basement membrane at the dermal epidermal junction. Bar = 3.0 microns (Inset Bar = 0.5 microns).

Electron microscopy

Electron microscopic evaluation of the white vitiliginous skin confirmed that melanocyte/melanoblasts were not present or were dramatically reduced in number or, if present, were not identifiable by the many techniques employed for electron microscopy of the epidermis (Breathnach *et al.* 1966; Moellmann *et al.* 1982; Koh *et al.* 1983; Le Poole *et al.* 1997). In lesional skin, basal epithelial cells resting on the basement membrane of the dermal/epidermal junction predominantly resembled keratinocytes. Only occasionally were melanocytes or Langerhans cells present in this area (Fig. 5.2). Reports of melanocytes occasionally present in the vitiliginous lesion describe them as exhibiting ultrastructural abnormalities resembling those expressed by melanocytes at the border of the lesion (as described below) (Morohashi *et al.* 1977; Koh *et al.* 1983).

Immunocytochemistry

The histological, histochemical, and ultrastructural assessments of vitiliginous skin, as described above, provided evidence that melanocytes, either functional or inactive, are absent from vitiliginous lesions. However, concern still exists as to whether melanocytes of less differentiated stages, lacking morphologic indicators and the tyrosinase enzyme, remained in the vitiligo epidermis. To address this concern a histochemical study was undertaken by LePoole *et al.* (Le Poole *et al.* 1993) using a panel of antibodies reactive against melanocytic cells. The investigators utilized immunoperoxidase staining on frozen sections of control and vitiliginous skin. In addition to using antibodies that recognized pigmentation association antigens, these investigators also included antibodies that recognized melanocyte-expressed molecules unrelated to the synthesis of melanin or the melanosome. The results of this study confirmed that melanocytes were indeed absent in the lesions of vitiligo patients. Recently, Dippel *et al.* (Dippel *et al.* 1995) demonstrated that the c-kit receptor, a molecule expressed early in melanocyte differentiation (Grichnik *et al.* 1996; Boissy & Nordlund 1997), was undetectable in vitiligo skin. This finding is also consistent with the current hypothesis that nonfunctional melanocytes are absent from vitiligo lesions.

It should be noted that, in all the observations described in this section, an occasional melanocyte does remain in vitiligo skin. However, these melanocytes are morphologically aberrant. This suggests that the underlying pathophysiology in vitiligo does not necessarily require complete and total destruction of all melanocytes and may be incomplete, and that some melanocytes do survive the destruction and/or removal processes at play in vitiligo. This idea is most consistent with the clinical observation that vitiligo can be trichrome or pentachrome, the clinical equivalent of destruction of some but not all melanocytes. If persisting cells can repair the damage, they might serve as a reservoir for repigmentation.

The histology of the border between the lesion and normal skin

Histological observations on the margins of a vitiligo lesion have been performed in attempts to observe active processes responsible for the loss of pigmentation occurring in vitiligo. Frequently there is a clear line of demarcation between the amelanotic lesion that contains no functional melanocytes and the pigmented interface that contains morphologically normal melanocytes (Bleehen 1979). However, a few reports have shown key histological differences at this marginal site. Several reports demonstrate that in the peripheral zone surrounding the lesion, melanocytes are markedly reduced in number and morphologically different by light microscopy (Hu *et al.* 1959; Mishima *et al.* 1972; Le Poole *et al.* 1993; Abdel-Naser *et al.* 1994) and by electron microscopy (Breathnach *et al.* 1966; Morohashi *et al.* 1977). These melanocytes appear to have larger cell bodies and their dendrites are more arborized than normal melanocytes. In addition, melanocyte fragmentation was also noted in this area. In contrast, some reports have described the melanocytes at the border to be normal histologically (Bleehen 1979) and healthy ultrastructurally (Moellmann *et al.* 1982). This discrepancy in melanocyte condition at the border of a vitiligo lesion has never been correlated with the state of the lesion, i.e. a progressing as opposed to dormant lesion. It is possible that the destructive events in vitiligo are arrested when the lesion is not advancing.

We have occasionally noticed that melanocytes in the normally pigmented skin immediately outside of an amelanotic lesion from patients with vitiligo exhibit morphologic indicators of apoptosis (R.E. Boissy & J.J. Nordlund, personal observations). Melanocytes in this perilesional area can exhibit cellular shrinkage and increased nuclear heterochromatin (Fig.5.3), both morphologic indicators of cells in the initial stages of apoptosis. Apoptosis is a process of programmed cell death that prevents damaged/dying cells from instigating an immune response (Savill *et al.* 1993; Martins & Earnshaw 1997). In this process, an apoptotic cell will fragment into small pieces that are phagocytosed by macrophages in the vicinity, without resulting in the stimulation of an antigenic mediated cellular and/or humoral immune response. Keratinocytes are very avid phagocytosing cells of the epidermis (Blois 1968; Wolff & Konrad 1971). In theory, keratinocytes could effectively phagocytose fragmented apoptotic vitiligo melanocytes and carry the debris with them as they migrate up the stratum corneum where they desquamate off the epidermis. This process may be histologically indistinguishable from the normal process of melanosome transfer to, and degradation in, the keratinocyte. Re-examination of histological specimens of vitiligo is now warranted with this hypothesis in mind. Removal of melanocytes undergoing apoptosis by the keratinocyte would be consistent with the lack of inflammation and immune response at the lesional borders of most patients with vitiligo.

Keratinocyte damage has also been demonstrated at the edge of the

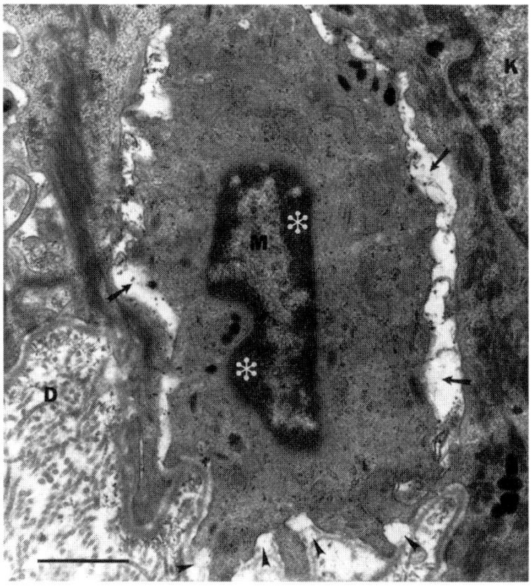

Fig. 5.3 Electron micrograph of a melanocyte (M) in normally pigmented skin 3 mm away from the edge of a lesion in a patient with vitiligo. The melanocyte (M) in the Stratum basalum of the epidermis exhibits morphological signs of the early stage in apoptosis including (1) extensive extracellular space (arrows) between it and both neighbouring keratinocytes (K) and the basement membrane at the dermal/epidermal junction (arrowheads) with condensation of the cytoplasm suggestive of cellular shrinkage; and (2) a dramatic increase in amount of nuclear heterochromatin (*). Absence of these morphological signs of the early stage in apoptosis are not present in tissue from control individuals (see Fig. 5.5b). D = dermis. Bar = 3.0 microns.

vitiligo lesion. Vacuolar degeneration of keratinocytes and the appearance of extracellular granular material (EGM) between the melanocytes and the keratinocytes, as well as between the keratinocytes themselves, suggests that the keratinocyte as well as the melanocyte is affected by the pathophysiological processes active in causing vitiligo (Moellmann *et al.* 1982). The EGM, that can be abundant at the border of a lesion (Fig. 5.4), resembles aggregates of free cytoplasmic ribosomes surrounding intracellular vacuoles in the periphery of keratinocytes. The authors of this observation implicated keratinocyte damage as the source of the EGM (Moellmann *et al.* 1982).

A prominent hypothesis for the aetiology of vitiligo is an autoimmune response against the melanocytes (see Chapter 16). The association of immunocytes with the loss of melanocytes in vitiligo has been assessed histologically. In most reports, a marked influx of lymphocytes in the skin of the amelanotic lesion and, more significantly at the border, was generally not observed in the noninflammatory form of vitiligo. However, a small subset of patients with vitiligo (i.e. ≅ 5%) present with an inflammation at the border of the lesion (Garb & Wise 1948; Buckley & Lobitz 1953; Michaelsson 1968). This form of vitiligo has been designated as inflammatory vitiligo (Boissy & Nordlund 1995). Several reports clearly demonstrate a dramatic abundance of lymphocytes present at the inflamed border of advancing lesion in inflammatory vitiligo (Gokhale & Mehta 1983; Abdel-Naser *et al.* 1991). In addition, epidermal infiltrates of lymphocytes or mononuclear cells other than Langerhans cells were identified ultrastructurally in some patients with vitiligo who were resistant to therapeutic treatment (Moellmann *et al.* 1982).

Recent immunocytochemical studies have begun to characterize the populations of lymphocytes that exist in this infiltrate (Abdel-Naser *et al.* 1994; Le Poole *et al.* 1996). This approach should help resolve how components of the cellular and humoral immune system are involved in the progression of vitiligo. Abdel-Naser *et al.* (1994) demonstrated that a few macrophages and cells with interleukin (IL)-2 and interferon (IFN)-γ receptors, but no significant natural killer (NK) cells, were immunocytochemically identifiable in the marginal skin of some patients with progressive, generalized (i.e. noninflammatory) vitiligo. However, in inflammatory vitiligo, the presence of T-cells has been immunocytochemically confirmed (Le Poole *et al.* 1996). Specifically, epidermal infiltrating T cells in the perilesional skin exhibited an increased CD8/CD4 ratio and in the cutaneous lymphocyte antigen and IL-2 receptor. In addition, $CD68^{+}OKM5^{-}$ macrophages were abundant in the dermis (Le Poole *et al.* 1996). The presence of B-cells in the border of vitiligo lesions has not been confirmed yet by immunocytochemistry. This is important to assess in light of the prevalent reports demonstrating autoantibodies somewhat specific to melanocyte antigens in serum of patients with vitiligo (see Chapter 16).

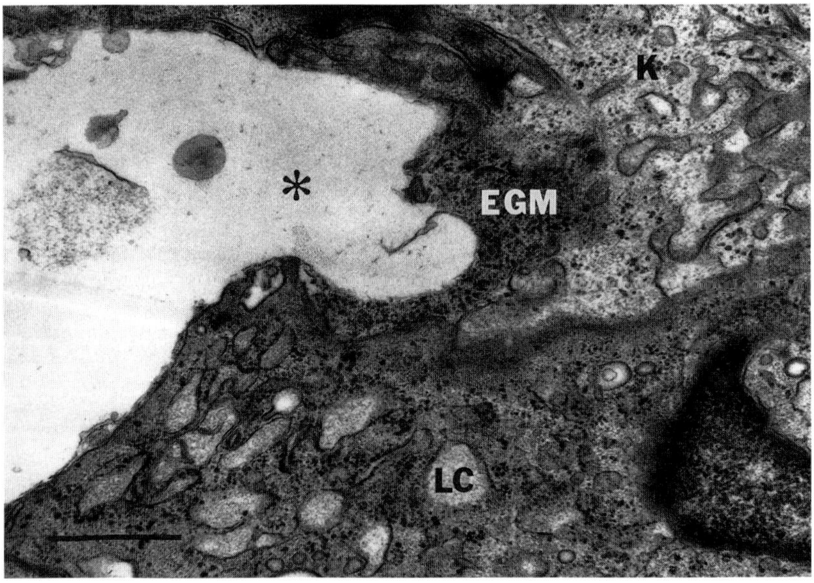

Fig. 5.4 Electron micrograph of extracellular granular material (EGM) between a keratinocyte (K), a Langerhans cell (LC), and an intracellular vacuole (*) within the epidermis at the pigmented border of a lesion in a patient with vitiligo. Bar = 1.0 microns.

The histology of the normally pigmented skin

In contrast to the vitiliginous lesion, the pigmented skin at distant sites from depigmented patches appears histologically unremarkable. Melanocytes appear normal in both their morphology and density. This suggests that the pigmented skin is normal and unaffected in vitiligo. However, under closer

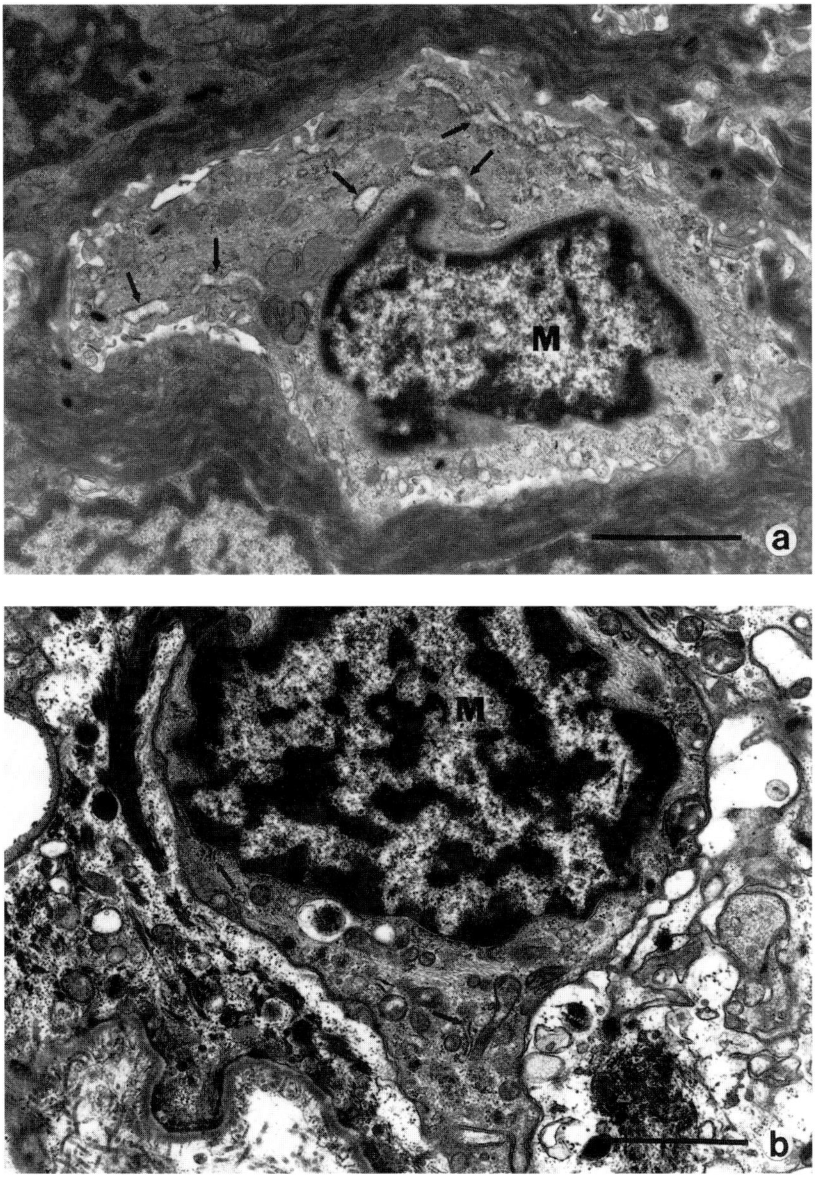

Fig. 5.5 Electron micrograph of melanocytes (M) in the Stratum basalum of the epidermis in (a) the normally pigmented skin 3 mm away from a lesion in a patient with vitiligo, and (b) a control Caucasian individual. The melanocyte in the patient with vitiligo (a) exhibits dilated profiles of rough endoplasmic reticulum (arrows) not present (arrows) in the melanocyte from a control individual (b). Bars = 3.0 microns.

scrutiny, some distinct histological variations were observed in the normal-appearing, pigmented skin. Intracellular vacuolization was observed histologically in semi thin sections in some specimens of normal skin from vitiligo patients (Moellmann *et al.* 1982). In addition, ultrastructural evaluations of pigmented skin have clearly demonstrated that this area of skin was indeed affected. Of great interest is the report by Moellmann *et al.* demonstrating that in the pigmented regions of patients with vitiligo, as far away from a lesion as 15 cm, ultrastructural evidence of cellular damage exists. Specifically, melanocytes as well as keratinocytes appeared vacuolated and the deposition of EGM had occurred. It has also been demonstrated that melanocytes in the pigmented skin of patients with vitiligo may exhibit a dilation of the rough endoplasmic reticulum (RER) not present in control skin (Fig. 5.5; Boissy *et al.* 1991). Dilated profiles of RER in vitiligo melanocytes were also apparent in micrographs published by Moellmann *et al.* (1982) and in melanocyte cultures developed from pigmented skin of patients with vitiligo (Boissy *et al.* 1991; Im *et al.* 1994; Jimbow *et al.* 1996). Therefore, the pigmented skin of patients with vitiligo may not be as healthy and unaffected as previously assumed. Such an observation may provide the explanation for the isomorphic (Koebner) response typical of skin from those with vitiligo.

Summary

The histological, histochemical, and immunocytochemical analysis of vitiligo has clearly defined the cellular profile of amelanotic epidermis. Of significance is the confirmation that melanocytes are absent from the lesions. In addition, it is clear that melanocyte and keratinocyte damage can occur at the margin of a vitiligo lesion, as well as within the normally pigmented skin. However, remaining unresolved are the cellular and molecular mechanisms underlying the removal of the vitiligo melanocytes from various areas of the patient's body. Recently, the understanding of the molecular mechanisms regulating programmed cell death and immunocytochemical markers available to assess this process, has expanded tremendously. Critical information regarding the selective melanocyte destruction/removal may be forthcoming from investigations of apoptosis in vitiligo.

References

Abdel-Naser, M.B., Gollnick, H. & Orfanos, C.E. (1991) Evidence for primary involvement of keratinocytes in vitiligo. *Archives of Dermatological Research—Archiv für dermatologische Forschung* **283**, 47 (Abstract).

Abdel-Naser, M.B., Kruger-Krasagakeis, S., Krasagakis, K., Gollnick, H. & Orfanos, C.E. (1994) Further evidence for involvement of both cell mediated and humoral immunity in generalized vitiligo. *Pigment Cell Research* **7**, 1–8.

Becker, S.W. Jr, Fitzpatrick, T.B. & Montgomery, H. (1952) Human melanogenesis:

cytology and histology of pigment cells (melanodendrocytes). *Archives of Dermatology and Syphilology* **65**, 511–523.

Birbeck, M.S., Breathnach, A.S. & Everall, J.D. (1961) an electron microscope study of basal melanocytes and high-level clear cells (Langerhans' cells) in vitiligo. *Journal of Investigative Dermatology* **37**, 51–63.

Bleehen, S.S. (1979) Histology of vitiligo. In: *Pigment Cell 5: Part II of Proceedings of the Xth International Pigment Cell Conference, Cambridge, Massachusetts, 1977* (ed. S.N.Klaus), pp. 54–61. S. Karger, Basel/New York.

Bloch, B. (1917) Das problem der Pigmentbildung in der Haut. *Archiv für Dermatologie und Syphilologie* **124**, 129–208.

Blois, M.S. (1968) Phagocytosis of melanin particles by human epidermal cells *in vitro*. *Journal of Investigative Dermatology* **50**, 336–337.

Boissy, R.E. & Nordlund, J.J. (1995) Biology of Vitiligo. In: *Cutaneous Medicine and Surgery: an Integrated Program in Dermatology* (eds K.A.Arndt, P.E.LeBoit, J.K.Robinson & B.U.Wintroub), pp. 1210–1218. W.B. Saunders Company, Philadelphia.

Boissy, R.E. & Nordlund, J.J. (1997) Molecular basis of congenital hypopigmentary disorders in humans: a review. *Pigment Cell Research* **10**, 12–24.

Boissy, R.E., Liu, Y.-Y., Medrano, E.E. & Nordlund, J.J. (1991) Structural aberration of the rough endoplasmic reticulum and melanosome compartmentalization in long-term cultures of melanocytes from vitiligo patients. *Journal of Investigative Dermatology* **97**, 395–404.

Breathnach, A.S. (1975) Ultrastructural features of vitiliginous skin. *Giornale Italiano Di Dermatologia* **110**, 116–121.

Breathnach, A.S., Bor, S. & Wyllie, L.M. (1966) Electron microscopy of peripheral nerve terminals and marginal melanocytes in vitiligo. *Journal of Investigative Dermatology* **47**, 125–140.

Buckley, W.R. & Lobitz, W.C. Jr (1953) Vitiligo with a raised inflammatory border. *Archives of Dermatology and Syphilology* **67**, 316–320.

Dippel, E., Haas, N., Grabbe, J., Schadendorf, D., Hamann, K. & Czarnetzki, B.M. (1995) Expression of the c-kit receptor in hypomelanosis: a comparative study between piebaldism, naevus depigmentosus and vitiligo. *British Journal of Dermatology* **132**, 182–189.

Garb, J. & Wise, F. (1948) Vitiligo with raised borders. *Archives of Dermatology and Syphilology* **58**, 149–153.

Gokhale, B.B. & Mehta, L.N. (1983) Histopathology of vitiliginous skin. *International Journal of Dermatology* **22**, 477–480.

Grichnik, J.M., Ali, W.N., Burch, J.A., Byers, J.D., Garcia, C.A., Clark, R.E. & Shea, C.R. (1996) KIT expression reveals a population of precursor melanocytes in human skin. *Journal of Investigative Dermatology* **106**, 967–971.

Hu, F., Fosnaugh, R.P. & Lesney, P.F. (1959) *In vitro* studies on vitiligo. *Journal of Investigative Dermatology* **33**, 267–280.

Im, S., Hann, S.K., Kim, H.I., Kim, N.S. & Park, Y.-K. (1994) Biologic characteristics of cultured human vitiligo melanocytes. *International Journal of Dermatology* **33**, 556–562.

Jarrett, A. & Szabo, G. (1956) Pathological varieties of vitiligo and response to treatment with meladinine. *British Journal of Dermatology* **68**, 313–326.

Jimbow, K., Chen, H. & Park, J. (1996) Molecular mechanisms for TRP-1 involvement in vitiligo/leukoderma pathogenesis. *Pigment Cell Research* **S5**, 81 (Abstract).

King, R.A., Hearing, V.J., Creel, D.J. & Oetting, W.S. (1994) Albinism. In: *The Metabolic and Molecular Bases of Inherited Disease*, Vol. II (eds C.R.Scriver, A.L.Beaudet, W.S.Sly & D.Valle), 7th edn, pp. 4353–4392. McGraw-Hill, New York.

Koh, H.K., Sober, A.J., Nakagawa, H., Albert, D.M., Mihm, M.C. & Fitzpatrick, T.B. (1983) Malignant melanoma and vitiligo-like leukoderma: an electron microscopic study. *Journal of the American Academy of Dermatology* **9**, 696–708.

Kugelman, T.P. & Van Scott, E.J. (1961) Tyrosinase activity in melanocytes of human albinos. *Journal of Investigative Dermatology* **37**, 73–76.

Le Poole, C. & Boissy, R.E. (1997) Vitiligo. In: *Seminars in Cutaneous Medicine and Surgery*,

Vol. 16 (eds K.A.Arndt, P.E.Le Boit, J.K.Robinson & B.U.Wintroub), pp. 3–14. W.B. Saunders Company, Philadelphia.

Le Poole, I.C., van den Wijngaard, R.M.J.G.J., Westerhof, W., Dutrieux, R.P. & Das, P.K. (1993) Presence or absence of melanocytes in vitiligo lesions: an immunohistochemical investigation. *Journal of Investigative Dermatology* **100**, 816–822.

Le Poole, I.C., van den Wijngaard, R.M.J.G.J., Westerhof, W. & Das, P.K. (1996) Presence of T cells and macrophages in inflammatory vitiligo skin parallels melanocyte disappearance. *American Journal of Pathology* **148**, 1219–1228.

Martins, L.M. & Earnshaw, W.C. (1997) Apoptosis: alive and kicking in 1997. *Trends in Cell Biology* **7**, 111–114.

Masson, P. (1948) *Pigment Cells in Man*. New York Academy of Sciences Special Publication 4, 15–51.

Michaelsson, G. (1968) Vitiligo with raised borders. Report of two cases. *Acta Dermato-Venereologica (Stockholm)* **48**, 158–161.

Mishima, Y., Kawasaki, H. & Pinkus, H. (1972) Dendritic cell dynamics in progressive depigmentations. Distinctive cytokinetics of dendritic cells revealed by electron microscopy. *Archives of Dermatological Research—Archiv für dermatologische Forschung* **243**, 67–87.

Moellmann, G., Klein-Angerer, S., Scollay, D., Nordlund, J.J. & Lerner, A.B. (1982) Extracellular granular material and degeneration of keratinocytes in the normally pigmented epidermis of patients with vitiligo. *Journal of Investigative Dermatology* **79**, 321–330.

Morohashi, M., Hashimoto, K., Goodman, T.F. Jr, Newton, D.E. & Rist, T. (1977) Ultrastructural studies of vitiligo, Vogt–Koyanagi syndrome, and incontinentia pigmenti achromians. *Archives of Dermatology* **113**, 755–766.

Okun, M.R., Edelstein, L.M., Niebauer, G. & Hamada, G. (1969) The histochemical tyrosine-DOPA reaction for tyrosinase and its use in localizing tyrosinase activity in mast cells. *Journal of Investigative Dermatology* **53**, 39–45.

Quevedo, W.C. Jr & Holstein, T.J. (1998) General biology of mammalian pigmentation. In: *The Pigmentary System. Physiology and Pathophysiology* (eds J.J.Nordlund, R.E.Boissy, V.J.Hearing, R.A.King & J.-P.Ortonne), pp. 43–58. Oxford University Press, New York.

Savill, J., Fadok, V., Henson, P. & Haslett, C. (1993) Phagocyte recognition of cells undergoing apoptosis. *Immunology Today* **14**, 131–136.

Wolff, K. & Konrad, K. (1971) Melanin pigmentation: an *in vivo* model for studies of melanosome kinetics within keratinocytes. *Science* **174**, 1034–1035.

6: Clinical Features of Generalized Vitiligo

SEUNG-KYUNG HANN AND JAMES J. NORDLUND

Introduction

Vitiligo is a relatively common depigmenting disorder affecting approximately 0.5–2% of the general population (Lerner 1959). The diagnostic lesion of vitiligo is characterized by discrete, pale-white macules, few or many in number, which tend to enlarge centrifugally over time. All races and ethnic groups seem to be affected equally. Vitiligo is not contagious, nor does it contribute to the loss of general health. However, it can be troublesome, especially to brown and black people but also to white people who tan deeply (skin types 2, 3 and 4). Many patients are socially embarrassed and experience psychological turmoil (Porter *et al.* 1978, 1986, 1987; Porter 1989; Porter & Beuf 1988, 1991; Moscher 1993) (see Chapter 13). It should be noted that even those with very fair complexions are distressed by the onset of vitiligo although the disorder might not be apparent to others.

Reports from a few investigators suggest that females are more commonly involved than males. More recent studies suggest that the prevalence is the same in both genders (Nordlund & Majumder 1997). This discrepancy probably can be attributed to the inclination of women to seek dermatological assistance because of their concern about cosmesis and appearance (see Chapter 13). Vitiligo is often associated with a family history of first or distant relatives affected by vitiligo. Up to 30% of patients with vitiligo report that another family member is affected (Majumder *et al.* 1988, 1993; Nath *et al.* 1994; Nordlund & Majumder 1997) (see Chapter 4).

Age of onset

Vitiligo may appear any time from shortly after birth to senescence, although an onset between 5 and 30 years of age is most common. Congenital vitiligo has been reported on one or two occasions (Song *et al.* 1994). The average age of onset is around 20 years (Nordlund & Majumder 1997). In the latter study, the mean and median ages of onset, 20 and 21 years, respectively, were similar.

Many reports have suggested that the mean age of onset is younger in females than in males. Levai (1958) found the average age of onset in India to be 18 years for females and 26 years for males. Howitz *et al.* (1977), working in Denmark, found virtually no difference in age of onset for the two genders, e.g. a mean of 36.7 years for females and 38.7 years for males. Results of a study by Song *et al.* (1994) showed that the mean age of onset was 21.9 years (male: 20.7, female: 22.9), and the minimal and maximal ages of onset were at birth and 68 years, respectively. It does seem probable that females seek medical assistance for treatment of vitiligo sooner after onset than do males. That women have a heightened concern about the appearance of their skin contributes to an early sensibility of the condition and earlier presentation to a dermatologist for treatment.

Precipitating factors

Patients with vitiligo often attribute the onset of their disease to a specific life event such as a crisis or an illness. However there is no factor that has been proven to cause or initiate vitiligo. From 10% to 76% of patients with vitiligo implicate a precipitating antecedent such as a physical injury, sunburn, emotional trauma, illness or pregnancy (Behl & Bhatia 1972; Koo *et al.* 1996). However, such events are very common and are easily blamed by the patient and physicians for initiating a disorder like vitiligo. That such events are very common makes it difficult for the investigator to prove that they are in fact involved in causing or precipitating vitiligo. On the other hand, the possibility of a chance association does not negate the possibility that they might precipitate vitiligo. Regardless, these factors reputed by patients or physicians to cause vitiligo must be considered anecdotal and theoretical until the actual pathogenesis of vitiligo is known.

The development of vitiligo at the site of a physical injury such as a cut or abrasion is referred to as the Koebner or isomorphic phenomenon. Song *et al.* (1994) reported that 324 patients (24.6%) among a total of 1315 patients attributed a multiplicity of events to be involved in precipitating vitiligo. Physical injury was the most common preceding factor (44.1%), possibly as a manifestation of the isomorphic response. Other factors implicated in initiating vitiligo were emotional tension (26.2%), sunburn (11.7%), pregnancy and parturition (2.8%). Frequent sites where vitiligo tended to spread during pregnancy were the breasts and abdomen. Distension of skin and striae formation on the breasts and abdomen might be considered a form of physical trauma. Vitiligo in the United States and Europe appears to be more commonly observed in areas exposed to the sun such as the hands and face. Thus sunburn has been implicated in initiating the expression of vitiligo in predisposed individuals. However, in other parts of the world, such as East Africa which is sun drenched because of its location near the equator, vitiligo is less commonly seen on the exposed skin and affects principally the covered skin. Many patients have noted good repigmentation from sun exposure. Possibly this discrepancy about the harm or usefulness of sunlight is explained by the amount of exposure, so that exposure without burn prevents or restores pigment, sun exposure with burn aggravates vitiligo. Therapeutic radiation has been reported to induce vitiligo. Koo *et al.* (1996) reported on two patients who developed vitiligo on the chest where radiation had been given for treatment of breast cancer.

Characteristics of lesions

The typical lesion of vitiligo is a discrete, well circumscribed, chalk white macule. There may be one, several, or up to hundreds of macules that may be small to large in size. As vitiligo evolves over time, the macules enlarge, coalesce, and form a patch with sharp, convex margins which are usually easily distinguishable from other disorders of hypopigmentation such as piebaldism or naevus depigmentosus (Berg & Tarnowski 1974; Kang & Hann 1996; Nordlund *et al.* 1998) (see Chapter 14). An early lesion may be a slightly white, hypopigmented macule with an indistinct border. Poorly defined lesions are easily detected by Wood's light examination. While vitiligo macules are characteristically chalk white in colour, in those with darker coloured skin, there may be trichrome or multichrome pigmentation which takes on a tan colour intermediate between the normally pigmented skin and the typically white vitiligo macule (Seghal 1974; Fargnolic & Bolognia 1995). Confetti-sized (2–4 mm) macules, which are typically white in colour may occur randomly over the integument or may be located in the perifollicular skin.

Distribution of vitiligo

Vitiligo can exhibit two general patterns, i.e. it can be either unilateral or bilateral (see the section on classification below). Bilateral vitiligo has several distinguishable subpatterns. Vitiligo lesions may be localized or generalized, the latter being more common. Localized vitiligo is restricted to a few small areas on both sides of the trunk. The spots are not segmental in distribution. Generalized vitiligo implies more widespread distribution of lesions involving larger and more numerous areas of the integument. Unilateral or segmental involvement only very rarely coexists with generalized vitiligo, which is classified as mixed type (see Chapter 7).

Although vitiligo may occur on any part of the integument, there are characteristic patterns of involvement. The most frequently involved sites are the face and dorsum of the hands, the axillae, umbilicus, nipples, sacrum, and inguinal regions. Song *et al.* (1994) reported that the most common sites of involvement were the face (24.5%), neck (18.8%), and scalp (11.2%). Many of the most common sites of occurrence are areas subjected to repeated trauma or irritation. Such common sites include the bony prominences, extensor forearm, ventral wrists, dorsal hands and digital phalanges. One explanation for this distribution is that these sites represent a manifestation of the Koebner phenomenon. Involvement of the palms and soles is common but has not been appreciated. Palm and sole involvement in light skinned people is difficult to detect without the use of a Wood's

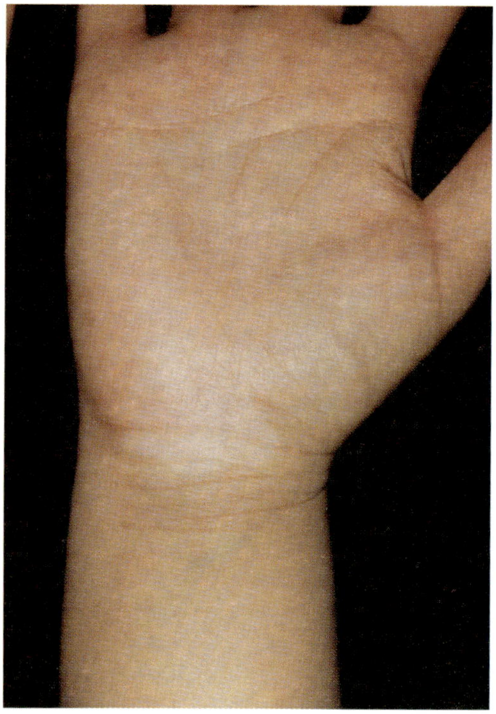

Fig. 6.1 Vitiligo distributed on the ventral wrist.

light. Involvement of the ventral wrist may be linked to vitiligo of the palms (Figs 6.1 & 6.2). The interfollicular epidermis of the scalp frequently is overlooked as a site of depigmentation although the melanocytes in the hair follicles are spared. The involvement of the skin of the scalp usually is conspicuous in those with dark skin.

Mucous membrane involvement in vitiligo is not mentioned or is said to be rare. The mucous membranes of Caucasians are pink in colour and loss of pigment is very difficult to detect even with a Wood's lamp. In contrast the mouth of those with darker skin is pigmented and the patchy loss of pigmentation is readily apparent to the attentive observer. In a study of 45 patients living in Tanzania, 75% had patchy loss of pigment from the gums or mucosa of the inner lips. We speculate that Michael Jackson, the popular singer, first began wearing lipstick to cover the onset of vitiligo involving his lips and mucous membranes and later wore a glove to cover vitiligo on his hands. In addition to the mucous membranes of the mouth, vitiligo often occurs on the genitals, areolae and nipples (Song *et al.* 1994).

Involvement of body and scalp hair

Depigmentation of body and scalp hair occurs in 9–45% of those patients with vitiligo (Dutta & Mandal 1969; Howitz *et al.* 1977; Song *et al.* 1994). The perifollicular and/or interfollicular skin often is affected. Vitiligo of the follicles on the scalp usually presents as scattered white hairs. The appearance

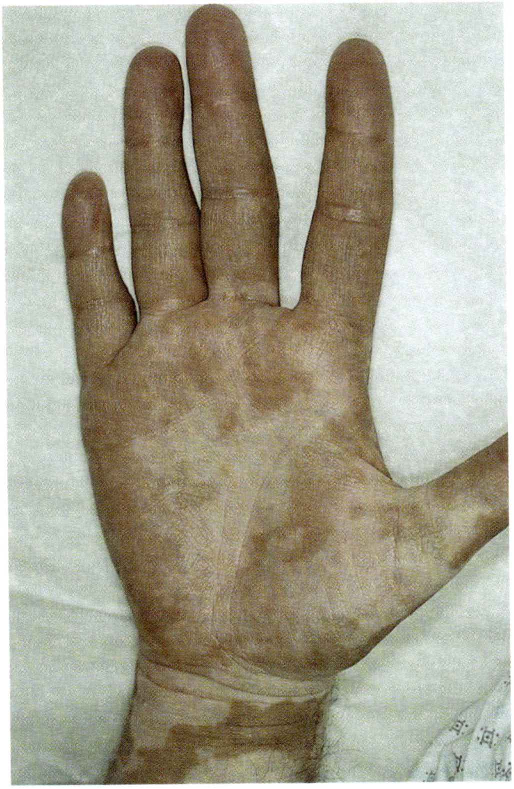

Fig. 6.2 Vitiligo on the palms.

of the scalp sometimes is described as salt and pepper colour. Very rarely total depigmentation of all the hair of the scalp occurs. Song *et al.* (1994) noted 355 patients (27%) out of 1350 patients with vitiligo had some leukotrichia. Scalp involvement was the most frequent (63.7%), followed by eyebrow (13.8%), pubic hair (8.4%) and axilla (2%). Leukotrichia is a marker for poor prognosis in regard to repigmentation (Dutta & Mandal 1969) because of the need for a reservoir of melanocytes for successful therapy (see Chapter 20). In addition to the leukotrichia, premature greying of hair has been observed in up to 37% of those with vitiligo (Moscher 1993). White, depigmented hairs must be distinguished from grey hairs that retain melanin that is distributed in an aberrant fashion.

Clinical classification of vitiligo

There have been many attempts to classify types of vitiligo, often with confusing results. One simple classification is presented here.

Localized

Focal. One or more macules in one area, but not clearly in a segmental or zosteriform distribution (Fig. 6.3).

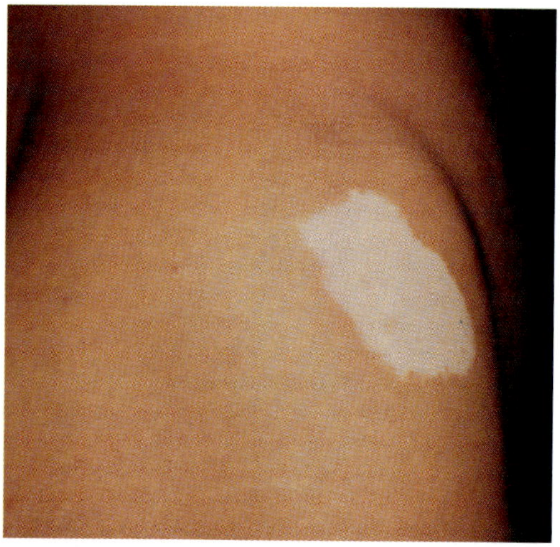

Fig. 6.3 Focal vitiligo.

Segmental. One or more macules involving a unilateral segment of the body, i.e. part of the face, part of the trunk and extremity or one extremity (Koga 1977). The lesions stop abruptly at the midline of the affected segment (Figs 6.4, 6.5 and see Fig. 7.1).

Mucosal. Vitiligo of the mouth and mucous membranes (Fig. 6.6), vitiligo on the genitalia (Fig. 6.7).

Generalized

Acrofacial. Distal parts of the extremities and face (Fig. 6.8).

Vulgaris. Scattered macules (Fig. 6.9).

Mixed. Acrofacial and vulgaris, or segmental and acrofacial and/or vulgaris.

Universal

Complete or nearly complete depigmentation. The incidence of each type of vitiligo using this classification varies from study to study. Generalized type of vitiligo varies from 50–90% (Howitz *et al.* 1977; Moscher 1993; Song *et al.* 1994). Song *et al.* (1994) reported on 1315 patients. There were 660 cases (50.2%) of generalized type which consisted of acrofacial (14.4%) and vulgaris (35.8%) varieties. There were 654 cases (49.7%) of localized type consisting of focal (33.7%), segmental (15.4%), and mucosal (0.6%) forms and one case of universal type. Localized types of vitiligo, with the exception of segmental type, may be an intermediary stage and evolve into the generalized or, rarely, into the universal type. Segmental vitiligo is never an intermediary stage of vitiligo. There are very few patients with both generalized

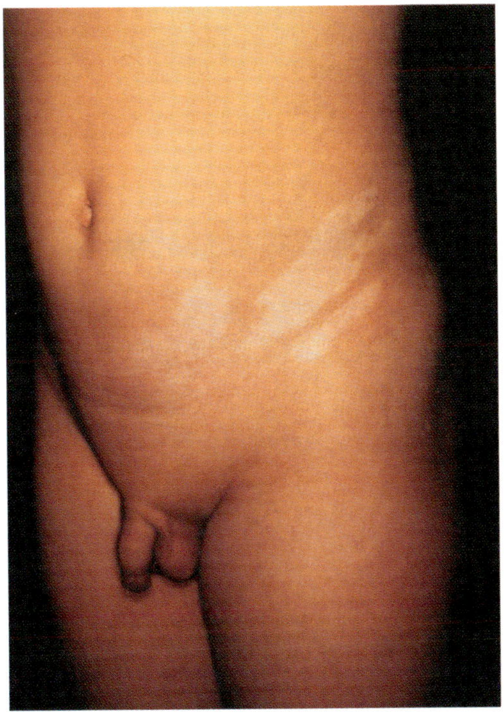

Fig. 6.4 Segmental vitiligo on the flank.

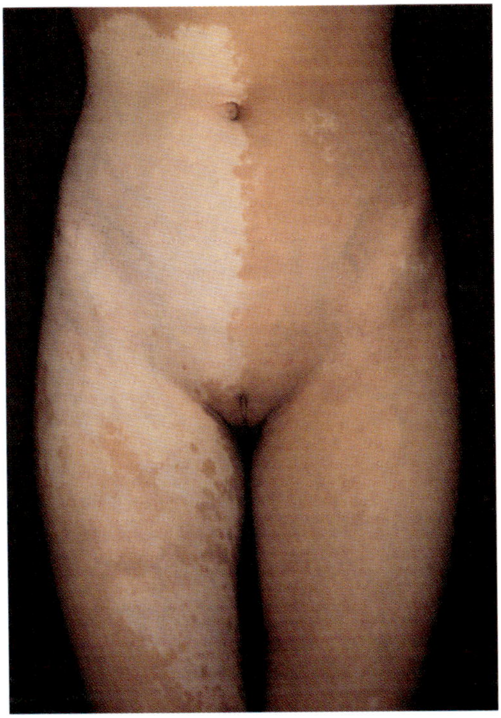

Fig. 6.5 Segmental vitiligo involving right side of the trunk and right leg.

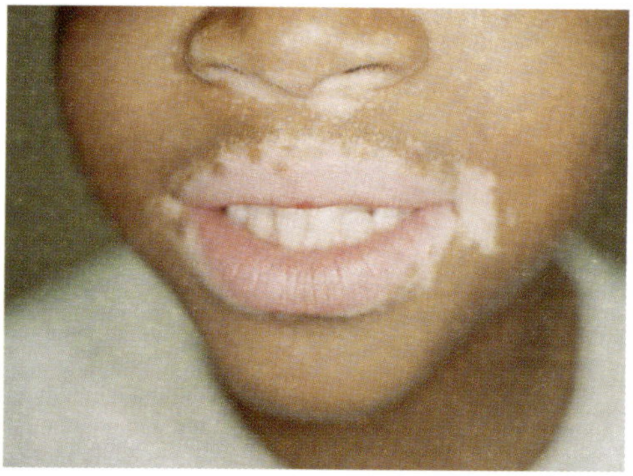

Fig. 6.6 Mucosal vitiligo on the mouth.

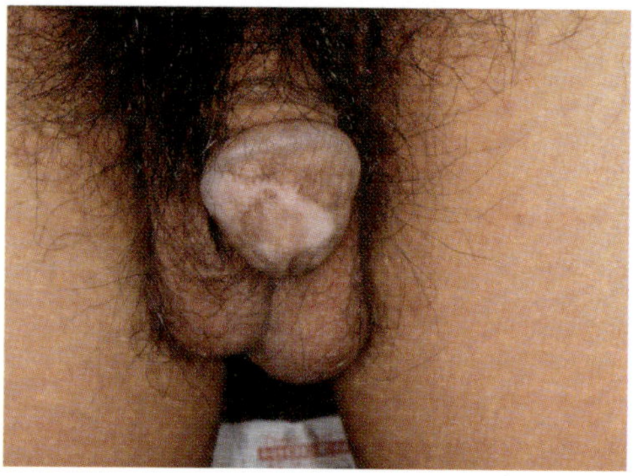

Fig. 6.7 Mucosal vitiligo on the genitalia.

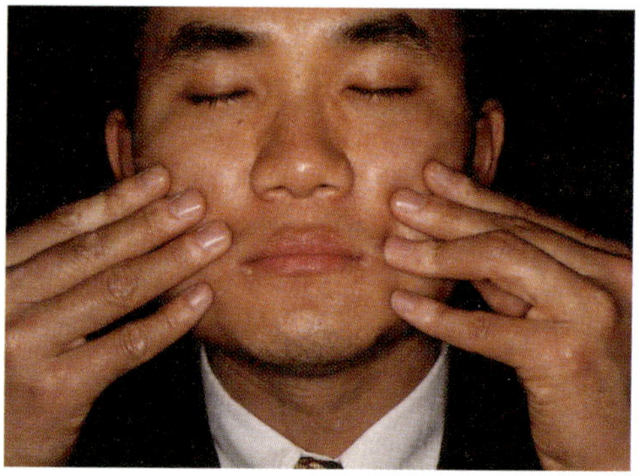

Fig. 6.8 Acrofacial vitiligo on the fingertips and around the mouth.

and segmental vitiligo. The authors know of two such individuals and they seem to have two different types of vitiligo.

Vitiligo can also be classified into three major clinical types, segmental nonsegmental and mixed, as follows:

1 segmental (unilateral);

2 nonsegmental (bilateral):

(a) focal

(b) mucosal

(c) acrofacial

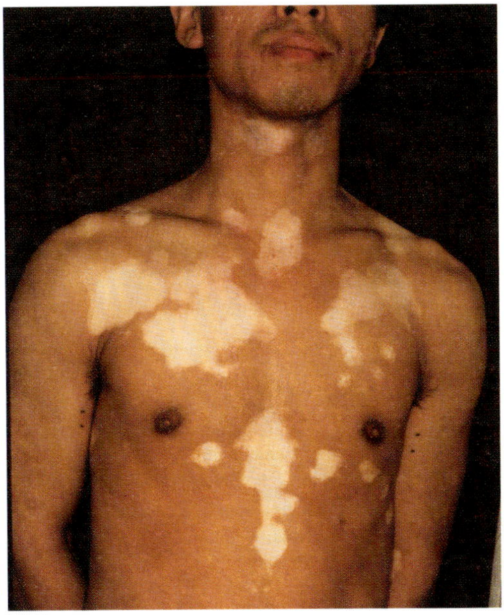

Fig. 6.9 Vitiligo vulgaris.

(d) vulgaris
(e) universal;

3 mixed, segmental and nonsegmental.

Segmental vitiligo represents lesions distributed on one side of the body in a pseudodermatomal pattern. In segmental vitiligo, depigmented patches are confined to a particular patch of skin (see Chapter 7). The central border of this type of vitiligo does not cross the midline (Barona *et al.* 1995).

Course of vitiligo

The course of vitiligo is often unpredictable. The natural course of the disease is usually one of slow progression, but it may stabilize or exacerbate rapidly. Vitiligo spreads either by appearance of new depigmented macules, by centrifugal enlargement of pre-existing lesions or both. On rare occasions, there is rapid or galloping vitiligo that leads to extensive depigmentation over a few days to weeks, a condition that is called vitiligo fulminans. The reverse also happens but not often enough. Vitiligo can spontaneously repigment but usually only partially. Spontaneous repigmentation is noted in about 10–20% of patients with vitiligo, most frequently in sun-exposed areas and is usually minimal in extent.

Focal or generalized vitiligo spreads progressively to involve small or large portions of the integument on any part of the body without any predictable pattern. Chun and Hann (1997) reported the progression pattern of bilateral vitiligo and its implications on prognosis. In the study, the body surface was divided into 9 topographical areas to record the distribution of lesions. They were the face, neck, anterior trunk, posterior trunk, genital

Table 6.1 Initial sites and progression rates of nonsegmental vitiligo.

		Progression rate (%)	
Initial site	Incidence (%)	One site[1]	Two sites[2]
Face	124 (39.0)	81 (64.8)	65 (52.4)
Neck	33 (10.4)	28 (84.8)	22 (66.7)
Anterior trunk	75 (23.6)	61 (81.3)	55 (73.3)
Posterior trunk	31 (9.1)	28 (90.3)	25 (80.6)
Genitalia	5 (1.6)	4 (80.0)	3 (60.0)
Upper extremity	10 (3.1)	6 (60.0)	6 (60.0)
Lower extremity	18 (5.7)	12 (66.7)	12 (66.7)
Hands	20 (6.3)	19 (95.0)	17 (85.0)
Feet	2 (0.6)	2 (100.0)	2 (100.0)
Total	318	241 (75.8)	207 (65.1)

[1] One site means involvement of at least one body surface area in addition to the initial site.
[2] Two sites means involvement of at least two body surface areas in addition to the initial site.

area, upper extremities, lower extremities, hands and feet. The progression rate was assessed by applying the following formula:

Progression = Number of patients whose vitiligo started from a particular site but progressed to another site) ÷ (total number of patients whose vitiligo started from a particular site).

The progression rate of bilateral vitiligo according to the initial sites was studied (Table 6.1). When the face was the initial site, the progression of vitiligo was less common than for other sites of onset. Facial vitiligo was followed by spread to one additional site in 64.8% of those involved and to two sites in 52.4%. The average rates of progression for more than one and two sites were 75.8% and 65.1%, respectively. When the posterior trunk, hands, or feet were the initial sites, there was progression of vitiligo in over 90% of patients.

The progression pattern of bilateral vitiligo starting from the face, neck, anterior trunk, posterior trunk, and hands has been studied (Table 6.2). The percentages indicate the respective progression rates from the initial sites to other specific body surface areas. The body surface areas contiguous to the initial sites usually showed the highest rates of progression. However, when the hands were the initial site, vitiligo most commonly progressed to the face. The progression of nonsegmental vitiligo had significant differences according to the site of the initial lesions. When the initial sites were the posterior trunk, hands or feet, there was more widespread progression to other body areas, while there was less progression when the initial sites were the face and upper or lower extremities. These results indicate that the prognosis of vitiligo may be predicted by the location of the initial lesions. The progression pattern of nonsegmental vitiligo was usually contiguous to the initial site regardless of the location. This was interesting because nonsegmental vitiligo is usually associated with autoimmune diseases (Norris

Table 6.2 The progression pattern of nonsegmental vitiligo from initial sites.

Initial sites	Face	Neck	AT	PT	Hands
Spreading sites	(124)[1]	(33)	(75)	(31)	(20)
Face	. . . . . .	7 (25.0%)	13 (21.3%)	3 (11.1%)	9 (45.0%)
Neck	25[2] (30.9%)	. . . . . .	7 (11.5%)	1 (3.7%)	1 (5.0%)
Anterior trunk (AT)	24 (29.6%)	14 (50.0%)	. . . . . .	12 (44.5%)	3 (15.0%)
Posterior trunk (PT)	9 (11.1%)	2 (7.1%)	18 (29.5%)	. . . . . .	0 0
Genitalia	5 (6.2%)	0 0	6 (9.8%)	3 (11.1%)	0 0
Upper extremity	4 (4.9%)	0 0	7 (11.5%)	0 0	2 (10.0%)
Lower extremity	6 (7.4%)	1 (3.6%)	7 (11.5%)	3 (11.1%)	3 (15.0%)
Hands	8 (9.9%)	4 (14.3%)	3 (4.9%)	5 (18.5%)	. . . . . .
Feet	0 0	0 0	0 0	0 0	2 (10.0%)

[1] The number of patients whose initial site is the face.
[2] The number of patients whose second involved site is the neck.

et al. 1988; Harning *et al.* 1991) and one would expect a generalized, haphazard progression if autoimmune mechanisms were involved in its pathogenesis. When the hands were the initial site, vitiligo most commonly progressed to the face. This could be explained clinically by the fact that 1/3 of the patients whose vitiligo started from the hands were of the acrofacial type.

Factors affecting progression of vitiligo

Factors that are claimed to aggravate vitiligo include emotional shock, physical illness, sunburn, and pregnancy (Dutta & Mandal 1969; Behl & Bhatia 1972; Song *et al.* 1994). These subjective experiences vary from one patient to another and cannot be used with certainty by the dermatologist to advise patients. Objective clinical characteristics such as gender, family history, clinical type, onset age, duration, Koebner's phenomenon, leukotrichia, and mucous membrane involvement may be important. Various clinical characteristics and their significance in the progression of vitiligo were evaluated by Hann *et al.* (1997). The summary of clinical characteristics of progressive and nonprogressive vitiligo is presented in Table 6.3. There were no differences between the sexes where progression of vitiligo was concerned. Patients with no progression were relatively

Table 6.3 Summary of clinical characteristics of progressive and nonprogressive vitiligo.

Clinical parameter	Progressive vitiligo (N = 355)	Nonprogressive vitiligo (N = 45)	*P* value
Sex			>0.05
Male	137	15	
Female	218	30	
Family History			<0.05
Present	51	1	
Absent	304	44	
Clinical Type			<0.05
Segmental	66	16	
Nonsegmental	289	29	
Onset Age (yr)	20.2	16.5	>0.05
Duration (yr)	8.1	4.2	<0.05
Koebner's phenomenon			<0.05
Present	80	4	
Absent	275	41	
Leukotrichia			>0.05
Present	158	16	
Absent	197	29	
Mucosal involvement			<0.05
Present	255	41	
Absent	100	4	

younger, an observation that might be expected since childhood vitiligo is associated with a higher incidence of segmental vitiligo and consequently a better prognosis (Halder *et al.* 1987; Hann & Lee 1996).

The duration of the disease was important in evaluating the progression of vitiligo. Patients with longer duration demonstrated a significant progression of vitiligo. Koebner's phenomenon refers to the development of vitiligo or other skin diseases after a physical injury such as a cut, burn or abrasion and it is present in at least one-third of vitiligo patients (Moscher 1993). The results of one study demonstrated that patients with Koebner's isomorphic phenomenon were more likely to have progressive vitiligo. Leukotrichia is reported as a marker for a poor prognosis in repigmentation (Dutta & Mandal 1969). However, vitiligo with leukotrichia did not progress more significantly than in patients without leukotrichia. Significant progression of vitiligo in patients with mucosal involvement indicates that it is a poor prognostic factor.

Clinical characteristics of bilateral vitiligo

Bilateral vitiligo comprises all types of vitiligo other than segmental. Confetti type vitiligo or vitiligo fulminans may appear initially as generalized type. Clinically, today's focal vitiligo can change to a generalized type tomorrow. Therefore, prevention of spreading is an important management strategy of bilateral vitiligo. When focal vitiligo appears initially as a single lesion, it may not be easy to determine the type of vitiligo. When a single white macule appears on the areola unilaterally, the diagnosis most often will be focal vitiligo. However, it can often spread in a linear fashion, very slowly manifesting the features of segmental vitiligo. Areolar or nipple involvement in nonsegmental vitiligo usually appears bilaterally as a late manifestation.

Focal vitiligo is a starting point leading to other types of vitiligo. Although early treatment does not always prevent spread of vitiligo, focal vitiligo frequently spreads to the whole body without treatment. From Moon *et al.'s* study (1995) systemic steroid effectively prevents the spreading of vitiligo, not only focal type but also generalized type. It is not known what percentage of focal vitiligo progresses to other types of vitiligo.

Conclusion

Vitiligo has various clinical features. Understanding these characteristics can give us valuable information in differentiating vitiligo from other hypopigmentary disorders, in treating vitiligo with the proper methods and in predicting the prognosis of vitiligo to some extent.

References

Barona, M.I., Arrunategui, A., Falabella, R. & Alzate, A. (1995) An epidemiologic case-control study in a population with vitiligo. *Journal of the American Academy of Dermatology* **33**, 621–625.

Behl, P.N. & Bhatia, R.K. (1972) 400 cases of vitiligo: a clinico-therapeutical analysis. *Indian Journal of Dermatology* **17**, 51–55.

Berg, M. & Tarnowski, W. (1974) Nevus depigmentosus. *Archives of Dermatology* **109**, 920–921.

Chun, W.H. & Hann, S.K. (1997) The progression of nonsegmental vitiligo: clinical analysis of 318 patients. *International Journal of Dermatology* **36**, 908–910.

Dutta, A.K. & Mandal, S.B. (1969) Clinical study of 650 vitiligo cases and their classification. *Indian Journal of Dermatology* **14**, 103–115.

Fargnolic, M.C. & Bolognia, J.L. (1995) Pentachrome vitiligo. *Journal of the American Academy of Dermatology* **33**, 853–856.

Halder, R.M., Grimes, P.E., Cowan, C.A., Enterline, J.A., Chakrabarti, S.G. & Kenny, J.A. Jr (1987) Childhood vitiligo. *Journal of the American Academy of Dermatology* **16**, 948–954.

Hann, S.K. & Lee, H.J. (1996) Segmental vitiligo: clinical findings in 208 patients. *Journal of the American Academy of Dermatology* **35**, 671–674.

Hann, S.K., Chun, W.H. & Park, Y.K. (1997) Clinical characteristics of progressive vitiligo. *International Journal of Dermatology* **36**, 353–355.

Harning, R., Cui, J. & Bystryn, J.C. (1991) Relation between the incidence and level of pigment cell antibodies and disease activity in vitiligo. *Journal of Investigative Dermatology* **97**, 1078–1080.

Howitz, J., Brodthagen, H., Schwartz, M. *et al.* (1977) Prevalence of vitiligo: epidemiologic survey on the Isle of Borholm, Denmark. *Archives of Dermatology* **113**, 47–52.

Kang, I.K. & Hann, S.K. (1996) Vitiligo coexistent with nevus depigmentosus. *Journal of Dermatology* **23**, 187–190.

Koga, M. (1977) Vitiligo: a new classification and therapy. *British Journal of Dermatology* **97**, 255–261.

Koo, S.W., Suh, C.O. & Hann, S.K. (1996) Vitiligo following radiotherapy for carcinoma of breast. *British Journal of Dermatology* **135**, 752–853.

Lerner, A.B. (1959) Vitiligo. *Journal of Investigative Dermatology* **32**, 285–310.

Levai, M. (1958) A study of certain contributory factors in the development of vitiligo in South Indian patients. *Archives of Dermatology* **78**, 364–370.

Majumder, P.P., Das, D.K. & Li, C.C. (1988) A genetical model for vitiligo. *American Journal of Human Genetics* **43**, 119–125.

Majumder, P.P., Nordlund, J.J. & Nath, S.K. (1993) Pattern of familial aggregation of vitiligo. *Archives of Dermatology* **129**, 994–998.

Moon, T.K., Im, S., Hann, S.K., Cho, S.H. & Park, Y.K. (1995) The effect of small doses of oral corticosteroids in vitiligo patients. *Korean Journal of Dermatology* **33**, 880–885.

Moscher, D.B. (1993) Vitiligo: etiology, pathogenesis, diagnosis, and treatment. In: *Dermatology in General Medicine,* Vol I (eds T.B. Fitzpatrick, A.Z. Eisen, K. Wolff, I.M. Freedberg & K.F. Austen) 4th edn., pp. 923–933. McGraw-Hill, New York.

Nath, S.K., Majumder, P.P. & Nordlund, J.J. (1994). Genetic epidemiology of vitiligo: multilocus recessivity cross-validated. *American Journal of Human Genetics* **55**, 981–990.

Nordlund, J.J. & Majumder, P.P. (1997) Recent investigations on vitiligo vulgaris. (Review). *Dermatologic Clinics* **15**, 69–78.

Nordlund, J.J., Boissy, R.E., Hearing, V.J., King, R.A. & Ortonne, J.-P., eds. (1998) *The Pigmentary System: Physiology and Pathophysiology*. Oxford University Press, New York.

Norris, D.A., Kissinger, R.M. & Naughton, G.M. (1988) Evidence for immunologic mechanisms in human vitiligo: patients' sera induce damage to human melanocytes in vitro by complement-mediated damage and antibody-dependent cellular toxicity. *Journal of Investigative Dermatology* **90**, 783–789.

Porter, J. (1989) Psychosocial effects of skin disease. *Medical and Health Annual*, pp. 388–390. Encyclopedia Britannica, Chicago.

Porter, J. & Beuf, A. (1988) Response of older people to impaired appearance: the effect of age on disturbance by vitiligo. *Journal of Aging Studies* **2**, 167–181.

Porter, J.R. & Beuf, A.H. (1991) Racial variation in reaction to physical stigma: a study of degree of disturbance by vitiligo among black and white patients. *Journal of Health Social Behavior* **32**, 192–204.

Porter, J., Beuf, A., Nordlund, J.J. & Lerner, A.B. (1978) Personal responses of patients to vitiligo: the importance of the patient–physician interaction. *Archives of Dermatology* **114**, 1384–1385.

Porter, J.R., Beuf, A.H., Lerner, A.B. & Nordlund, J.J. (1986) Psychosocial effect of vitiligo: a comparison of vitiligo patients with 'normal' control subjects, with psoriasis patients, and with patients with other pigmentary disorders. *Journal of the American Academy of Dermatology* **15**, 220–224.

Porter, J., Beuf, A.H., Lerner, A.B. & Nordlund, J.J. (1987) Response to cosmetic disfigurement: patients with vitiligo. *Cutis* **39**, 493–494.

Seghal, V.N. (1974) A clinical evaluation of 202 cases of vitiligo. *Cutis* **14**, 439–445.

Song, M.S., Hann, S.K., Ahn, P.S., Im, S. & Park, Y.K. (1994) Clinical study of vitiligo: comparative study of type A and type B vitiligo. *Annals of Dermatology* **6**, 22–30.

7: Clinical Features of Segmental Vitiligo

SEUNG-KYUNG HANN

Introduction

The classification of vitiligo into two types, generalized and localized, is widely used. Localized lesions in a dermatomal distribution that do not cross the midline are called segmental or unilateral vitiligo. Koga (1977) divided vitiligo into two varieties, type A which is characterized as the bilateral, non segmental vitiligo; and type B, the segmental form. The clinical features of bilateral vitiligo have been frequently reported (Lerner 1959; Seghal 1974; Hann *et al.* 1991), but few studies on segmental vitiligo have been completed. The clinical features of segmental vitiligo differ markedly from those of nonsegmental vitiligo. Segmental vitiligo usually has an onset early in life and spreads rapidly within the affected area which is limited to one segment of the integument. The course of the segmental type can arrest and the depigmented patches can persist unchanged for the life of the patient. This feature differs very strikingly from the chronic progressive course of bilateral, nonsegmental vitiligo (Koga & Tango 1988; Hann & Lee 1996).

Incidence

The incidence of segmental type is not well established but the percentage of those with vitiligo having the segmental form has been reported. El Mofty and El Mofty (1980) reported 5% of those with vitiligo had the segmental type, while Koga and Tango (1988) indicated that as many as 27.9% had this type of depigmentation. Results of Korean studies suggested a range between 5.5 and 16.1% (Park *et al.* 1988; Song *et al.* 1994).

Age of onset

Vitiligo develops at all ages, but usually occurs in younger people between the ages of 5 and 30 years (Seghal 1974). Koga & Tango (1988) reported that the onset of segmental vitiligo generally affected young children whereas nonsegmental vitiligo occurred at any age. In Hann and Lee's report (1996), segmental vitiligo developed before 30 years of age in 87.0% of patients, and 41.3% were younger than 10 years. These observations are in accord with Koga and Tango's report (1988) that segmental vitiligo occurs in young

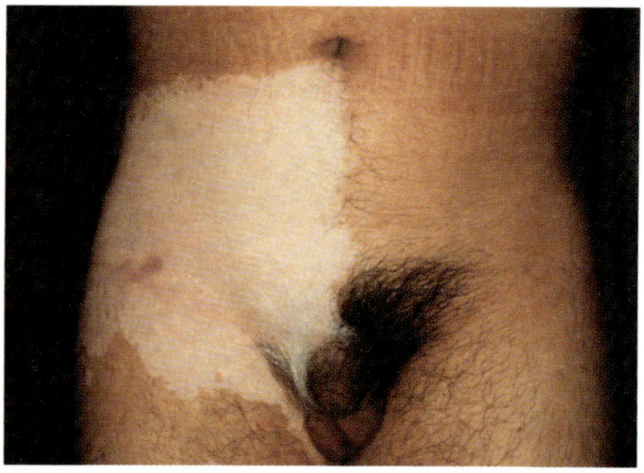

Fig. 7.1 Segmental vitiligo distributed along thoracic and lumbar dermatomes.

people before age 30 years. The mean age of onset was 15.6 years in Hann and Lee's study (1996), which is younger than the 23.1 years reported by Levai (1958) and the 24.2 years reported by Seghal (1974).

Site of involvement

In Hann and Lee's study (1996) of segmental vitiligo, the face was the most common site of involvement regardless of the gender of the patient. The trunk, neck, extremities and scalp were involved in descending frequency in males (Fig. 7.1.) In females the neck was more frequently involved than the extremities (Table 7.1). Lerner (1959) reported that segmental vitiligo occurs as a single lesion in 75% of patients, a finding confirmed by the study of Hann and Lee. They found that 87% of patients had a single lesion (1996). Among the 31 patients with segmental vitiligo studied by Park *et al.* 1988, the abdomen, neck, face, and chest, in descending order of frequency, were the most commonly involved sites. The results in this report differ from those of Hann and Lee's study (1996).

Involvement of body and scalp hair

Poliosis, known to be associated with vitiligo in 8.9–45% of cases (Lerner 1959; Dutta & Mandal 1969; Lerner 1971; Howitz *et al.* 1977), occurred in 48.6% of cases of segmental vitiligo (Hann & Lee 1996). The eyebrows and scalp hair were mostly involved (46.7%). Due to the fact that segmental vitiligo tends to involve the face, neck and scalp, poliosis of the eyebrows and scalp hair is commonly present. White hair indicates that the reservoir for repigmentation has been destroyed (see Chapter 20). Leukotrichia of the eyebrows can be treated by undergoing epidermal grafting and receiving PUVA (Hann *et al.* 1992).

Distribution of lesions

From Hann and Lee's study (1998), the distribution of segmental vitiligo on the face was classified into five patterns (Table 7.2). Type 1a represents the

Table 7.1 Site of segmental vitiligo.

Site	Male (%)	Female (%)	Total (%)
Head&Neck	57(62.6)	87(65.9)	144(64.6)
Face	49(53.8)	65(49.2)	114(51.1)
Neck	7(7.7)	20(15.2)	27(12.1)
Scalp	1(1.1)	2(1.5)	3(1.4)
Trunk	21(23.1)	34(25.8)	55(24.7)
Chest & Abdomen	17(18.7)	31(23.5)	48(21.5)
Back	4(4.4)	3(2.3)	7(3.1)
Extremities	13(14.3)	11(8.3)	24(10.8)
Upper limbs	7(7.7)	7(5.3)	14(6.3)
Lower limbs	6(6.6)	4(3.0)	10(4.5)
Total	91	132	223

Table 7.2 Classification of segmental vitiligo on the face.

	Site		
Type	Left(%)	Right(%)	Total(%)
I	51(1a)(26.7)	89(1b)(4.2)	59(30.9)
II	12(6.3)	18(9.4)	30(15.7)
III	24(12.6)	18(9.4)	42(22.0)

lesion which initiates from the right side of the forehead and crosses the midline of the face and spreads down to the eyeball, nose and cheek on the left side of the face (Fig. 7.2). Type 1b shows a mirror image of 1a. The lesion starts from the left side of the face and spreads down the right side of the face, crossing the midline (Fig. 7.3). In type 2, the lesion starts from the area between the nose and lip, then arches to the preauricular area (Fig. 7.4). In type 3, the lesion initiates from the lower lip and spreads down to the chin and neck (Fig. 7.5). In type 4, the lesion originates from the right side of the forehead and spreads down to the eyeball, nose and cheek areas without crossing the midline (Fig. 7.6). In type 5, the lesion is confined to the left cheek area (Fig. 7.7). Some segmental vitiligo on the face cannot be classified by this system. Type 1 was the most common (30.9%) and type 5 was the least common (9.4%). This classification of facial segmental vitiligo can provide some indication on the future distribution of early lesions if they have begun to spread.

Studies on the distribution of segmental vitiligo revealed that the skin innervated by the trigeminal nerve was most frequently involved, followed by the thoracic, cervical, lumbar and sacral nerves (Table 7.3) (Hann & Lee 1996). Although the skin is innervated by certain sensory nerves, the actual distribution of the depigmentation did not

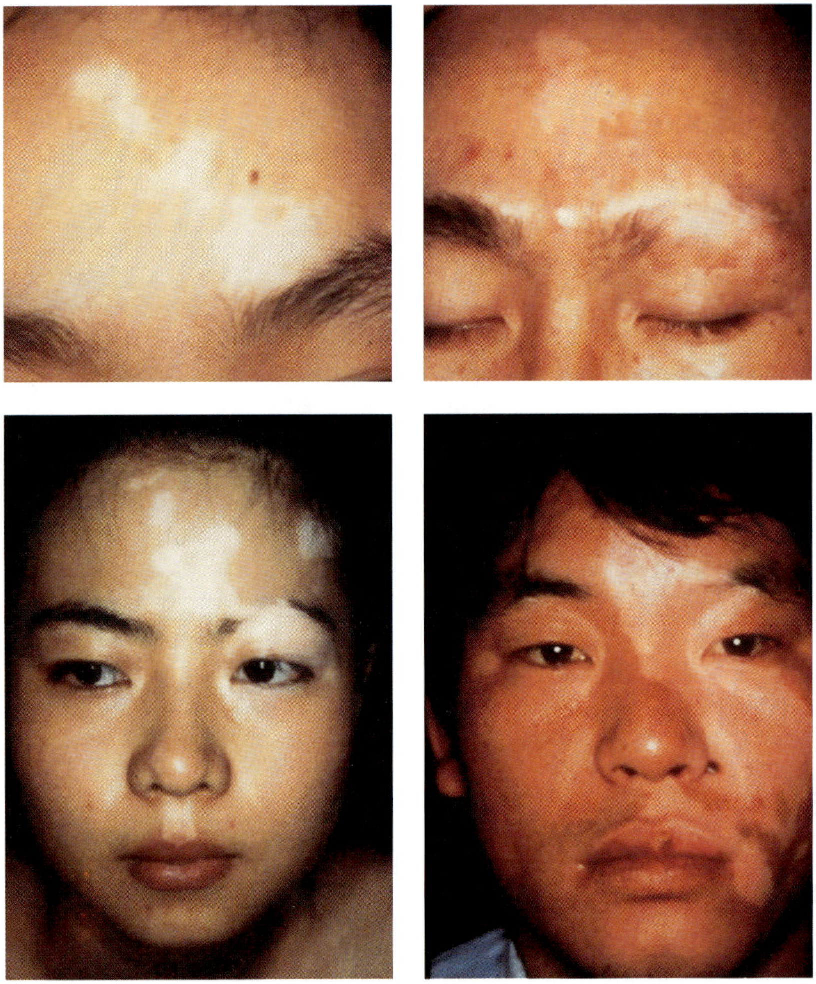

Fig. 7.2 Type 1a represents the lesion which initiates from the right side of the forehead and crosses the midline of the face and spreads down to the eyeball, nose and cheek of the left side of the face.

Table 7.3 Dermatomal distribution of segmental vitiligo.

Dermatome	Male(%)	Female(%)	Total(%)
Trigeminal	49(53.9)	65(50.8)	114(52.1)
Cervical	12(13.2)	26(20.3)	38(17.4)
Thoracic	19(20.9)	31(24.2)	50(22.8)
Lumbar	10(11.0)	4(3.1)	14(6.4)
Sacral	1(1.1)	2(1.6)	3(1.4)
Total	91	128	219

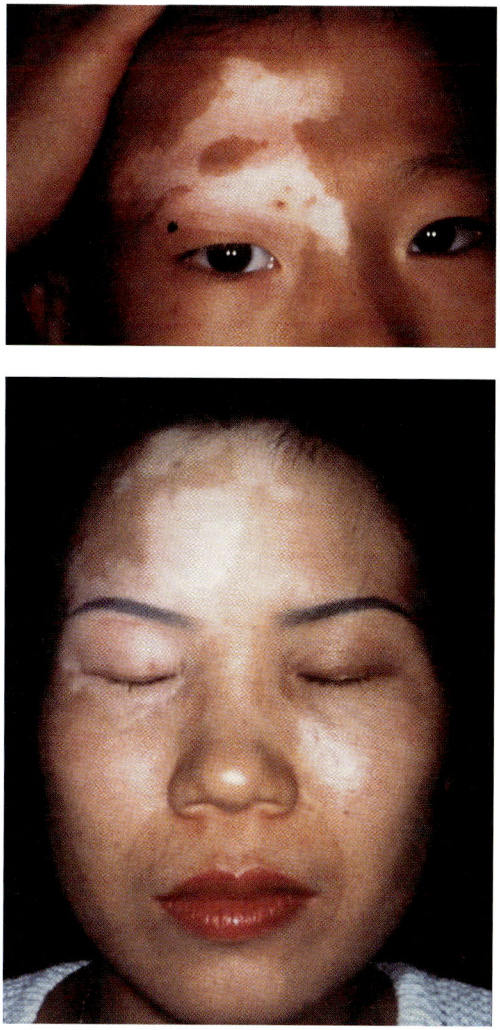

Fig. 7.3 Type 1b shows a lesion that started from the left side of the face and spread down to the right side of the face, crossing over the midline.

correspond very well to a true dermatome such as is seen in other disorders like herpes zoster. Most of the patterns of segmental vitiligo listed above did not follow a dermatomal distribution. For example, type 4 segmental vitiligo (Fig. 7.6) cannot be explained by dermatomal distribution. The chin is innervated by the mandibular branches of the trigeminal nerve and the neck is innervated by cervical nerves. It has been suggested that segmental vitiligo might follow Blaschko's lines or acupuncture lines (Bolognia *et al.* 1994). The distribution of segmental vitiligo possibly follows an unknown pathway which may be a group of identical clonal cells.

Hann and Lee (1996) studied whether hand dominance had any relation with vitiligo affecting the right or left side of the body, but there was no significant relationship between these two factors. They observed that left side involvement (104 patients: male 41; female 63) was almost the same as right side involvement (102 patients: male 47; female 55). Of the 133 patients who

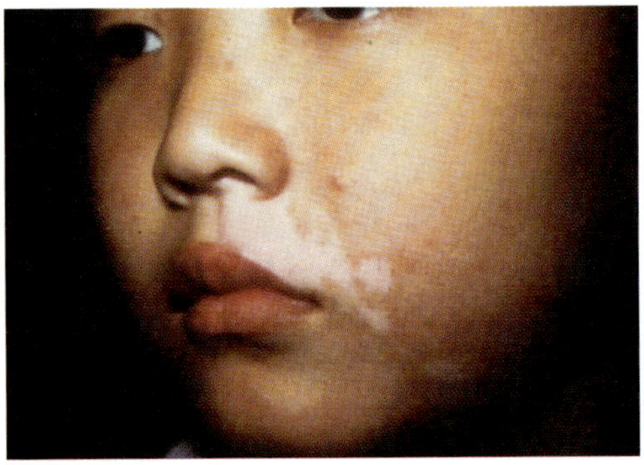

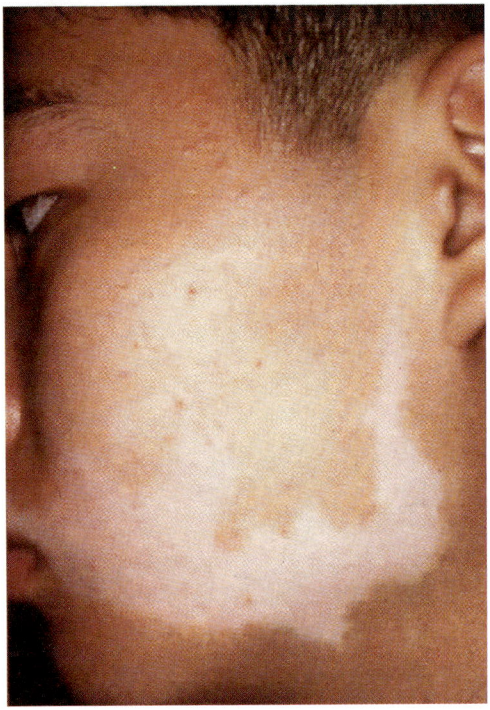

Fig. 7.4 Type 2 shows a lesion that started from the area between the nose and lip, arching to the preauricular area.

mentioned their dominant hand, eight were left-handed and 125 were right-handed. The right side was involved in 57 of 125 right-handed patients, whereas in left-handed patients four had left-side involvement and four had right-side involvement. Both sides were involved in two patients. Seven patients had lesions in two different unilateral dermatomes.

Progression of lesions

Most segmental vitiligo usually persist unchanged for the rest of the patient's life after rapid spreading in the affected dermatomal area. However, rarely it can progress again after being quiescent for several years. Segmental vitiligo usually spreads over the affected area, so the

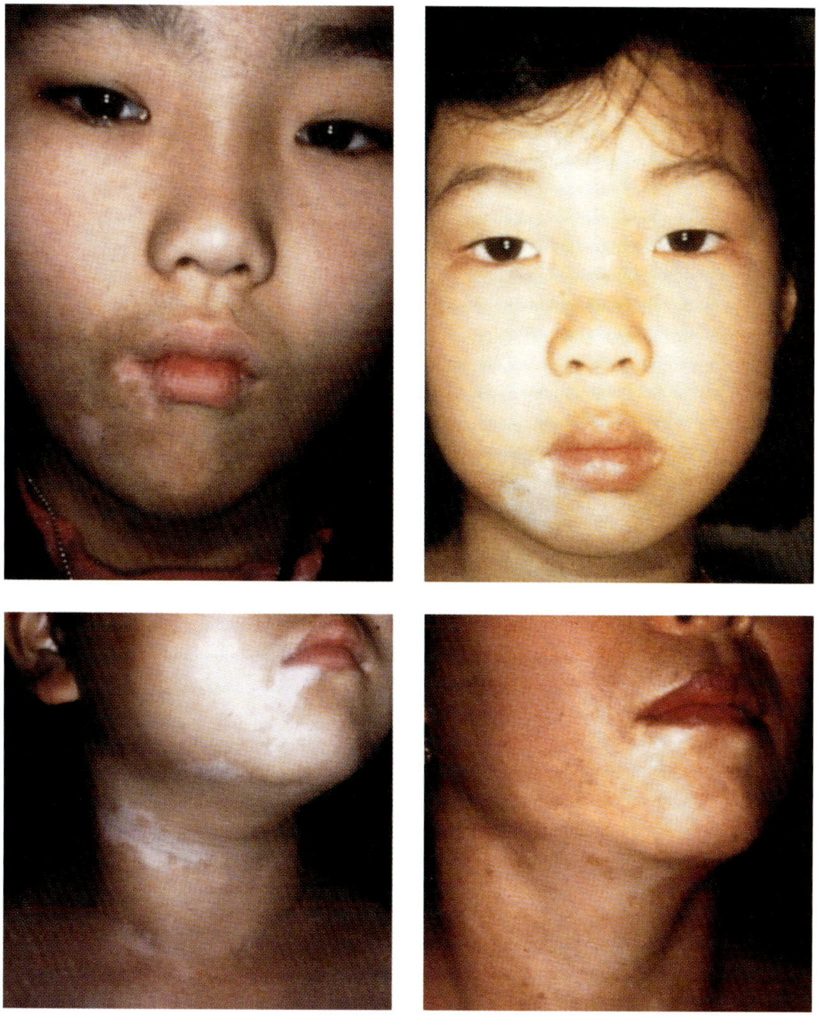

Fig. 7.5 Type 3 shows a lesion that initiated from the lower lip and spread down to the chin and neck.

progression pattern can be easily predicted. However, in very rare patients, lesions may become bilateral and generalized. This type of vitiligo is called mixed type. Early segmental vitiligo usually appears as a single oval shaped white macule or patch which is difficult to differentiate from focal type vitiligo until a typical distribution of lesions has appeared. A white macule on the nipple or areola appearing as the initial lesion can be assumed to be an early sign of segmental vitiligo (Fig. 7.8). Nipple or areolar involvement as the initial lesion in nonsegmental vitiligo is very rare and is frequently bilateral.

Precipitating factors

Physical trauma, sunburn, psychological stress, inflammation, pregnancy and contraceptives are said to be the precipitating factors of vitiligo. But

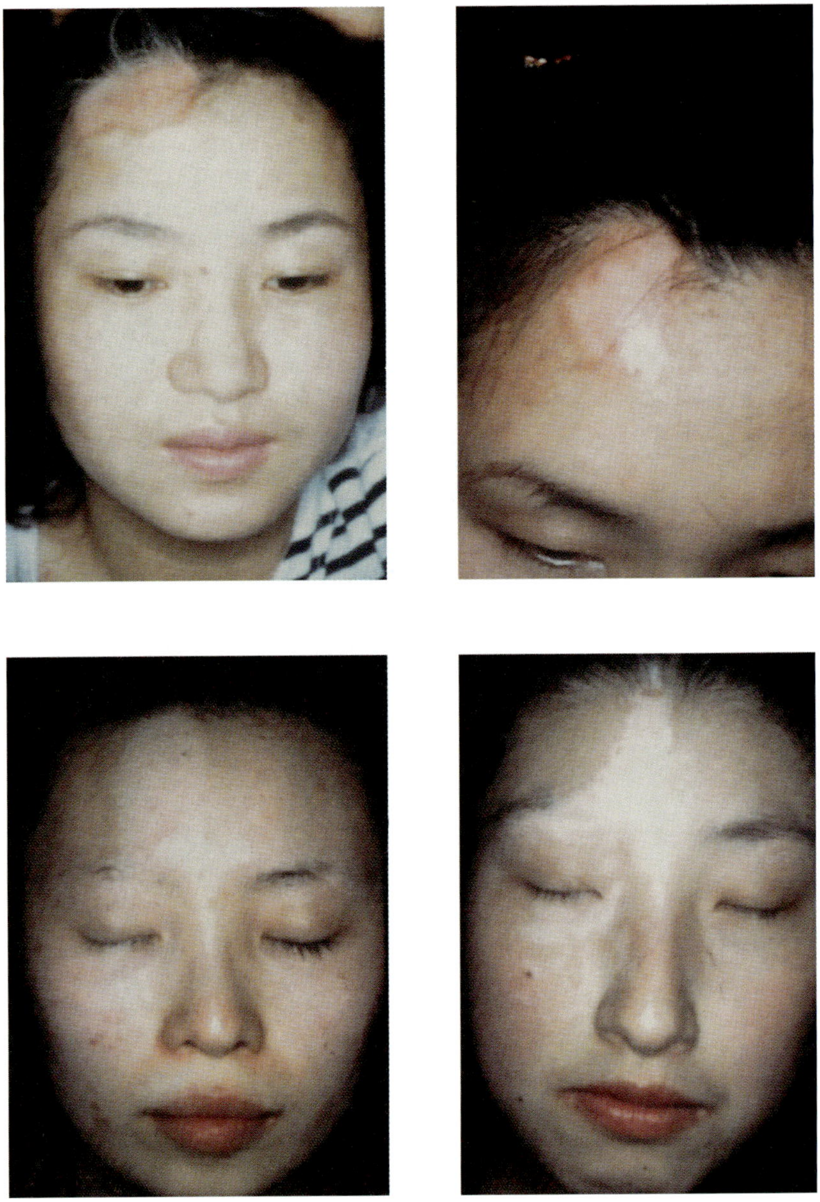

Fig. 7.6 Type 4 shows a lesion that originated from the right side of the forehead and spread down to the eyeball, nose and cheek areas without crossing over the midline.

unlike others, Park *et al.* (1988) and Hann and Lee (1996) reported that sunburn, trauma or pregnancy were considered aggravating factors in only 10 (4.8%) out of 208 patients with segmental vitiligo.

Family history

Family history of vitiligo was reported by 11.5% of the patients in Hann and Lee's report (1996), similar to that of nonsegmental vitiligo. Park *et al.* (1988)

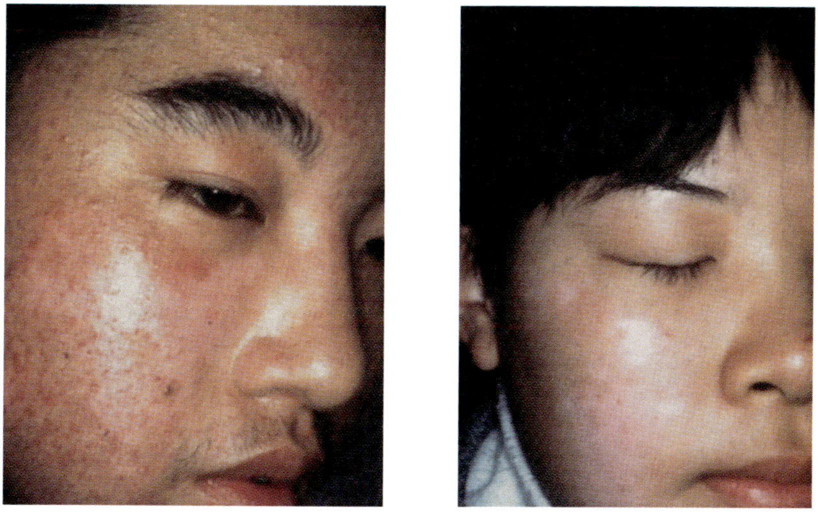

Fig. 7.7 Type 5 shows a lesion that is usually confined to the cheek area.

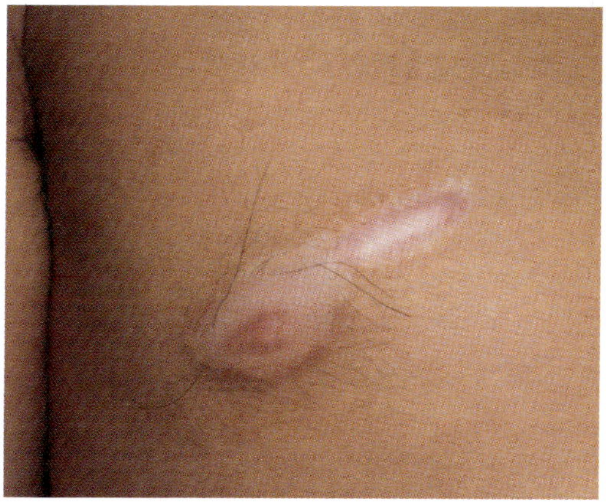

Fig. 7.8 A white macule on areola or nipple often progresses to segmental vitiligo.

reported a family history of vitiligo in 7.4% of his patients with segmental vitiligo.

Koebner's phenomenon

Koga and Tango (1998) reported that Koebner's phenomenon, the appearance of vitiligo after scratches or trauma, was not found in 134 patients with segmental vitiligo. However, Koebner's phenomenon was observed in 5.3% in Hann and Lee's study (1996).

Associated disease

El Mofty and El Mofty (1980) claimed that segmental vitiligo is not associated with other autoimmune diseases, but Park *et al.* (1988) found that they

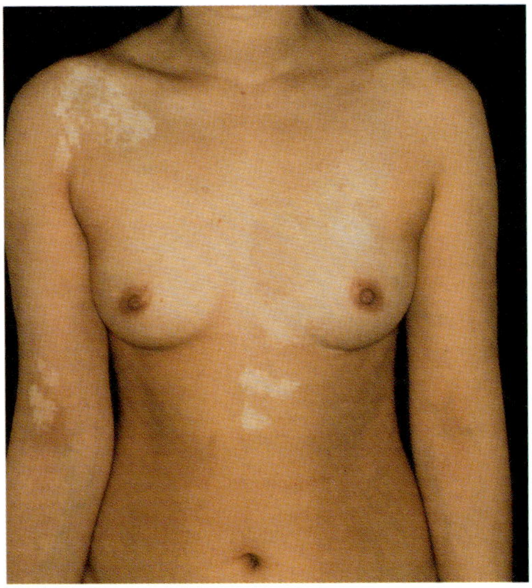

Fig. 7.9 Bilateral segmental vitiligo distributed in a linear pattern on both the right and left thoracic dermatome. The right side lesions are located on the shoulder and arm, while the left side lesions are located at the lower chest and upper abdomen, which do not cross the midline.

were associated in about 9.5% of cases. Koga and Tango (1988) asserted that an autoimmune disease associated with vitiligo occurred more significantly in nonsegmental vitiligo than in segmental vitiligo and that this difference might be due to different pathogenic mechanisms. In Hann and Lee's study (1996), association with thyroid diseases, diabetes mellitus, pernicious anaemia and halo naevus, which frequently accompany vitiligo, was seen in 3.4% of patients with segmental vitiligo, a figure lower than other reports (Koga & Tango 1988; Park *et al.* 1988). The prevalence of autoimmune disorders in the general population is reported to be as high as 15% in European countries.

Bilateral segmental vitiligo

Hann *et al.* (1997) reported that 5 out of 240 patients who had segmental vitiligo exhibited two different depigmented segments on the same or opposite sides of the body (Fig. 7.9). The clinical characteristics of bilateral segmental vitiligo are shown in Table 7.4. The clinical course of bilateral segmental vitiligo seems to be the same as unilateral segmental vitiligo

Table 7.4 Clinical characteristics of bilateral segmental vitiligo.

Patient Sex/Age (yrs)	Duration	Distribution: Left	Distribution: Right	Treatment
F/4	2 months	Chest, back, arm	Chest, arm	Systemic steroid
F/6	4 years	Chest, back, arm	Buttock, thigh	Topical steroid
F/8	2 years	Chest, back, arm	Chest, back, arm	Topical steroid
F/27	3 years	Chest, back, arm	Chest, back, arm	Systemic PUVA
F/12	2 years	Chest, arm	Chest, back, arm	Systemic PUVA

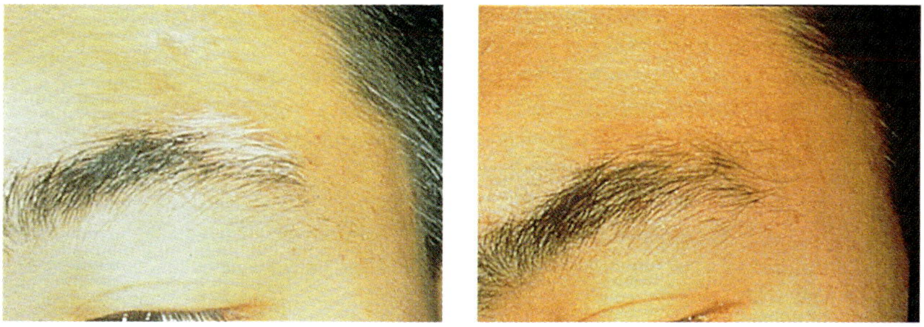

Fig. 7.10 Black eyebrow is shown after epidermal grafting and subsequent PUVA.

although only 5 cases have been followed for up to a maximum of 3 years. PUVA therapy and steroid treatment could induce repigmentation or stop progression of vitiliginous lesions in bilateral segmental vitiligo.

Treatment

Segmental vitiligo is said to be resistant to treatment. Recent studies (Hann *et al.* 1995; Moon *et al.* 1995) showed good results in the treatment of segmental vitiligo if done correctly. The most frequently involved site is the face where it can be easily detected and treated at an early stage with steroid or PUVA therapy (Moon *et al.* 1995) (see Chapters 21 and 22). Because segmental vitiligo often causes leukotrichia in as many as half of the patients with segmental vitiligo, it cannot always respond to medical therapies for repigmentation (see Chapter 20). Stable segmental vitiligo with leukotrichia can be cured with epidermal grafting and subsequent PUVA (Hann *et al.* 1995) (Fig. 7.10) (see Chapter 24). Segmental vitiligo has an excellent prognosis for cure because it responds well either to medical or surgical therapies.

Conclusion

Segmental vitiligo has clinical features that are different from those of bilateral vitiligo. Understanding these characteristics can give us valuable information in differentiating segmental vitiligo from nonsegmental vitiligo, in treating vitiligo with the proper methods and in predicting the prognosis of vitiligo.

References

Bolognia, J.L., Orlow, S.J. & Gilck, S.A. (1994) Lines of Blaschko. *Journal of the American Academy of Dermatology* **31**, 157–190.

Dutta, A.K. & Mandal, S.B. (1969) Clinical study of 650 vitiligo cases and their classification. *Indian Journal of Dermatology* **14**, 103–115.

El Mofty, A.M. & El Mofty, M. (1980) Vitiligo: a symptom complex. *International Journal of Dermatology* **19**, 238–247.

Hann, S.K. & Lee, H.J. (1996) Segmental vitiligo: clinical findings in 208 patients. *Journal of the American Academy of Dermatology* **35**, 671–674.

Hann, S.K., Song, M.S., Park, Y.K. & Ahn, S.K. (1991) Childhood vitiligo: clinical study compared with adult vitiligo. *Annals of Dermatology* **3**, 112–118.

Hann, S.K., Im, S., Park, Y.K. & Hur, W. (1992) Repigmentation of leukotrichia by epidermal grafting and systemic psoralen plus UV-A. *Archives of Dermatology* **128**, 998–999.

Hann, S.K., Im, S., Bong, H.W. & Park, Y.K. (1995) Treatment of stable vitiligo with autologous epidermal grafting and PUVA. *Journal of the American Academy of Dermatology* **32**, 943–948.

Hann, S.K., Park, Y.K. & Chun, W.H. (1997) Clinical features of vitiligo. *Clinics in Dermatology* **15**, 891–897.

Howitz, J., Brodthagen, H., Schwartz, M. & Thomsen, K. (1977) Prevalence of vitiligo: epidemiologic survey on the Isle of Borholm, Denmark. *Archives of Dermatology* **113**, 47–52.

Koga, M. (1977) Vitiligo: a new classification and therapy. *British Journal of Dermatology* **97**, 255–261.

Koga, M. & Tango, T. (1988) Clinical features and course of type A and type B vitiligo. *British Journal of Dermatology* **118**, 223–228.

Lerner, A.B. (1959) Vitiligo. *Journal of Investigative Dermatology* **32**, 285–310.

Lerner, A.B. (1971) On the etiology of vitiligo and gray hair. *American Journal of Medicine* **51**, 147–156.

Levai, M. (1958) A study of certain contributory factors in the development of vitiligo in South Indian patients. *Archives of Dermatology* **78**, 364–370.

Moon, T.K., Im, S., Hann, S.K., Cho, S.H. & Park, Y.K. (1995) The effect of small doses of oral corticosteroids in vitiligo patients. *Korean Journal of Dermatology* **33**, 880–885.

Park, K.C., Youn, J.I. & Lee, Y.S. (1988) Clinical study of 326 cases of vitiligo. *Korean Journal of Dermatology* **26**, 200–205.

Seghal, V.N. (1974) A clinical evaluation of 202 cases of vitiligo. *Cutis* **14**, 439–445.

Song, M.S., Hann, S.K., Ahn, P.S., Im, S. & Park, Y.K. (1994) Clinical study of vitiligo: comparative study of type A and type B vitiligo. *Annals of Dermatology* **6**, 22–30.

8: Childhood Vitiligo: Clinical Spectrum and Therapeutic Approaches

PEARL E. GRIMES AND MAVIS BILLIPS

Introduction

Vitiligo is a common idiopathic disorder characterized by multiple white patches of skin. Many investigators now regard the disorder as a heterogeneous disease with multiple aetiologies (Grimes 1996). There are only a few published studies which address the clinical spectrum of vitiligo in children. Halder *et al.* (1987) assessed 82 children with vitiligo. Their patients had an increased frequency of segmental vitiligo and strong family history of autoimmune disease compared to adults. Other studies (Koga & Tango 1988; Hann & Lee 1996) have also reported an increased frequency of segmental vitiligo in paediatric patients with vitiligo. Finco *et al.* (1991) demonstrated an increased frequency of HLA-DR5, DQW3, BfS, C4A3 and C4B1 in the paediatric form of vitiligo. In addition, Schallreuter *et al.* (1994) assessed 101 children with vitiligo and reported an increased frequency of a positive family history of vitiligo, the presence of Koebner's phenomenon, halo naevi and premature greying. This article will address the clinical spectrum of paediatric vitiligo and review therapeutic approaches.

Spectrum of disease

Childhood vitiligo encompasses a unique subgroup of patients. Previous studies (Lerner 1959; Halder *et al.* 1987) have reported that 50% of patients develop vitiligo prior to age 20 years. In contrast, recent studies of 448 patients evaluated at our Vitiligo Institute demonstrated that 29% reported the onset of vitiligo prior to age 20 and 14% prior to age 10 years.

Data were reviewed in vitiligo patients less than 15 years of age evaluated at the Vitiligo and Pigmentation Institute of Southern California. Extensive histories and physical examinations were performed on each patient to determine the duration of disease, family history, age of onset, clinical type, extent of vitiligo, and the presence of autoimmune disease. The patients ranged in age from 6 months to 15 years. Their mean age was 9 years. One hundred and four (69%) were females and 48 (31%) were males. The predominance of females is consistent with the results from other studies (Halder *et al.* 1987; Schallreuter *et al.* 1994). Our patients comprised a racially diverse group. There were 35 (23%) African Americans, 30 (20%) Caucasians, 58 (38%) Hispanics and 29 (19%) comprising other racial/ethnic groups. Hispanics probably predominate our patient population because of the population demographics of Los Angeles. However, studies do not support any racial predisposition for vitiligo. The mean duration of disease was 3 years. Percentage of cutaneous surface involvement ranged from 1% to 80% with a mean severity of 16%.

Table 8.1 demonstrates the clinical types of vitiligo observed in children as compared with the types observed in an adult vitiligo group. The generalized pattern of vitiligo is the most common clinical type reported in children (Fig. 8.1). As reported in previous studies (Halder *et al.* 1987; Koga & Tango 1988), the frequency of segmental vitiligo in our study was significantly increased in children (Fig. 8.2). No statistically significant differences were observed in the frequency of other types of vitiligo such as the acral/acrofacial and localized varieties. Jaisankar *et al.* (1992) reported the most common location for the appearance of vitiligo in children included face and neck 50%, lower extremities 28%, trunk 18%, upper extremities 17% and perineum 6%.

The frequency of associated diseases in children with vitiligo is significantly less than observed in the adult vitiligo population (Table 8.2). However, as with adult vitiligo patients, the most frequently identified other diseases were thyroid disorders and alopecia areata. Schallreuter *et al.* (1994) reported an increased frequency of thyroid disease in children with vitiligo. Halder *et al.* (1987) reported two cases of alopecia areata in 82 children with vitiligo. None had thyroid disorders or other autoimmune/endocrine disorders.

In contrast to adults, children with vitiligo in our patient population demonstrated a statistically significant increased frequency of autoimmune diseases in first- and second-degree relatives compared to adults (82% vs. 52% $P < 0.01$).

The frequency of autoantibodies did not differ significantly in children compared to adults in our patient population. Of the 152 paediatric patients, 15% had antinuclear antibodies and 15% had thyroid microsomal antibodies. Of the adult population, 21% had positive antinuclear antibody tests and 22% had thyroid antibodies. The increased frequency of autoantibodies in our paediatric patients with vitiligo corroborates previous studies by Halder and Grimes (1987).

Table 8.1 Distribution of the clinical types of vitiligo.

Type	Number of cases (534)	Children (119) No.	Children (119) (%)	Adults (415) No.	Adults (415) (%)
Generalized	316	54	45	262	63
Acrofacial/acral	99	19	16	80	19
Segmental	71	34*	29	37	9
Localized	48	12	10	36	9

* $P < 0.0001$.

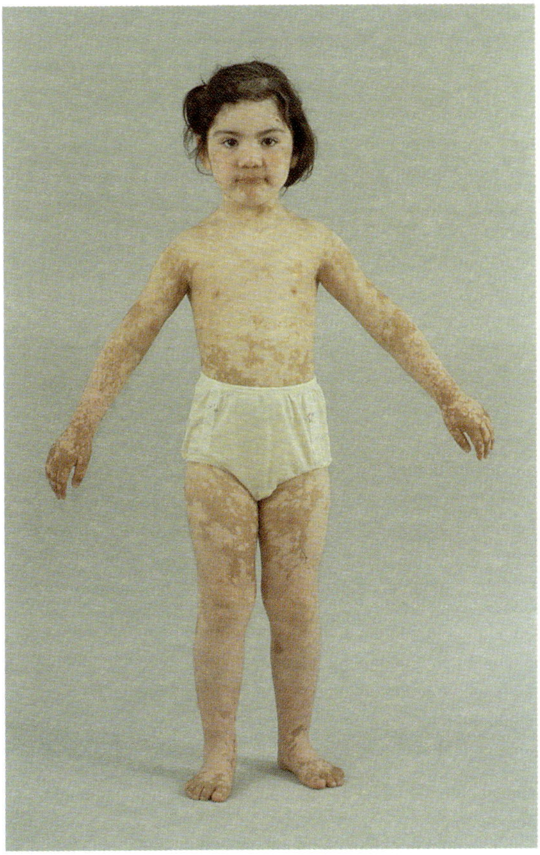

Fig. 8.1 Five-year-old female with extensive generalized vitiligo.

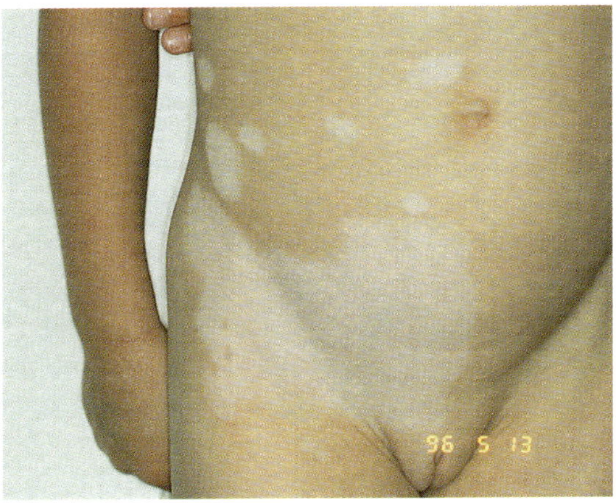

Fig. 8.2 Four-year-old female with segmental vitiligo.

Therapeutic approaches

Several studies have assessed therapeutic responses in paediatric patients with vitiligo. Halder (1987) initially reported poor therapeutic responses in 82 children with vitiligo treated primarily with topical photochemotherapy

Table 8.2 Frequency of associated diseases in vitiligo patients.

	Children (N = 152)		Adults (N = 465)	
	No.	(%)	No.	(%)
Hyperthyroidism	2	1	20	4
Hypothyroidism	5	4	51	11
Diabetes	2	1	27	6
Rheumatoid arthritis	1	1	20	4
Alopecia areata	6	4	34	8
Pernicious anaemia	0	0	6	1

*$p < 0.01$.

Table 8.3 Therapeutic responses.

Therapeutic modality	No. of children	Mean repigmentation (%)	No. of adults	Mean repigmentation (%)
Topical steroids	30	54	57	41
Topical PUVA	44	63	134	45
Topical/PUVA/ sunlight (PUVASOL)	40	78	28	50
PUVASOL/Topical steroids	16	58	33	43
Oral PUVA	14	69	128	45
Autologous grafting	9	75	35	73

(PUVA). However, a subsequent study by Halder (1997) reported response rates of 45%, 58% and 71%, respectively, using topical steroids, topical PUVA, and systemic PUVA, respectively. In addition, Schulpis *et al.* (1989) treated 13 children with vitiligo using L-phenylalanine and exposure to UVA. Of the 13 patients, 3 had complete repigmentation of all areas, 6 had 50% to 90% improvement and 4 showed no improvement. None experienced side-effects.

Table 8.3 summarizes and compares repigmentation responses in 130 children and 415 adults with vitiligo treated at the Vitiligo and Pigmentation Institute of Southern California. Therapies included topical steroids using mid to high potency preparations; topical PUVA (in office); topical photochemotherapy with sunlight (PUVASOL), combination therapy using PUVASOL and topical steroids, systemic photochemotherapy and autologous grafting. Children demonstrated an enhanced therapeutic response to each modality assessed (Figs 8.3 & 8.4). For all therapies overall mean repigmentation was 61% for children compared to 50% for adults.

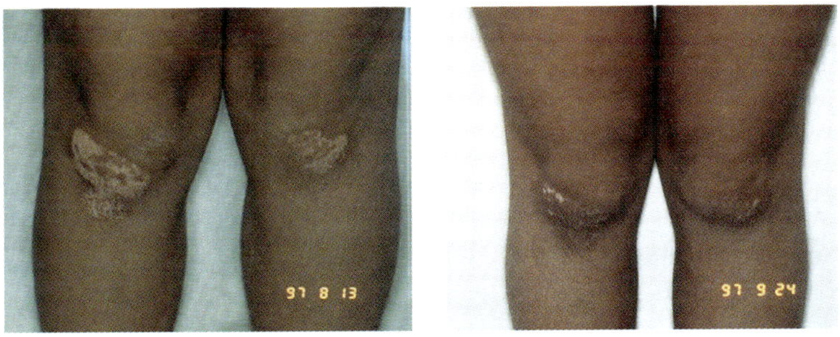

(a) (b)

Fig. 8.3 (a) Localized vitiligo. (b) Excellent repigmentation of the knees achieved with Class I topical steroid therapy.

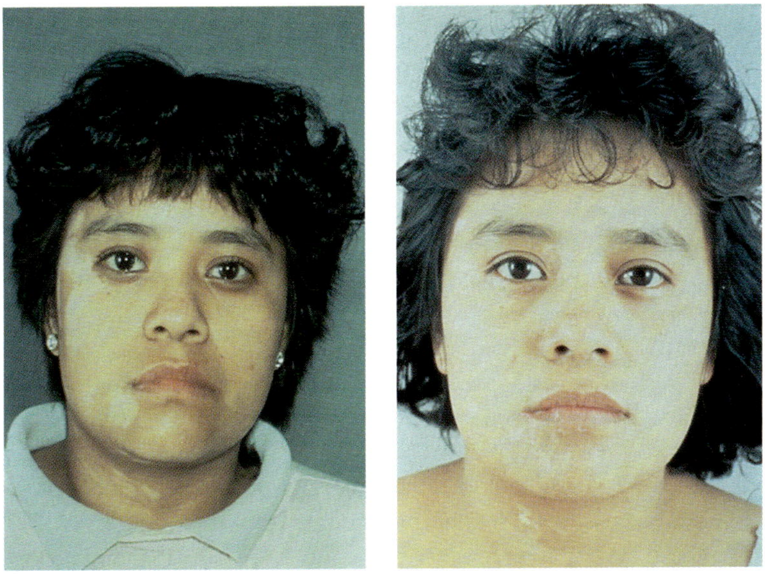

(a) (b)

Fig. 8.4 (a) Segmental vitiligo. (b) 90% repigmentation achieved with oral PUVA.

In general, children less than 2 years of age are treated with topical steroids. Children greater than 2 years of age are treated with mid to high potency topical steroids or topical PUVA or topical PUVASOL. Children greater than 9 years with more than 25% cutaneous surface involvement are treated with oral PUVA (Grimes 1997). Therapeutically recalcitrant areas are sometimes treated by autologous grafting in older children.

Topical steroid therapy

Topical steroids should be considered in the initial treatment phases of children with limited (less than 10%) vitiligo. These preparations can also be used in children less than 2 years of age, who are too young for PUVA therapy. Low potency to mid potency topical steroids are used in young children. High potency topical steroids can be used in older children. Class I steroids are applied once or twice daily for the first month or two, then tapered to lower potency preparations. They should be applied to very limited or localized areas of involvement. Patients must be monitored closely to avoid steroid-induced side-effects, including atrophy, striae, and telangiectasia. Because of case reports of steroid-induced glaucoma, mid potency to high potency topical steroids should be used with caution when treating periorbital areas of depigmentation. Short courses of systemic steroids may be indicated in patients with rapidly progressive vitiligo.

Topical photochemotherapy (out-patient)

Topical photochemotherapy is also an option for children with limited involvement (less than 20% of the body surface). It avoids many of the systemic side-effects associated with oral psoralens. A thin coat of 0.1% methoxsalen ointment is routinely used for out-patient topical PUVA. Oxsoralen solution 1% (ICN Pharmaceuticals, Costa Mesa, CA) is diluted to a concentration of 0.1% in Aquaphor or petrolatum. A thin coat of this preparation is applied to vitiliginous areas 30 minutes prior to UVA exposure. The initial UVA dose is 0.12–0.25 J and is increased by increments of 0.12–0.25 J weekly according to the patient's response. After moderate asymptomatic erythema is achieved, the UVA dosage should be maintained at a dosage sufficient to retain erythema. The treated areas should be washed with soap and water immediately after the UVA exposure followed by application of a broad-spectrum sunscreen. Treatments are administered weekly. The major side-effect of topical photochemotherapy using this regimen is a severe phototoxic or blistering reaction and perilesional hyperpigmentation. Patients should be made cognisant of these side-effects prior to initiating therapy. Oxsoralen ointment 0.1% with sunlight as a UVA source should be avoided because of the increased potential of developing severe phototoxic reactions. The major advantages of out-patient topical photochemotherapy include its lower cumulative UVA dose and its lack of systemic and ocular toxicity when compared with systemic PUVA.

Topical photochemotherapy wth sunlight

In light of the difficulties of out-patient PUVA for many patients and their families (time and cost), a modified topical PUVA protocol can be used to allow for daily or alternate day sunlight exposure as the UVA light source by using a very dilute (0.001%) concentration of Oxsoralen. It is recommended for children with less than 10% cutaneous surface involvement. A thin coat of 0.001% Oxsoralen ointment is applied to lesional skin 30 minutes prior to sun exposure. The affected areas are exposed to sunlight for 15–30 minutes between 10:00 a.m. and 4:00 p.m. After 2 weeks, exposure time can be increased to 45 minutes to 1 hour if mild erythema has not occurred. Following sun exposure, the treated areas are washed with soap and water, followed by application of a broad-spectrum sunscreen. This treatment approach minimizes the adverse reactions routinely associated with out-patient topical photochemotherapy. Costs are minimal, and it provides increased therapeutic accessibility to larger segments of the paediatric population.

Systemic photochemotherapy

Systemic photochemotherapy is reserved for children with more extensive involvement. A dosage of 0.3–0.4 mg kg^{-1} of 8-methoxypsoralen (8-MOP) (Oxsoralen-Ultra, ICN Pharmaceuticals) is ingested with food 1.5 hours prior to UVA exposure. The initial UVA dose should be in a range of 1–2 J, with increments of 1 joule on every other visit until moderate asymptomatic erythema is achieved. The UVA dosage can then be maintained at a level necessary to retain 1+ or 2+ erythema of vitiliginous lesions. As with the topical protocols, a broad-spectrum sunscreen should be applied to exposed areas prior to leaving the treating facility. Protective UVA sunglasses should be worn indoors and outdoors ideally for 18–24 hours after ingestion of 8-MOP but at least until night time. Treatments are given twice weekly and never on 2 consecutive days. Oral psoralens should not be used in children younger than 9 years. Ocular defects, including cataracts, and abnormal liver function tests are contraindications for oral PUVA and, in general, photosensitivity disorders contraindicate the use of oral or topical PUVA. Trisoralen, which is less phototoxic and associated with fewer gastrointestinal side-effects, may be used as an alternative drug.

Side-effects of oral photochemotherapy include nausea and vomiting, pruritus, erythema and oedema, hypertrichosis, diffuse hyperpigmentation, xerosis, premature ageing, skin cancer, cataracts, and immunological defects. In contrast to psoriasis, studies have not documented a PUVA-induced increase in skin cancer in vitiligo. Compared with topical PUVA, the major advantages of oral PUVA therapy include its effectiveness in limiting the progression of actively spreading vitiligo, its lower frequency of blistering reactions, and its superiority as a repigmenting agent in patients with skin Types I and II.

Autologous grafting

This procedure can easily be performed for small, stable areas of vitiligo which have been recalcitrant to other therapeutic modalities in children 10–15 years of age. In brief, 2 mm punch grafts are harvested from the buttock area. Two-millimeter punch grafts are removed from the recipient site. The donor 2 mm punch grafts are placed 5–8 mm apart at the recipient site. Pigmentation can be observed migrating from the grafts into the areas of depigmentation 3–4 weeks after the procedure (Grimes 1993) (see Chapter 24).

Adjunctive therapy

Montes *et al.* (1992) reported excellent repigmentation in 15 patients after 1–2 years of treatment with oral folic acid, ascorbic acid and parental B_{12}. In general, most paediatric patients treated at the Vitiligo and Pigmentation Institute of Southern California are placed on vitamin and mineral supplementation which includes ascorbic acid, 250–500 mg daily and a multivitamin which contains vitamin E, vitamin B_6, folic acid, vitamin B_{12}, biotin, pantothenic acid, calcium, iron, zinc, copper and magnesium.

Summary

Our findings suggest that children indeed constitute a unique subgroup of patients with vitiligo. They typically demonstrated an increased frequency of segmental vitiligo. As observed in adults the most frequently observed autoimmune diseases are thyroid disorders and alopecia areata. Children, however, have a significantly higher frequency of first- and second-degree relatives with autoimmune disease. In addition, children with vitiligo demonstrate an increased frequency of autoantibody production suggesting a propensity for autoimmune disease. In contrast to previous studies, our paediatric patient population showed enhanced repigmentation to all therapeutic modalities. In light of these enhanced repigmentation responses, early therapeutic intervention is indeed indicated.

References

Finco, O., Cuccia, M., Martinetti, M., Ruberto, G., Orecchia, G. & Rabbiosi, G. (1991) Age of onset in vitiligo: relationship with HLA supratypes. *Clinical Genetics* **39**, 48–54.

Grimes, P.E. (1993) Vitiligo. An overview of therapeutic approaches. *Dermatologic Clinics* **11**, 325–338.

Grimes, P.E. (1996) Diseases of hypopigmentation. In: *Principles and Practice of Dermatology* (eds U.M.Sams & P.J.Lynch), 2nd edn, pp. 873–885. Churchill-Livingstone, New York.

Grimes, P.E. (1997) Psoralen photochemotherapy for vitiligo. *Clinics in Dermatology* **15**, 899–906.

Halder, R.M. (1997) Childhood vitiligo. *Clinics in Dermatology* **15**, 899–906.

Halder, R.M., Grimes, P.E., Cowan, C.A., Enterline, J.A., Chakrabarti, S.G. & Kenney, J.A. Jr (1987) Childhood vitiligo. *Journal of the American Academy of Dermatology* **16**, 948–954.

Hann, S.K. & Lee, H.J. (1996) Segmental vitiligo: clinical findings in 208 patients. *Journal of the American Academy of Dermatology* **35**, 671–674.

Jaisankar, T.J., Baruah, M.C. & Garg, B.R. (1992) Vitiligo in children. *International Journal of Dermatology* **31**, 621–623.

Koga, M. & Tango, T. (1988) Clinical features and course of type A and type B vitiligo. *British Journal of Dermatology* **118**, 223–228.

Lerner, A.B. (1959) Vitiligo. *Journal of Investigative Dermatology* **32**, 285–310.

Montes, L.F., Diaz, M.L., Lajous, J. & Garcia, N.J. (1992) Folic acid and vitamin B_{12} in vitiligo: a nutritional approach. *Cutis* **50**, 39–42.

Schallreuter, K.U., Lemke, R., Brandt, O., Schwartz, R., Westhofen, M., Montz, R. &

Berger, J. (1994) Vitiligo and other diseases: coexistence or true association? Hamburg study on 321 patients. *Dermatology* **188**, 269–275.

Schulpis, C.H., Antoniou, C., Michas, T. & Strarigos, J. (1989) Phenylalanine plus ultraviolet light: Preliminary report of a promising treatment for childhood vitiligo. *Pediatric Dermatology* **6**, 332–335.

9: Special Features of Vitiligo

JEAN-PAUL ORTONNE

Trichrome vitiligo

The terms 'trichrome vitiligo' (Fitzpatrick 1964) or 'vitiligo gradata' (vitiligo by steps) (Siemens 1954) were used to describe lesions that show a tan zone of varying width between the normal and the totally depigmented skin. This intermediate zone is not a gradual gradation of colour from white to normal, but rather a fairly uniform intermediate hue, particularly accentuated in those who tan deeply (Fig. 9.1). The colour is generally uniform from macule to macule in a given patient. This results in three shades of colour, i.e. medium brown (unaffected skin), tan and white in the same patient.

Trichrome has also been described as an isomorphic Koebner's phenomenon. In one patient, trichrome concentric rings or lines surrounding an achromic line corresponding to former scratches were observed (Dupre & Christol 1978). The significance of trichrome is unknown but several reports suggest it is part of a dynamic process. A reasonable interpretation is that trichrome corresponds to a gradual centrifugal spread of hypomelanosis or stepwise depigmentation. However, the sharp demarcation between the three areas is inconsistent with such an active centrifugally spreading lesion.

'Quadrichrome vitiligo' is another variant of vitiligo that reflects the presence of a fourth colour, dark brown at sites of perifollicular repigmentation (Mosher *et al.* 1987). The term 'quadrichrome vitiligo' was also used to describe a 'trichrome vitiligo' in which the intermediate hue was surrounded peripherally by a hyperpigmented border resulting in four shades of colour—medium brown (unaffected skin), dark brown, tan and white (Ortonne *et al.* 1983) (Fig. 9.2). A case of 'pentachrome vitiligo' with five shades of colour—black, dark-brown, medium brown (unaffected skin), tan, white—has also been described in an untreated patient (Concetta-Fargnoli & Bolognia 1995). The depigmented areas showed a complete absence of melanocytes, whereas the most hyperpigmented areas had an increase in epidermal pigment and number of melanocytes.

The isomorphic response

One of the manifestations of vitiligo is the isomorphic Koebner's phenomenon (IKP). This phenomenon is defined as the development of vitiligo macules at sites of specific trauma such as a cut, burn or abrasion. Epidemiological studies indicate that this IKP occurs in a majority of patients ranging from 21% to more than 60% (Schallreuter *et al.* 1994; Barona *et al.* 1995; Hann *et al.* 1997). A significantly higher incidence of the IKP has been reported in childhood vitiligo (45.5% vs. 35.2% in adolescent vitiligo and 27.8% in adult vitiligo) (Schallreuter *et al.* 1994). At least two studies conclude that the IKP is significantly more common in patients with progressive vitiligo (Schallreuter *et al.* 1994; Hann *et al.* 1997). The IKP is observed in both bilateral and unilateral vitiligo (Barona *et al.* 1995).

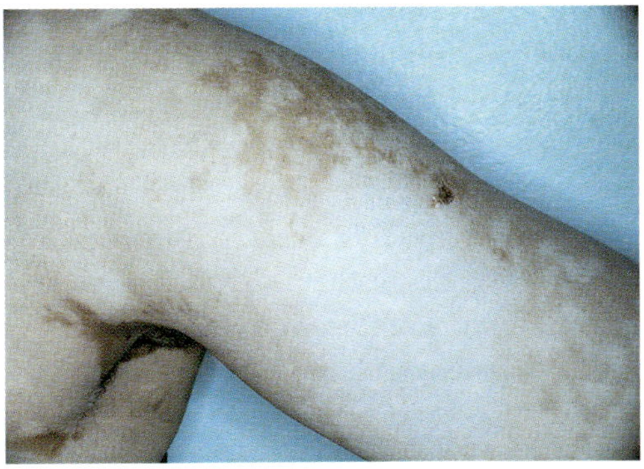

Fig. 9.1 Trichrome vitiligo.

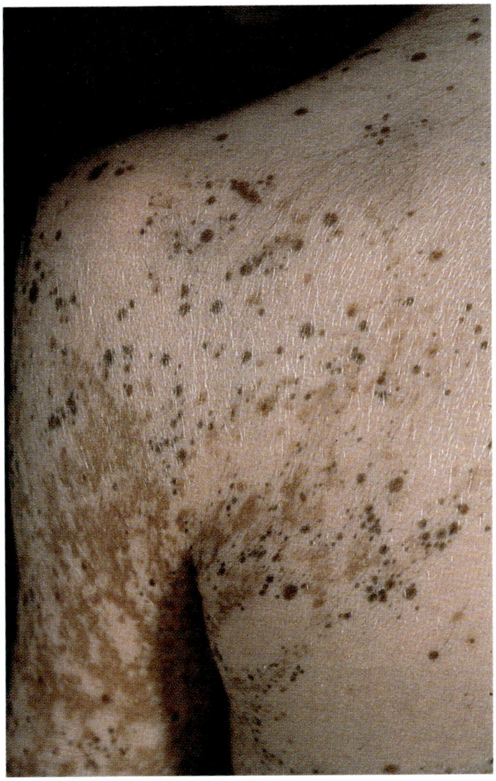

Fig. 9.2 Quadrichrome vitiligo.

Clinically, the IKP depigmented lesions are easily recognizable by their artefactual or elongated 'streak-line' shape. Trichrome IKP may be observed (Dupre & Christol 1978). The IKP may follow the trauma or may occur on an ancient scar once the vitiligo develops (Sweet 1978). Typical vitiligo following an inflammatory dermatosis such as psoriasis or a generalized figurate erythematosquamous eruption of unknown origin and involving the same sites have been described (Powell & Dicken 1983; Arata & Abe-Matsuura 1994). These cases could be considered as examples of the IKP in a broad sense. The clinical significance of the IKP is still a matter of discussion. Vitiligo occurs commonly in areas exposed to pressure or microtraumas. Pressure from a sari tightening at the waist or cutaneous excoriations resulting from scratching are considered as inducers of the IKP (Levaï 1958). There appears to be a minimal threshold of injury required for the IKP to occur (Gopinathan 1965). Epidermal stripping was ineffective in inducing depigmentation of uninvolved skin in vitiligo patients, whereas epidermodermal scarification did in a majority of patients. The induction of the IKP was more commonly observed in the skin adjacent to the lesions than at distant sites, suggesting a difference in reactivity of uninvolved skin to epidermal trauma in the same patient (Gopinathan 1965). These observations are inconsistent with the hypothesis that superficial and/or minor traumas such as clothes friction and washing, in the absence of deep injury, play an important role in the induction of vitiligo lesions (Gauthier 1995). This hypothesis must be substantiated before the early removal of all the factors suspected to lead to the IKP is recommended.

The IKP should be explained in detail to the patients and taken into consideration when they decide to undergo surgical or cosmetic procedures such as electrolysis dermabrasion or laser surgery (Sommer & Dicken 1998) (Fig. 9.3). It may also limit the use of grafting techniques to repigment vitiligo skin. One recent study suggests that the therapeutic success of epidermal grafting in generalized vitiligo is limited by the Koebner phenomenon (Hatchome *et al.* 1990). The IKP may be a good explanation for onset or spread of vitiligo as a consequence of severe sunburn. For the same risk, phototoxic reactions should be avoided in patients undergoing phototherapy or photochemotherapy.

Vitiligo with raised borders

Generally, vitiligo macules have distinct margins. However, raised borders have, on a few occasions, been observed at the margins of the depigmented borders. This is a rare macroscopic presentation of vitiligo and only few cases have been reported (Michaelsson 1968; Eng 1970; Ortonne *et al.* 1979) (Fig. 9.4). Vitiligo with raised borders has been reported in males and females at any age.

The red, raised borders may be present from the onset of vitiligo or may appear several months or years later. A mild pruritus may be present. Histological features of the raised borders show eczematous changes in the epi-

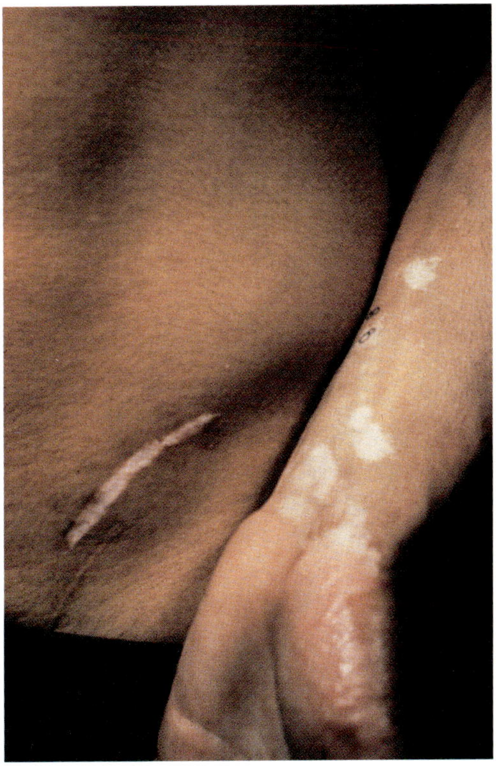

Fig. 9.3 Isomorphic Koebner's phenomenon on a surgical scar.

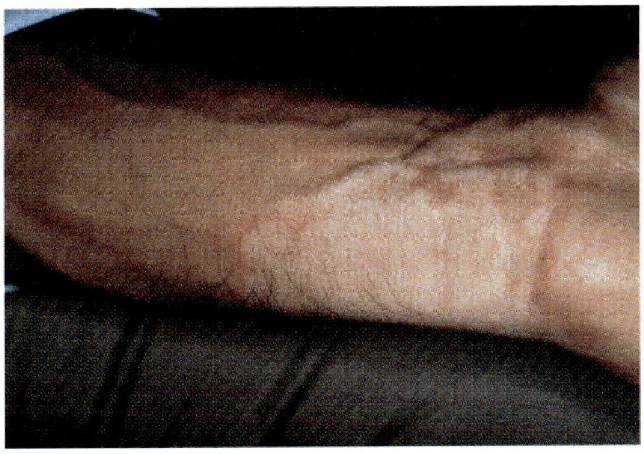

Fig. 9.4 Vitiligo with red, raised borders.

dermis with absence or decrease of melanin pigmentation and fairly dense lymphocytic and histiocytic infiltrate in the upper dermis. Complete regression of the red, raised borders is reported in several patients either spontaneously or after topical corticotherapy.

The significance of this localized inflammatory reaction is unknown. According to several histological studies, the presence of a mild lymphocytic infiltrate at the border of active vitiligo may be observed even in the absence of clinical inflammation. Thus, the occurrence of red, raised borders could represent simply an amplification of the 'usual' inflammatory process occurring in vitiligo (Eng 1970).

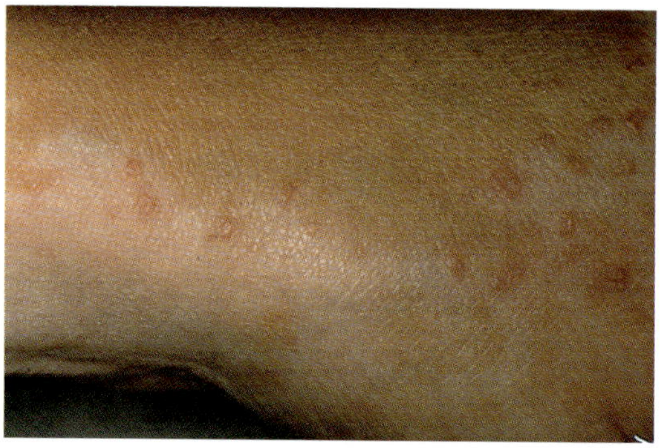

Fig. 9.5 Lichen planus papules at the border of vitiligo macules.

In a few cases of coexisting vitiligo and lichen planus (LP), typical polygonal papules of LP were distributed on the pigmented border of some vitiligo macules, but did not give the typical aspect of a red, linear rim delineating the junction of involved and uninvolved skin (Fig. 9.5) (Baran *et al.* 1997).

Inflammatory vitiligo macules with an oedematous border and slight scaliness are very unusual. As the inflammatory component disappears, the skin becomes depigmented. It has been suggested that this inflammatory pattern occurs in atopics (Macmillan & Rook 1971).

Blue vitiligo

The blue colouration of vitiligo macules has been observed in a patient already affected by post-inflammatory hyperpigmentation in whom vitiligo developed. Histological examination of the 'blue vitiligo' lesions showed an absence of epidermal melanocytes and numerous melanophages in the dermis. The blue colouration subsequently disappeared with follicular repigmentation typical of resolving vitiligo (Ivker *et al.* 1994).

Vitiligo ponctué

This unusual clinical presentation of vitiligo is characterized by small confetti or tiny, discrete, hypomelanotic macules occurring either on otherwise normal skin or on a hyperpigmented macule (Sidi 1957).

References

Arata, J. & Abe-Matsuura, Y. (1994) Generalized vitiligo preceded by a generalized figurate erythematosquamous eruption. *Journal of Dermatology* **21**, 438–441.

Baran, R., Ortonne, J.P. & Perrin, C.H. (1997) Vitiligo associated with a lichen planus border. *Dermatology* **194**, 199.

Barona, M.I., Arrunategui, A., Falabella, R. & Alzate, A. (1995) An epidemiologic case-control study in a population with vitiligo. *Journal of the American Academy of Dermatology* **33**, 621–625.

Concetta-Fargnoli, M. & Bolognia, L. (1995) Pentachrome vitiligo. *Journal of the American Academy of Dermatology* **33**, 853–856.

Dupre, A. & Christol, B. (1978) Cockade-like vitiligo and linear vitiligo a variant of fitzpatrick's trichrome vitiligo. *Archives of Dermatological Research—Archiv für Dermatologische Forschung* **262**, 197–203.

Eng, A.M. (1970) Marginal inflammatory vitiligo. *Cutis* **6**, 1005–1008.

Fitzpatrick, T.B. (1964) Hypomelanosis. *Southern Medical Journal* **57**, 995–1005.

Gauthier, Y. (1995) The importance of Koebner's phenomenon in the induction of vitiligo vulgaris lesions. *European Journal of Dermatology* **5**, 704–708.

Gopinathan, T. (1965) A study of the lesion of vitiligo. *Archives of Dermatology* **91**, 397–404.

Hann, S.-K., Chun, W.H. & Park, Y.-K. (1997) Clinical characteristics of progressive vitiligo. *International Journal of Dermatology* **36**, 353–355.

Hatchome, N., Kato, T. & Tagami, H. (1990) Therapeutic success of epidermal grafting in generalized vitiligo is limited by the Koebner phenomenon. *Journal of the American Academy of Dermatology* **22**, 87–91.

Ivker, R., Goldaber, M. & Buchness, M.R. (1994) Blue vitiligo. *Journal of the American Academy of Dermatology* **30** (2), 829–831.

Levaï, M. (1958) The relationship of pruritus and local skin conditions to the development of vitiligo. *Archives of Dermatology* **78**, 372–377.

Macmillan, A. & Rook, A. (1971) Vitiligo with a raised rim in atopic subjects. *British Journal of Dermatology* **85**, 491.

Michaelsson, G. (1968) Vitiligo with raised borders. Report of two cases. *Acta Dermato-Venereologica (Stockholm)* **48**, 158–161.

Mosher, D.B., Fitzpatrick, T.B., Ortonne, J.P. *et al*. (1987) Vitiligo. In: *Dermatology in General Medicine* (eds T.B. Fitzpatrick, A.Z. Eisen, K. Wolff), 3rd edn, pp. 810–821. McGraw-Hill, New York.

Ortonne, J.P., Baran, R. & Civatte, J. (1979) Vitiligo à bordure inflammatoire. A propos de 2 observations avec revue de la littérature (18 cas). *Annals of Dermatology and Venereology* **106**, 613–615.

Ortonne, J.-P., Mosher, D.B. & Fitzpatrick, T.B. (1983) *Vitiligo and Other Hypomelanoses of Hair and Skin*. Plenum Medical Book Company, New York.

Powell, F.C. & Dicken, C.H. (1983) Psoriasis and vitiligo. *Acta Dermato-Venereologica (Stockholm)* **63**, 246–249.

Schallreuter, K.U., Lemke, R., Brandt, O., Schwartz, R., Westhofen, M., Montz, R. & Berger, J. (1994) Vitiligo and other diseases: coexistence or true association? Hamburg study on 321 patients. *Dermatology* **188**, 269–275.

Sidi, E. (1957) Dyschromies et Vitiligo. *Expansion Scientifique Française*. Expansion, Paris.

Siemens, H.W. (1954) Vitiligo gradata (Stufenvitiligo). *Dermatologica* **109**, 228 (Abstract).

Sommer, S. & Dicken, C.Y. (1998) The Koebner phenomenon in vitiligo following treatment of a port-wine stain naevus by pulsed dye laser. *British Journal of Dermatology* **138**, 200–201.

Sweet, R.D. (1978) Vitiligo as a Koebner phenomenon. *British Journal of Dermatology* **99**, 223–224.

10: Depigmentation of Hair and Mucous Membranes

JEAN-PAUL ORTONNE

Melanocytes are present in the oral and genital mucosae. Like epidermal and follicular melanocytes, they may be affected by vitiligo.

Oral vitiligo

In caucasoid subjects, the oral mucosa and the lips most often do not exhibit signs of melanin pigmentation, despite the presence of melanocytes in oral epithelium, in variable numbers, occurring as groups or isolated cells in the basal layer. Physiological oral pigmentation is seen most regularly in dark-skinned races and the sites most consistently showing this pigmentation are the buccal and labial aspects of the gingiva. This may explain that oral vitiligo has long been considered uncommon if not rare. Furthermore the oral cavity of vitiligo patients is very seldom examined. Lip involvement is a common feature in dark-skinned vitiligo patients (Seghal 1974; Coondoo *et al.* 1976). Several epidemiological studies show that the incidence of vitiligo of the lip may be more than 50% (Seghal 1974; Coondoo *et al.* 1976) (Fig. 10.1). Lip vitiligo may be isolated and is equally distributed among men and women. Much less is known about the incidence of vitiligo of the oral mucosa, but patchy loss of melanin pigment from the buccal mucosa, gingiva and gum line is invariably observed in patients with vitiligo (Dummet 1959) (Fig. 10.2). A case of complete clinical depigmentation of the oral mucosa in an African-American has even been reported (Dummet 1959). Wood's light examination is most useful to detect lip and oral vitiligo. It demonstrates that this site is very commonly involved in light-skinned individuals.

Genital involvement is also documented (Jayle & Aubry 1921; Moss & Stevenson 1981; Gaffoor 1984). It occurs in both males and females, but is apparently more common in males. Involvement of the glans penis is not a rare finding. Only a few cases of vitiligo of the vulva and vaginal mucosa have been reported (Jayle & Aubry 1921). It is possible that the mucous membranes covering the vaginal vault are depigmented, but this feature has not been specifically studied and examination of the genital tract is not performed on a regular basis in female vitiligo patients.

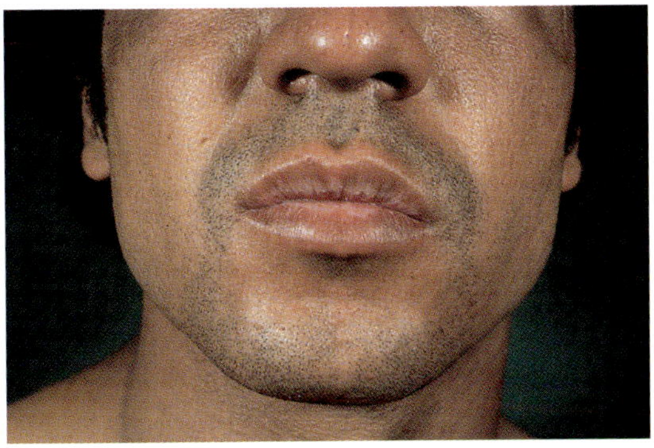

Fig. 10.1 Vitiligo of the lips.

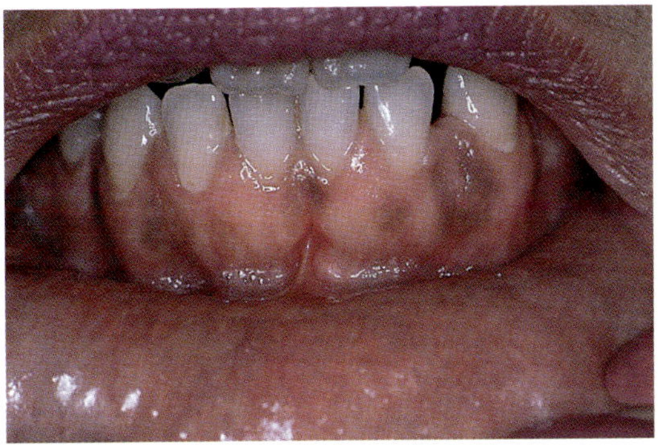

Fig. 10.2 Vitiligo of the gums.

Depigmentation of hair

Melanocytes of the hair bulb are responsible for hair colour. They transfer their melanosomes to the surrounding hair keratinocytes. In the hair follicles, melanin granules are mainly in the cortex, their long axes parallel to the hair surface.

Involvement of hair in vitiligo macules is variable, indicating that the follicular compartment of the melanocyte organ may be spared while the epidermal compartment is destroyed by the 'vitiligo' process. This dissociated behaviour of epidermal and follicular melanocytes is very common in vitiligo.

The incidence of body leukotrichia in the different series of the literature varies from 10% to more than 60% (Dutta & Mandal 1969; Seghal 1974). Poliosis occurs in both patients with bilateral or unilateral vitiligo. Its incidence has been estimated at 48.6% in a group of 101 patients with segmental vitiligo (Hann & Lee 1996). A few or all body hair of a single macule may be amelanotic and not all macules are uniformly involved. Presence of leukotrichia has been accorded special significance. In these instances, transplantation of melanocytes is required for repigmentation.

The occurrence of leukotrichia is not correlated to disease activity. A recent study demonstrates that the disease does not progress more significantly in patients with leukotrichia than in patients with normal hair pigmentation (Hann *et al.* 1997).

Vitiligo of the scalp usually presents as a localized patch of white or grey hair, but total depigmentation of all scalp hair may happen (Fig.10.3). On the contrary, only a few follicles may be involved leading to a scattering of white hairs on the scalp (Fig. 10.4) (Lerner & Nordlund 1978). The interfollicular scalp epidermis may be involved with or without associated leukotrichia (Fig. 10.5). Isolated early greying or whitening before 30 years of age has also been suggested to represent a form of vitiligo. Histological and ultrastructural studies suggest that in greying or whitening of hair resulting from the ageing process, abnormal melanocytes are still present in the follicle, whereas in white hair of vitiligo, all melanocytes have been lost.

All hairy areas of the body may be involved, including eyebrows, eyelashes and pubic hair (Figs 10.6 & 10.7). Spontaneous repigmentation of depigmented hair in vitiligo does not occur .

Until recently, little attention was paid to vitiligo leukotrichia. This clinical feature has been accorded special significance. It is considered as a sign that the involved area will not repigment with medical therapies because it indicates that the melanocyte reservoir within the hair follicle has been destroyed. This statement implies that spontaneous or therapy-

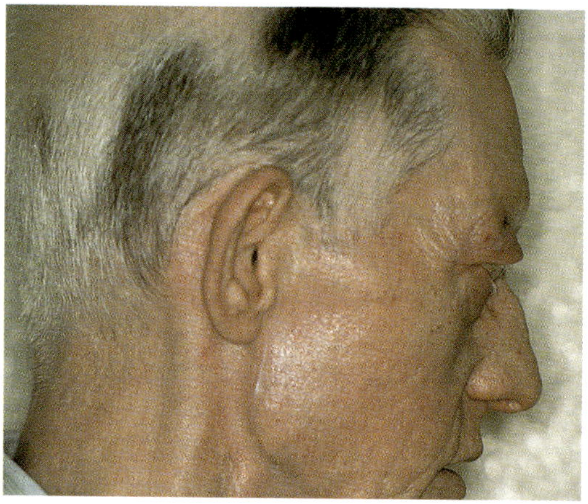

Fig. 10.3 Extensive vitiligo of the scalp.

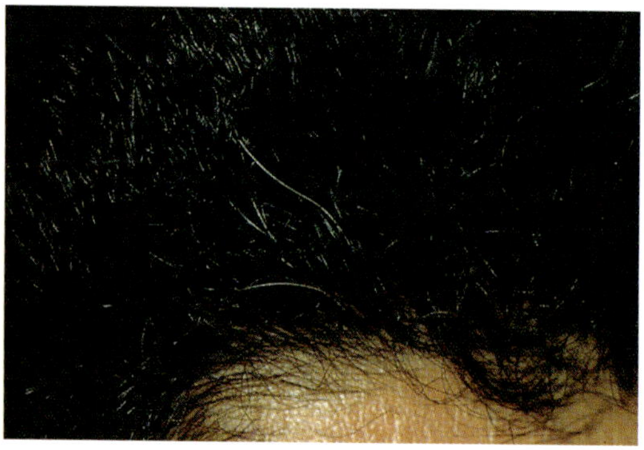

Fig. 10.4 Single hair involvement in a patient with vitiligo.

induced repigmentation of vitiligo leukotrichia is very unlikely. Three vitiligo patients undergoing epidermal grafting and PUVA therapy showing repigmentation of leukotrichia in the eyebrows have been reported (Hann *et al.* 1992). Repigmentation of vitiligo hair after dermabrasion and split thickness skin grafting of vitiligo macules over hair-bearing areas has also been observed. These isolated reports have been confirmed by a systemic study demonstrating that surgical (dermabrasion and thin split thickness skin grafting) repigmentation of vitiligo could be achieved, partial to nearly total, in seven out of eight patients (Agrawal & Agrawal 1995).

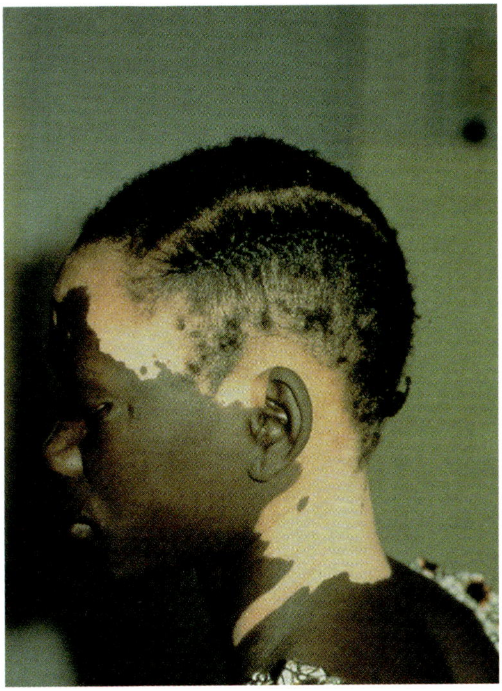

Fig. 10.5 Depigmentation of the scalp skin without changes of hair colour.

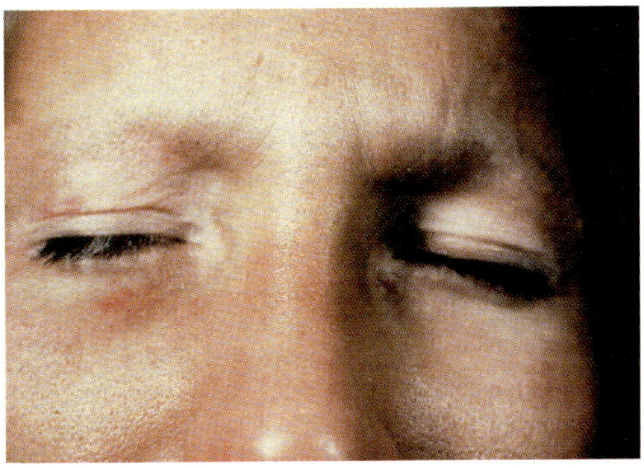

Fig. 10.6 Poliosis of the eyelids.

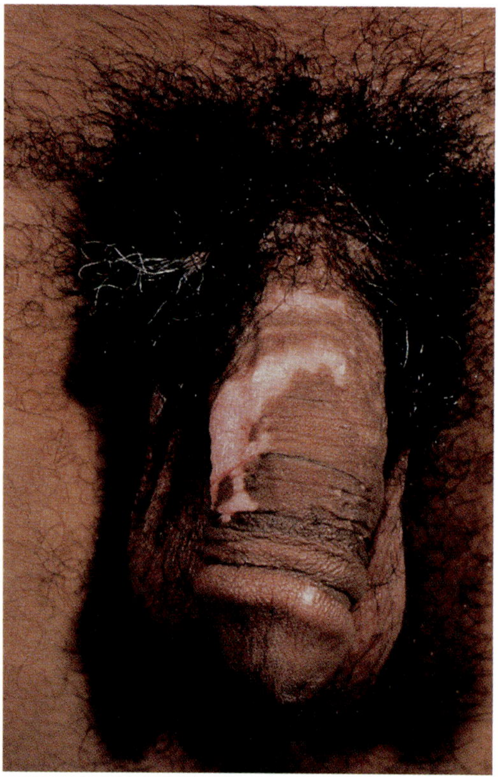

Fig. 10.7 Vitiligo macule on the external genitalia including the glans penis. Localized depigmentation of pubic hair.

References

Agrawal, K. & Agrawal, A. (1995) Vitiligo: surgical repigmentation of leukotrichia. *Dermatologic Surgery* **21**, 711–715.

Coondoo, A., Sen, N. & Panja, R.K. (1976) Leucoderma of the lips. A clinical study. *Indian Journal of Dermatology* **21**, 29–33.

Dummet, C.O. (1959) The oral tissues in vitiligo. *Oral Surgery, Oral Medicine, and Oral Pathology* **12**, 1073–1079.

Dutta, A.K. & Mandal, S.B. (1969) A clinical study of 650 vitiligo cases and their classification. *Indian Journal of Dermatology* **14**, 103–111.

Gaffoor, P.M. (1984) Depigmentation of the male genitalia. *Cutis* **34**, 492–494.

Hann, S.K. & Lee, H.J. (1996) Segmental vitiligo: clinical findings in 208 patients. *Journal of the American Academy of Dermatology* **35**, 671–674.

Hann, S.K., Im, S., Park, Y.K. & Hur, W. (1992) Repigmentation of leukotrichia by epidermal grafting and systemic psoralen plus UV-A (letter). *Archives of Dermatology* **128**, 998–999.

Hann, S.-K., Chun, W.H. & Park, Y.-K. (1997) Clinical characteristics of progressive vitiligo. *International Journal of Dermatology* **36**, 353–355.

Jayle, F. & Aubry, H. (1921) Le vitiligo génital et abdominal chez la femme. *Revue Francaise de Gynocologie et D'obstetrique (Paris)* **16**, 193–225.

Lerner, A.B. & Nordlund, J.J. (1978) Vitiligo. What is it? Is it important? *JAMA* **239**, 1183–1187.

Moss, T.R. & Stevenson, C.J. (1981) Incidence of male genital vitiligo. Report of a screening programme. *British Journal of Venereal Diseases* **57**, 145–146.

Seghal, V.N. (1974) A clinical evaluation of 202 cases of vitiligo. *Cutis* **14**, 439–445.

11: Ocular and Otic Findings in Vitiligo

MONTE D. MILLS AND DANIEL M. ALBERT

Introduction

The eye, as a pigmented organ, is susceptible to many congenital and acquired abnormalities of pigmentation which affect the skin and other pigmented tissues. The eye contains two populations of pigmented cells:

1 the pigment epithelial layers of the retina, ciliary body and iris, and
2 the melanocytes of the uvea.

The latter resemble the melanocytes of the skin. In patients with vitiligo both types of pigmented cells of the eye, as well as the melanocytes in periocular cutaneous tissues, may be affected, presumably by the same pathophysiological mechanism affecting the skin. Various forms of intraocular depigmentation have been observed in patients with cutaneous vitiligo. Most importantly, inflammatory ocular abnormalities including the Vogt–Koyanagi–Harada syndrome (VKH) and nonspecific idiopathic uveitis have been associated with cutaneous vitiligo. Other autoimmune diseases thought to be associated with vitiligo, including Graves' disease and diabetes mellitus, may also affect the eyes. Pigmented cells are also found in the inner ear, and sensorineural hearing loss may be seen in patients with VKH as well as those with non-VKH vitiligo. The purposes of this chapter are to review the ocular and otic abnormalities which have been reported in association with vitiligo, and discuss the possible pathophysiological mechanisms for eye and ear involvement in this pigmentary disorder.

Vitiligo and ocular disease

The most significant ocular abnormality associated with vitiligo is ocular inflammation, or uveitis. Uveitis seen with vitiligo may occur across a spectrum of severity and anatomical location. Anterior uveitis, or iridocyclitis, is inflammation of the anterior chamber, iris, and ciliary body at the front of the eye. Posterior uveitis, or chorioretinitis, is inflammation of the pigmented choroid and retina of the ocular fundus. The most severe form of uveitis associated with vitiligo is the Vogt–Koyanagi–Harada syndrome.

Vogt–Koyanagi–Harada syndrome (VKH) is a multisystem disorder characterized by idiopathic uveitis, central nervous system abnormalities and cutaneous signs including vitiligo. VKH is a common cause of uveitis in Japan and other Asian countries (Ohno *et al.* 1977; Sugiura 1978). In the

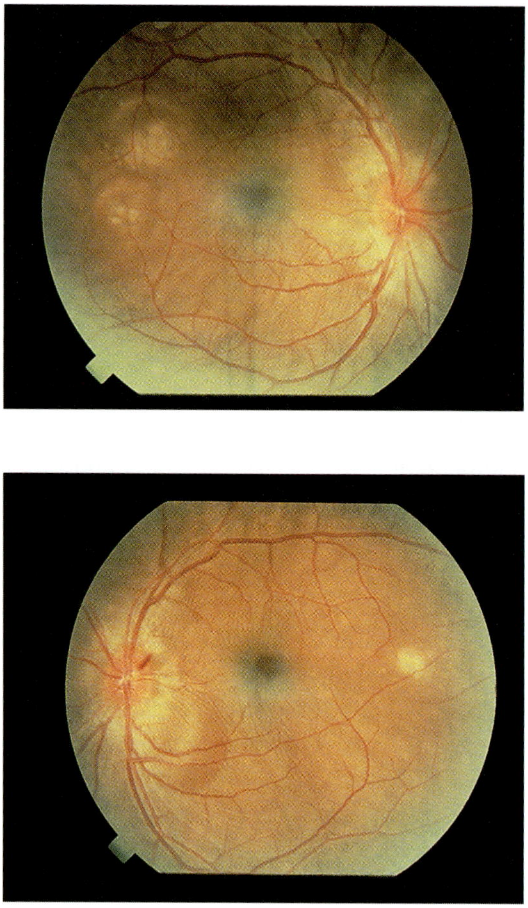

Fig. 11.1 The ocular fundi of a patient with acute VKH in the uveitic phase. Retinal striae, exudative retinal detachments, focal depigmentation of the retinal pigment epithelium and choroid, optic disc oedema, and optic disc haemorrhage are evidence of the posterior uveitis.

United States, VKH is most frequently seen in patients of Asian, Hispanic, African or American Indian descent, and is a rare cause of uveitis in non-Hispanic white patients. Women are slightly more frequently affected than men, and most patients are in the second to fifth decade at the time of diagnosis. The diagnosis of VKH is made on the basis of clinical criteria, including bilateral chronic iridocyclitis, posterior uveitis which may include exudative retinal detachment (Fig. 11.1) and central nervous system (CNS) symptoms including meningismus, headache or dysacousia, and cutaneous manifestations (Table 11.1). There are no specific diagnostic tests, although examination of cerebrospinal fluid may demonstrate a sterile pleocytosis. Laboratory evaluation is also useful to exclude other possible causes of severe bilateral uveitis, including syphilis, tuberculosis, Lyme disease, and systemic lupus erythematosus. A history of penetrating eye trauma or surgery may be the only clinical feature to distinguish VKH from sympathetic ophthalmia, a similar bilateral autoimmune uveitis.

The typical course of VKH includes the abrupt onset of symptoms which may include nausea, fever, and neurological signs (Table 11.2). The uveitic stage follows within one week, with both anterior and posterior

Table 11.1 Diagnostic criteria for the Vogt–Koyanagi–Harada Syndrome (VKH). Adapted from Snyder & Tessler (1980).

1 No history of ocular trauma
2 At least three of the following:
  (a) bilateral chronic iridocyclitis
  (b) posterior uveitis, including exudative retinal detachment and optic disc oedema
  (c) neurological signs including tinnitus, neck stiffness, cranial nerve, or central nervous system impairment or cerebrospinal fluid pleocytosis
  (d) alopecia, poliosis or vitiligo

Table 11.2 Clinical course of Vogt–Koyanagi–Harada Syndrome. Adapted from Sugiura (1978) and Moorthy (1995).

Prodromal stage: symptoms

Uveitic stage: exudative retinal detachment

Convalescent stage: progressive uveitis and retinal inflammation, Dalen–Fuchs nodules, Sugiura's sign, vitiligo

Recurrent stage: anterior uveitis, retinal pigment changes

ocular inflammation. Treatment of VKH primarily consists of topical and systemic steroid medications to suppress ocular and CNS inflammation, although some patients may require immunosuppressive agents including cyclophosphamide, azathioprine, cyclosporin or FK 506 to control ocular inflammation. Depending on treatment, resolution of inflammation may occur over weeks to months. Relapses of uveitis, primarily anterior uveitis or iridocyclitis, may occur and are a primary source of the long-term sequelae which may threaten vision, including cataract, glaucoma, and subretinal neovascularization. With treatment, the visual prognosis is generally favourable, with 2/3 of affected eyes retaining vision of at least 20/40 (Moorthy *et al.* 1995). However, many eyes will develop cataract, glaucoma, or subretinal neovascularization which may require intervention.

A late sequelae of VKH is depigmentation and scarring of the ocular fundus, occurring in the convalescent phase (Fig. 11.2). Clinically, the fundus may appear to have diffuse depigmentation with increased visibility of the choroidal vasculature, known as the 'sunset-glow' fundus appearance, or may have focal geographical depigmentation. Small, round, focal areas of depigmentation of the choroid are known as Dalen–Fuchs nodules. Histopathologically, the few reported cases examined have demonstrated diffuse or focal granulomatous inflammation of the choroid, similar to the inflammation seen in sympathetic ophthalmia (Perry & Font 1977; Rao & Marak 1983). Choroidal melanocytes are reduced in number throughout the fundus. Skin biopsies from involved areas in patients with VKH-associated vitiligo demonstrate inflammatory characteristics similar to non-VKH vitiligo, with mononuclear infiltration consisting primarily of CD4+ (helper-inducer) lymphocytes, suggesting a prominent role for cell-mediated immunity in these skin lesions (Okada *et al.* 1996).

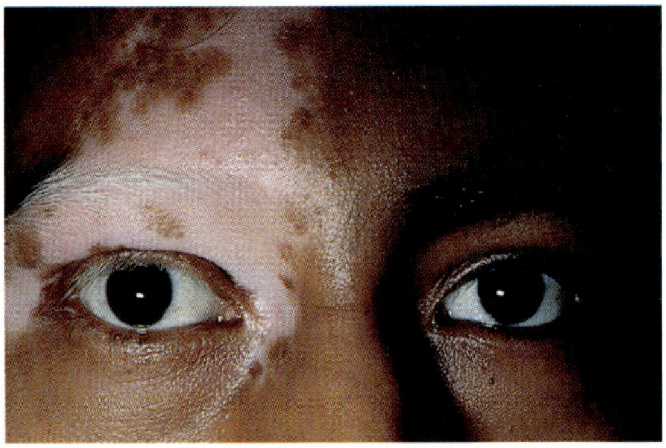

(a)

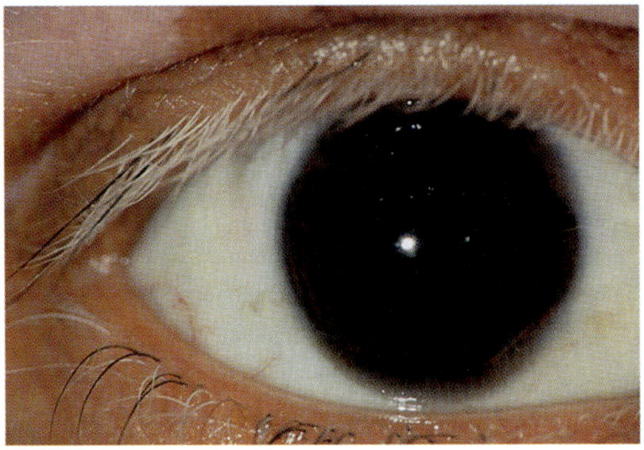

(b)

Fig. 11.2 Periocular depigmentation in a patient with VKH. Poliosis of the eyelashes and eyebrows, cutaneous depigmentation (a), and depigmentation of the limbal conjunctiva (Sugiura's sign) (b) are seen in the convalescent phase of VKH.

Vitiligo is seen in as many as 63% of VKH patients (Sugiura 1978; Moorthy *et al.* 1995), usually during the convalescent stage of the syndrome (Fig 11.3). It is rare for vitiligo to precede the uveitis in VKH. Depigmentation is frequently seen in periocular skin including the eyelids, and a distinctive focal depigmentation of the perilimbal conjunctiva (adjacent to the cornea), known as Sugiura's sign, has been recorded in 95% of Asian patients (Sugiura 1978). The reported incidence of poliosis of the eyelashes, eyebrows and scalp in VKH varies widely, from less than 10% to 90%, and may depend on racial background (Sugiura 1978; Barnes 1988; Moorthy *et al.* 1995). Focal alopecia similar to alopecia areata is also seen. The cutaneous manifestations of VKH may persist despite remission of uveitis.

Conversely, VKH is an uncommon cause of vitiligo, accounting for only 1–5% of patients attending vitiligo clinics (Table 11.3) (Albert *et al.* 1979, 1983; Cowan *et al.* 1986).

Less severe ocular inflammation, insufficient for the diagnosis of VKH, has been reported in 5% of vitiligo patients. Similarly, about 5% of patients with idiopathic uveitis, not meeting clinical criteria for the diagnosis of VKH, have been observed to have vitiligo or poliosis (Wagoner *et al.* 1983). The onset of vitiligo and uveitis were usually simultaneous or within weeks, although vitiligo may precede the onset of uveitis by years. Uveitis appears to be most common with vitiligo associated with cutaneous melanoma (19%) (Wagoner *et al.* 1983).

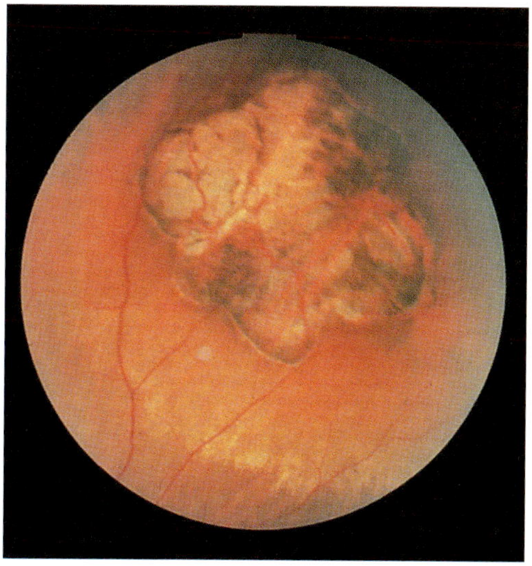

(a)

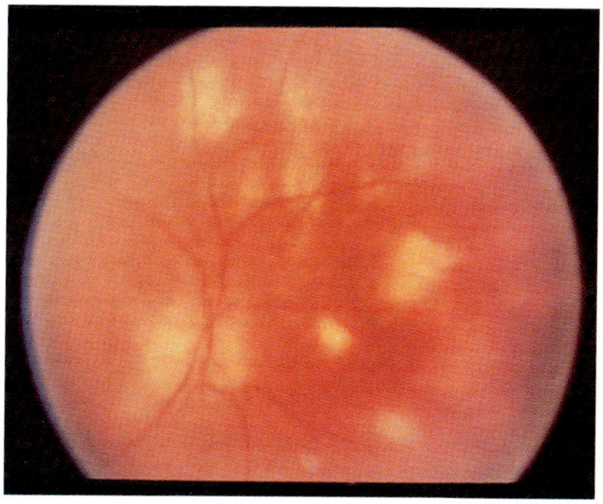

(b)

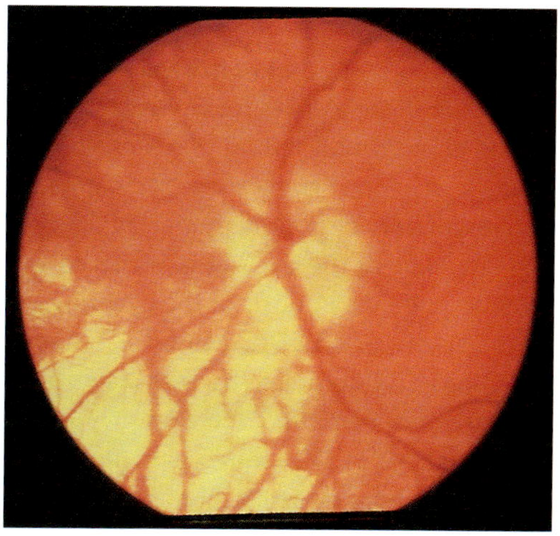

(c)

Fig. 11.3 Fundus depigmentation in non-VKH patients may include evidence of previous chorioretinal inflammation and scarring (a) or may show no evidence of inflammation (b). Diffuse depigmentation may also occur (c).

Table 11.3 Incidence of ocular and otic findings in vitiligo.

Abnormality	Patients with vitiligo (%)	Author
VKH syndrome	5.4	Albert *et al.* 1979
	1.3	Albert *et al.* 1983
	0.0	Cowan *et al.* 1986
Uveitis, non-VKH	2.7	Albert *et al.* 1979
	3.1	Wagoner *et al.* 1983
	18.5 (cutaneous melanoma-associated vitiligo	Wagoner *et al.* 1983
	1.8	Cowan *et al.* 1986
Fundus depigmentation	36.0	Albert *et al.* 1979
	30.9 (with scarring)	Wagoner *et al.* 1983
	26.9 (no scarring)	Wagoner *et al.* 1983
	7.0 (with scarring)	Cowan *et al.* 1986
	11.1 (no scarring)	Cowan *et al.* 1986
Periocular skin depigmentation	48.2	Albert *et al.* 1979
	63.0	Cowan *et al.* 1986
Iris transillumination	5.5 (Black)	Cowan *et al.* 1986
	23.3 (White)	Cowan *et al.* 1986
Poliosis of eyelashes	16.0	Albert *et al.* 1979
Poliosis of eyebrows	13.4	Albert *et al.* 1979
Reduced hearing	16.0	Tosti *et al.* 1987
	13.3	Nikiforidis *et al.* 1993

Sympathetic ophthalmia, a rare form of uveitis which is thought to be an autoimmune response to retinal antigens incited by eye trauma, has on occasion been associated with vitiligo and poliosis (Rao & Marak 1983). Clinically and histopathologically, sympathetic ophthalmia closely resembles VKH, with chorioretinitis and chronic granulomatous inflammation of the choroid (Perry & Font 1977; Lubin *et al.* 1982).

Noninflammatory depigmented lesions of the ocular fundus are observed in 18–31% of non-VKH vitiligo patients (Albert *et al.* 1979, 1983; Cowan *et al.* 1986), presumably representing focal areas of melanocyte loss in the choroid and retinal pigment epithelium. The depigmentation may include scarring, suggesting previous episodes of subclinical posterior uveitis, or may be noninflammatory depigmentation.

The skin of the eyelids is involved in as many as 48% of non-VKH vitiligo patients. Poliosis of the eyebrows and eyelashes is seen in 13–16% (Albert *et al.* 1979, 1983; Cowan *et al.* 1986).

Other autoimmune diseases have been reported in association with vitiligo, and may affect the eyes or vision. In a prospective survey of eye abnormalities in 112 vitiligo patients, 12% had thyroid disease (hyperthyroid, hypothyroid, or Hashimoto thyroiditis) which may cause proptosis, strabismus, and eyelid retraction (Albert *et al.* 1979). Diabetes mellitus, multiple myeloma, and mycosis fungoides have also been seen with increased frequency in vitiligo patients, and may cause significant visual symptoms (Mandry *et al.* 1996).

Vitiligo and otic disease

Dysacousia or tinnitus are prodromal symptoms in as many as 80% of patients with VKH. The cochlear dysfunction typically affects the high-frequency range, but may affect all frequencies and may be severe (up to 30 dB). Despite the frequency of vertigo, vestibular dysfunction is rarely persistent after the prodromal phase. The inner ear dysfunction usually improves during the convalescent phase over several months, although hearing may be permanently reduced (Sugiura 1978; Moorthy *et al.* 1995).

Abnormalities of hearing and brainstem auditory response have been measured in non-VKH vitiligo patients, and suggest that 13–16% of patients with vitiligo demonstrate abnormal sensorineural hearing loss (Tosti *et al.* 1987; Orecchia *et al.* 1989; Nikiforidis *et al.* 1993). Like ocular fundus depigmentation, these studies suggest subclinical involvement with VKH-like systemic involvement, but conclusions are limited by their retrospective nature. The role of the melanocytes within the inner ear is not understood well. Likewise, little is known concerning the histopathology or pathophysiology of the cochlear involvement in vitiligo. The presence of melanocytes within the cochlea is thought to play a role (Tosti *et al.* 1987).

Congenital and acquired deafness have been associated with vitiligo in certain kindreds (Thurmon *et al.* 1976; Tosti *et al.* 1986; Dereymaeker *et al.* 1989). The lack of molecular genetic evidence of a hereditary link between deafness and vitiligo in these cases limits our understanding of this phenomenon.

Conclusion

The ocular and otic associations of vitiligo suggest that vitiligo is a systemic disease affecting pigmented cells throughout the body, rather than a purely cutaneous problem. The inflammatory nature of the ocular diseases associated with vitiligo also supports the hypothesis of an antigen-specific inflammatory mechanism of melanocyte depletion in vitiligo (Ortonne & Bose 1993; Nordlund & Majumder 1997). The primary ocular association with vitiligo is the Vogt–Koyanagi–Harada syndrome. Patients with vitiligo have an increased incidence of more mild uveitis as well, and have been found to have evidence of subclinical inflammatory fundus depigmentation in many cases. Otic involvement, common in VKH but also reported in non-VKH vitiligo, may include permanent hearing loss.

References

Albert, D.M., Nordlund, J.J. & Lerner, A.B. (1979) Ocular abnormalities occurring with vitiligo. *Ophthalmology* **86**, 1145–1158.

Albert, D.M., Wagoner, M.D., Pruett, R.C., Nordlund, J.J. & Lerner, A.B. (1983) Vitiligo and disorders of the retinal pigment epithelium. *British Journal of Ophthalmology* **67**, 153–156.

Barnes, L. (1988) Vitiligo and the Vogt-Koyanagi–Harada syndrome. *Dermatologic Clinics* **6**, 229–239.

Cowan, C.L. Jr, Halder, R.M., Grimes, P.E., Chakrabarti, S.G. & Kenney, J.A. Jr (1986) Ocular disturbances in vitiligo. *Journal of the American Academy of Dermatology* **15**, 17–24.

Dereymaeker, A.M., Fryns, J.P., Ars, J., Andresescu, J. & van den Berghe, H. (1989) Retinitis pigmentosa, hearing loss and vitiligo: report of two patients. *Clinical Genetics* **35**, 387–389.

Lubin, J.R., Ni, C. & Albert, D.M. (1982) Clinicopathological study of the Vogt-Koyanagi–Harada syndrome. *International Ophthalmology Clinics* **22**, 141–156.

Mandry, R.C., Ortiz, L.J., Lugo-Somolinos, A. & Sanchez, J.L. (1996) Organ-specific autoantibodies in vitiligo patients and their relatives. *International Journal of Dermatology* **35**, 18–21.

Moorthy, R.S., Inomata, H. & Rao, N.A. (1995) Vogt-Koyanagi–Harada syndrome (review). *Survey of Ophthalmology* **39**, 265–292.

Nikiforidis, G.C., Tsambaos, D.G., Karamitsos, D.S., Koutsojannis, C.C. & Georgiou, S.V. (1993) Abnormalities of the auditory brainstem response in vitiligo. *Scandinavian Audiology* **22**, 97–100.

Nordlund, J.J. & Majumder, P.P. (1997) Recent investigations on vitiligo vulgaris. *Dermatologic Clinics* **15**, 69–78.

Ohno, S., Char, D.H., Kimura, S.J. & O'Connor, R. (1977) Vogt-Koyanagi–Harada syndrome. *American Journal of Ophthalmology* **83**, 735–740.

Okada, T., Sakamoto, T., Ishibashi, T. & Inomata, H. (1996) Vitiligo in Vogt-Koyanagi-Harada disease: immunohistological analysis of inflammatory site. *Graefe's Archive for Clinical and Experimental Ophthalmology* **234**, 359–363.

Orecchia, G., Marelli, M.A., Fresa, D. & Robiolio, L. (1989) Audiologic disturbances in vitiligo (letter to the editors). *Journal of the American Academy of Dermatology* **21**, 1317–1318.

Ortonne, J.-P. & Bose, S.K. (1993) Vitiligo: where do we stand? *Pigment Cell Research* **6**, 61–72.

Perry, H.D. & Font, R.L. (1977) Clinical and histopathological observations in severe Vogt-Koyanagi–Harada syndrome. *American Journal of Ophthalmology* **83**, 242–254.

Rao, N.A. & Marak, G.E. (1983) Sympathetic ophthalmia stimulating Vogt-Koyanagi-Harada's disease: a clinico-pathologic study of four cases. *Japanese Journal of Ophthalmology* **27**, 506–511.

Sugiura, S. (1978) Vogt-Koyanagi-Harada disease. *Japanese Journal of Ophthalmology* **22**, 9–35.

Thurmon, T.F., Jackson, J. & Fowler, C.G. (1976) Deafness and vitiligo. *Birth Defects: Original Article Series* **12**, 315–320.

Tosti, A., Bardazzi, F., De Padova, M.P., Veronesi, S. & Bergonzoni, C. (1986) Deafness and vitiligo in an Italian family (letter). *Dermatologica* **172**, 178–179.

Tosti, A., Bardazzi, F., Tosti, G. & Monti, L. (1987) Audiologic abnormalities in cases of vitiligo. *Journal of the American Academy of Dermatology* **17**, 230–233.

Wagoner, M.D., Albert, D.M., Lerner, A.B., Kirkwood, J.M., Forget, B.M. & Nordlund, J.J. (1983) New observations on vitiligo and ocular disease. *American Journal of Ophthalmology* **96**, 16–26.

12: The Association of Vitiligo with Disorders of Other Organ Systems

JAMES J. NORDLUND AND SEUNG-KYUNG HANN

Introduction

The aetiology of vitiligo remains an enigma but the most popular theory is based on an autoimmune mechanism. This idea that vitiligo and the destruction of melanocytes is caused by an autoimmune process seems to have been proposed first in the 1960s (Cunliffe *et al.* 1968) when the immune system was under intense study. Numerous reports have been published by investigators throughout the world to document an association of vitiligo with the immune system (reviewed in Nordlund *et al.* 1998). Other authors have attempted to link vitiligo with viral aetiologies, some with biochemical toxicity or genetic dysfunction.

Possibly the first report of vitiligo in association with another disorder was that of Thomas Addison (Addison 1855). He was interested in the cause of asthenia. He found two different causes, pernicious anaemia and adrenal insufficiency. He reported on 13 patients with adrenal insufficiency, all of whom had died and come to autopsy. He found that all 13 had a scrofulous or tuberculous destruction of the adrenal gland. One of these had vitiligo and it appears from the drawings in his book that another had halo naevi (Addison 1855).

Vitiligo and endocrine dysfunction

Polyglandular dysfunction

Polyglandular dysfunction is a syndrome in which a patient experiences end organ failure of many endocrine glands. The failure is due to atrophy of glands such as the thyroid, the islets of Langerhans, the adrenal gland, the gonads and often the gastric mucosa. The syndrome has been associated with a locus on chromosome 21 (Aaltonen *et al.* 1994). It is considered a prime example of an autoimmune disorder in which autoantibodies cause destruction of endocrine cells (Peserico *et al.* 1981; Bloch & Sowers 1985). All patients have failure of several, or rarely all, of the listed organs. Some of these individuals also have non-endocrine organs damaged by autoimmune processes. These include leukaemia, red cell hypoplasia (Mandel *et al.* 1989), neurological deficits, coeliac disease and sarcoid, and selective IgA deficiency (Torrelo *et al.* 1992). The pathogenesis of all of these disorders is thought to have some connection with the immune system.

Many patients with polyglandular dysfunction also have been noted to have vitiligo (Peserico *et al.* 1981; Bloch & Sowers 1985; Mandel *et al.* 1989; Sharma *et al.* 1990; Betterle *et al.* 1992; Csaszar & Patakfalvi 1992; Torrelo *et al.* 1992). Patients with polyglandular dysfunction have antibodies that seem to cause destruction of their endocrine system. A few have been reported to have antibodies to melanocytes although the type and nature of these antibodies is not well described (Peserico *et al.* 1981). Regardless, these syndromes of multiendocrine dysfunction associated with organ-specific antibodies are commonly associated with vitiligo. The association suggests that vitiligo, at least in these individuals, is an autoimmune disorder. It is not permissible simply to extrapolate these conclusions to other patients with isolated endocrine disorders.

Thyroid disorders

The first report of an association of vitiligo and thyroid dysfunction seems to have been published in 1968 (Cunliffe *et al.* 1968). Since that report many other authors have reported that those with vitiligo have a propensity to develop thyroid dysfunction, either hyper- or hypothyroidism (Godeau *et al.* 1973; Jacyk *et al.* 1976; Ortonne *et al.* 1976; Pal *et al.* 1980; Grimes *et al.* 1983; Lamartine de Assis *et al.* 1983; Midelfart *et al.* 1983; Korkij *et al.* 1984; Mullin & Eastern 1986; Ramanathan *et al.* 1989; Kumar *et al.* 1990; Nishida *et al.* 1990; Saban *et al.* 1991; Shong & Kim 1991; Auer-Grumbach & Stangl 1993; Hegedus *et al.* 1994; Zelissen *et al.* 1995). Thyroid dysfunction is thought to be caused in many individuals by an autoimmune process in which autoantibodies cause destruction of the thyroid parenchyma (Ramanathan *et al.* 1989; Prentice *et al.* 1990; Konno *et al.* 1993; Zelissen *et al.* 1995; Wang & Crapo 1997). That vitiligo occurs with an autoimmune process has been considered to be suggestive evidence for a common pathogenesis.

Unlike polyglandular dysfunction, thyroid disease is very common. As many as 15% or more of the population are thought to have thyroid disease, either overt or covert (Betterle *et al.* 1985; Ramanathan *et al.* 1989; Prentice *et al.* 1990; Konno *et al.* 1993; Wang & Crapo 1997). In a study of 460 subjects with vitiligo, 14% were found to have thyroid disorders (Nordlund & Majumder 1997). Others have found higher prevalence of thyroid dysfunction in those with vitiligo than those without cutaneous depigmentation (Pal *et al.* 1980; Grimes *et al.* 1983; Korkij *et al.* 1984; Shong & Kim 1991; Hegedus *et al.* 1994). Not all of these studies used appropriate controls for comparison. Regardless, it is difficult to draw definitive conclusions about the validity of the association of vitiligo with thyroid dysfunction or the presence of thyroid autoantibodies in the sera of those with vitiligo. At best the association is valid but might have little impact on understanding the aetiology of vitiligo. At the least it is a manifestation of the frequency of thyroid disease in the population, especially in females who tend to predominate in most studies on vitiligo.

Diabetes mellitus

The cause of diabetes mellitus also has escaped full elucidation. This endocrine disorder also has been considered an autoimmune disorder caused by autoantibodies destroying the islets of Langerhans. Investigators have tried to show that vitiligo is more common in those with diabetes or, vice versa, that diabetes is more common in those with vitiligo (Dawber 1968; Villaverde 1969; Dawber *et al.* 1971; Jacyk *et al.* 1976; Macaron *et al.* 1977; Gould *et al.* 1985; Pelosio *et al.* 1989). The validity of the association is not obvious from the data presented.

Other endocrine disorders

The first association of an endocrine failure and vitiligo seems to be the report of Addison who discovered adrenal failure. He reported on 13 patients with scrofulous infiltration of the adrenal gland. One of his patients had vitiligo (Addison 1855). However, his report is confined to individuals with tuberculosis. Other investigators have reported an incidental association of vitiligo with adrenal dysfunction as documentation of the autoimmune aetiology of vitiligo (Tadzhibaev 1971; Betterle *et al.* 1985; Mulligan & Sowers 1985; Zelissen *et al.* 1995). There are other reports of gonadal atresia, pernicious anaemia and haemolytic anaemia (Grunnet *et al.* 1970; Matsumoto *et al.* 1977; Sidi *et al.* 1978; Walters *et al.* 1978; Collen *et al.* 1979; Ruzicka 1981; Alper & Garner 1985; Pelosio *et al.* 1989; Gulden 1990; Held & Kohn 1990; Abraham *et al.* 1993; Duru *et al.* 1994). Little can be discerned from these reports that has not been more forcefully argued by the association of vitiligo with polyglandular dysfunction.

Vitiligo and haematological dysfunction

Similar analyses have been used to explain the occasional association of vitiligo and various forms of lymphomas and leukaemias (Alcalay *et al.* 1987; Walker *et al.* 1993). Many patients with lymphomas or leukaemias have a muted immune response. There are other reports of vitiligo developing in those infected with human immunodeficiency virus (HIV) (Alcalay *et al.* 1987; Walker *et al.* 1993). In each of these disorders, i.e. the malignancies and the viral infections, the immune system is dysregulated and might be predisposed to producing antibodies or cytotoxic lymphocytes against melanocytes. This theory remains highly speculative at this time. The observations seem neither to support nor refute the possible autoimmune origin of vitiligo.

Other associations

Vitiligo is a rather common disorder and might affect as many as 40 million people worldwide (reviewed in Nordlund *et al.* 1998). It is not surprising then that there is a long list of other disorders of many other organ systems that have been associated with vitiligo in an attempt to explain the cause for the destruction of melanocytes (Nordlund & Ortonne 1998). The list of disorders includes nail abnormalities (Barth *et al.* 1988), central nervous system abnormalities (Lison *et al.* 1981), dermatitis herpetiformis (Olholm-Larsen & Kavli 1980; Kavli *et al.* 1983), psoriasis (Moragas & Winkelmann 1970; Kubicz 1976; Koransky & Roenigk 1982; Mancuso & Gasponi 1983; Powell & Dicken 1983; Todes-Taylor *et al.* 1983; Iakovleva & Sen'kin 1984; Tham *et al.* 1987), lichen planus (Tan 1974; Brenner *et al.* 1979; Saha *et al.* 1979; Anstey & Marks 1993; Cecchi *et al.* 1994), collagen vascular disorders (Chowdhury & Berjee 1968; Durance & Hamilton 1971; Masutani *et al.* 1975; Abdusametova & Kolmakova 1977; Ramasastry *et al.* 1978; Collen *et al.* 1979; Goudie *et al.* 1979; Forestier *et al.* 1981; Khare *et al.* 1988; Gonggryp & Kalla 1992; Abraham *et al.* 1993) and alopecia areata (Thompson *et al.* 1974; Carter & Jegasothy 1976; Brenner *et al.* 1979; Korkij *et al.* 1984; De Padova *et al.* 1987; Valsecchi *et al.* 1989; Weitzner 1990; Shellow *et al.* 1992; Wang *et al.* 1994; Cho *et al.* 1995). Without very detailed surveys on each of these disorders and on vitiligo, it is difficult to use these data to form any conclusions about vitiligo or these diseases.

References

Aaltonen, J., Bjorses, P., Sandkuijl, L., Perheentupa, J. & Peltonen, L. (1994) An autosomal locus causing autoimmune disease: autoimmune polyglandular disease type 1 assigned to chromosome 21. *Nature Genetics* **8**, 83–87.

Abdusametova, Sh., R. & Kolmakova, A.N. (1977) Lupus erythematosus and porphyria in patients with vitiligo. *Vestnik Dermatologii I Venerologii* **7**, 58–59.

Abraham, Z., Rozenbaum, M., Gluck, Z., Feuerman, E.J., Lahat, N. & Kinarty, A. (1993) Vitiligo, rheumatoid arthritis and pernicious anemia. *Journal of Dermatology* **20**, 418–423.

Addison, T. (1855) *On the Constitutional and Local Effects of Disease of the Supra-Renal Capsules.* Samuel Highley, London.

Alcalay, J., David, M., Shohat, B. & Sandbank, M. (1987) Generalized vitiligo following Sezary syndrome. *British Journal of Dermatology* **116**, 851–855.

Alper, M.M. & Garner, P.R. (1985) Premature ovarian failure: its relationship to autoimmune disease. *Obstetrics and Gynecology* **66**, 27–30.

Anstey, A. & Marks, R. (1993) Colocalization of lichen planus and vitiligo (letter). *British Journal of Dermatology* **128**, 103–104.

Auer-Grumbach, P. & Stangl, M. (1993) Autoantibodies to nuclear mitotic apparatus in a patient with vitiligo and autoimmune thyroiditis. *Dermatology* **186**, 229–231.

Barth, J.H., Telfer, N.R. & Dawber, R.P. (1988) Nail abnormalities and autoimmunity. *Journal of the American Academy of Dermatology* **18**, 1062–1065.

Betterle, C., Caretto, A., De Zio, A., Pedini, B., Veller-Fornasa, C., Cecchetto, A., Accordi, F. & Peserico, A. (1985) Incidence and significance of organ-specific autoimmune disorders (clinical, latent or only autoantibodies) in patients with vitiligo. *Dermatologica* **171**, 419–423.

Betterle, C., Caretto, A., Pedini, B., Rigon, F., Bertoli, P. & Peserico, A. (1992) Complement-fixing activity to melanin-producing cells preceding the onset of vitiligo in a patient with type 1 polyglandular failure [letter]. *Archives of Dermatology* **128**, 123–124.

Bloch, M.H. & Sowers, J.R. (1985) Vitiligo and polyglandular autoimmune endocrinopathy. *Cutis* **36**, 417–419, 421.

Brenner, W., Diem, E. & Gschnait, F. (1979) Coincidence of vitiligo, alopecia areata, onychodystrophy, localized scleroderma and lichen planus. *Dermatologica* **159**, 356–360.

Carter, D.M. & Jegasothy, B.V. (1976) Alopecia areata and Down syndrome. *Archives of Dermatology* **112**, 1397–1399.

Cecchi, R., Giomi, A., Tuci, F., Bartoli, L. & Seghieri, G. (1994) Pityriasis rubra pilaris, lichen planus, alopecia universalis and vitiligo in a patient with chronic viral hepatitis C. *Dermatology* **188**, 239–240.

Cho, M., Cohen, P.R. & Duvic, M. (1995) Vitiligo and alopecia areata in patients with human immunodeficiency virus infection [Review]. *Southern Medical Journal* **88**, 489–491.

Chowdhury, D.S. & Berjee, A.K. (1968) Development of discoid lupus erythematosus in vitiligo. *Bulletin of the Calcutta School of Tropical Medicine* **16**, 111–112.

Collen, R.J., Lippe, B.M. & Kaplan, S.A. (1979) Primary ovarian failure, juvenile rheumatoid arthritis and vitiligo. *American Journal of Diseases of Children* **133**, 598–600.

Csaszar, T. & Patakfalvi, A. (1992) Treatment of polyglandular autoimmune syndrome with cyclosporin-A. *Acta Medica Hungarica* **49**, 187–193.

Cunliffe, W.J., Hall, R., Newell, D.J. & Stevenson, C.J. (1968) Vitiligo, thyroid disease and autoimmunity. *British Journal of Dermatology* **80**, 135–139.

Dawber, R.P. (1968) Vitiligo in mature-onset diabetes mellitus. *British Journal of Dermatology* **80**, 275–278.

Dawber, R.P., Bleehen, S.S. & Vallance-Owen, J. (1971) Vitiligo and diabetes mellitus. *British Journal of Dermatology* **84**, 600.

De Padova, M.P., Veronesi, S., Andriani, G.C. & Minghetti, G. (1987) Alopecia areata associated with onychodystrophy, vitiligo and lichen ruber planus. *Giornale Italiano Di Dermatologia E Venereologia* **122**, 191–192.

Durance, R.A. & Hamilton, E.B. (1971) Myasthenia gravis, rheumatoid arthritis, vitiligo, and autoimmune haemolytic anaemia. *Proceedings of the Royal Society of Medicine* **64**, 61–62.

Duru, F., Gurgey, A., Cetin, M., Kanra, T. & Altay, C. (1994) Chronic autoimmune hemolytic anemia in children: a report of four patients. *Journal of Medicine* **25**, 231–240.

Forestier, J.Y., Ortonne, J.P., Thivolet, J. & Souteyrand, P. (1981) Association of lupus erythematosus and vitiligo (author's translation). *Annales de Dermatologie et de Venereologie* **108**, 33–38.

Godeau, P., Herreman, G., Saltiel, H., Butler, J. & Alpern, J. (1973) Hyperthyroidism—thrombopenic purpura — vitiligo. *Annales de Medecine Interne* **124**, 327–331.

Gonggryp, L.A. & Kalla, A.A. (1992) Chloroquine-induced vitiligo in a patient with juvenile onset rheumatoid arthritis [letter]. *British Journal of Rheumatology* **31**, 790–791.

Goudie, R.B., Spence, J.C. & MacKie, R. (1979) Vitiligo patterns simulating autoimmune and rheumatic diseases. *Lancet* **2**, 393–395.

Gould, I.M., Gray, R.S., Urbaniak, S.J., Elton, R.A. & Duncan, L.J. (1985) Vitiligo in diabetes mellitus. *British Journal of Dermatology* **113**, 153–155.

Grimes, P.E., Halder, R.M., Jones, C., Chakrabarti, S.G., Enterline, J., Minus, H.R. & Kenney, J.A. Jr (1983) Autoantibodies and their clinical significance in a black vitiligo population. *Archives of Dermatology* **119**, 300–303.

Grunnet, I., Howitz, J., Reymann, F. & Schwartz, M. (1970) Vitiligo and pernicious anemia. *Archives of Dermatology* **101**, 82–85.

Gulden, K.D. (1990) Pernicious anemia, vitiligo, and infertility. *Journal of the American Board of Family Practice* **3**, 217–220.

Hegedus, L., Heidenheim, M., Gervil, M., Hjalgrim, H. & Hoier-Madsen, M. (1994) High frequency of thyroid dysfunction in patients with vitiligo. *Acta Dermato-Venereologica (Stockholm)* **74**, 120–123.

Held, J.L. & Kohn, S.R. (1990) Vitiligo and pernicious anemia presenting as congestive heart failure. *Cutis* **46**, 268–270.

Iakovleva, N.I. & Sen'kin, V.I. (1984) Case of alopecia associated with vitiligo and psoriasis. *Vestnik Dermatologii I Venerologii* **10**, 70–71.

Jacyk, W., Mazurek, W. & Baran, E. (1976) Acquired vitiligo, diseases of the thyroid gland and diabetes mellitus. *Przeglad Dermatologiczny* **63**, 59–64.

Kavli, G., Midelfart, K., Raa, J. & Volden, G. (1983) Phototoxicity from furocoumarins (psoralens) of Heracleum laciniatum in a patient with vitiligo. Action spectrum studies on bergapten, pimpinellin, angelicin and sphondin. *Contact Dermatitis* **9**, 364–366.

Khare, A.K., Singh, G. & Pandey, S.S. (1988) Vitiligo and disseminated discoid lupus erythematosus. *Indian Journal of Dermatology* **33**, 37–39.

Konno, N., Yuri, K., Taguchi, H., Miura, K., Taguchi, S., Hagiwara, K. & Murakami, S. (1993) Screening for thyroid disease in an iodine sufficient area with sensitive thyrotrophin assays, and serum thyroid autoantibody and urinary iodide determinations. *Clinical Endocrinology (Oxford)* **38**, 273–281.

Koransky, J.S. & Roenigk, H.H. Jr (1982) Vitiligo and psoriasis. *Journal of the American Academy of Dermatology* **7**, 183–189.

Korkij, W., Soltani, K., Simjee, S., Marcincin, P.G. & Chuang, T.Y. (1984) Tissue-specific autoantibodies and autoimmune disorders in vitiligo and alopecia areata: a retrospective study. *Journal of Cutaneous Pathology* **11**, 522–530.

Kubicz, J. (1976) Depigmentatio vitiligoidea in the course of psoriasis arthropatica. *Przeglad Dermatologiczny* **63**, 187–190.

Kumar, V., Shankar, V., Chaudhary, S., Bhatia, K.K., Mehta, L.K., Arora, N. & Arora, D.R. (1990) Radio-active iodine uptake in vitiligo. *Journal of Dermatology* **17**, 41–43.

Lamartine de Assis, J., Scaff, M., Nagahashi, S.K., Nobrega, J.P., Rodrigues-Alves, C.A., Monteiro, M.L., Sampaio, S.A. & Marchiori, P.E. (1983) Vitiligo, hyperthyroidism, periodic paralysis and myasthenia gravis. Report of a case. *Medicina Cutanea Ibero-Latino-Americana* **11**, 195–200.

Lison, M., Kornbrut, B., Feinstein, A., Hiss, Y., Boichis, H. & Goodman, R.M. (1981) Progressive spastic paraparesis, vitiligo, premature graying, and distinct facial appearance: a new genetic syndrome in 3 sibs. *American Journal of Medical Genetics* **9**, 351–357.

Macaron, C., Winter, R.J., Traisman, H.S., Kahan, B.D., Lasser, A.E. & Green, O.C. (1977) Vitiligo and juvenile diabetes mellitus. *Archives of Dermatology* **113**, 1515–1517.

Mancuso, G. & Gasponi, A. (1983) The vitiligo-psoriasis combination. Genetic and immunologic study. *Giornale Italiano Di Dermatologia E Venereologia* **118**, 369–372.

Mandel, M., Etzioni, A., Theodor, R. & Passwell, J.H. (1989) Pure red cell hypoplasia associated with polyglandular autoimmune syndrome type I. *Israel Journal of Medical Sciences* **25**, 138–141.

Masutani, M., Shoji, M., Taneda, A., Ogawa, H. & Miyazaki, H. (1975) A case of inflammatory vitiligo associated with lupus erythematosus (author's translation). *Nippon Hifuka Gakkai Zasshi—Japanese Journal of Dermatology* **85**, 525–531.

Matsumoto, T., Togawa, K., Yamamoto, M., Yamagami, Y. & Ogata, E. (1977) A case of idiopathic Addison's disease complicated with alopecia universalis, vitiligo vulgaris, superficial mycosis, pernicious anemia and bilateral medial longitudinal fasciculus syndrome (author's translation). *Nippon Naika Gakkai Zasshi—Journal of Japanese Society of Internal Medicine* **66**, 1588–1594.

Midelfart, K., Moseng, D., Kavli, G., Stenvold, S.E. & Volden, G. (1983) A case of chronic urticaria and vitiligo, associated with thyroiditis, treated with PUVA. *Dermatologica* **167**, 39–41.

Moragas, J.M. & Winkelmann, R.K. (1970) Psoriasis and vitiligo. *Archives of Dermatology* **101**, 235–237.

Mulligan, T.M. & Sowers, J.R. (1985) Hyperpigmentation, vitiligo, and Addison's disease. *Cutis* **36** (317–318), 322.
Mullin, G.E. & Eastern, J.S. (1986) Cutaneous signs of thyroid disease. *American Family Physician* **34**, 93–98.
Nishida, W., Mukai, M., Sumimoto, T., Hamada, M. & Hiwada, K. (1990) Vitiligo with primary hypothyroidism and hypoacusis: a case report. *Japanese Journal of Medicine* **29**, 66–70.
Nordlund, J.J. & Majumder, P. (1997) Recent investigations on vitiligo vulgaris. *Dermatologic Clinics* **15**, 69–78.
Nordlund, J.J., Boissy, R.E., Hearing, V.J., King, R.A. & Ortonne, J.-P., eds. (1998) *The Pigmentary System: Physiology and Pathophysiology*. Oxford University Press, New York.
Olholm-Larsen, P. & Kavli, G. (1980) Dermatitis herpetiformis and vitiligo. *Dermatologica* **160**, 41–44.
Ortonne, J.P., Perrot, H. & Thivolet, J. (1976) Clinical and statistical study of 100 patients with vitiligo. *Semaine Des Hopitaux* **52**, 679–686.
Pal, S.K., Ghosh, K.K. & Banerjee, P.K. (1980) Thyroid function in vitiligo. *Clinica Chimica Acta* **106**, 331–332.
Pelosio, A., Girelli, G., Arista, M.C., Galassi, A., Longhi, C. & Massini, R. (1989) Pernicious anemia, vitiligo and positive antiglobulin test: an unusual association. *Haematologica* **74**, 499–501.
Peserico, A., Rigon, F., Semenzato, G., Caretto, A., Pasini, C.V. & Betterle, C. (1981) Vitiligo and polyglandular autoimmune disease with autoantibodies to melanin-producing cells. A new syndrome? *Archives of Dermatology* **117**, 751–752.
Powell, F.C. & Dicken, C.H. (1983) Psoriasis and vitiligo. *Acta Dermato-Venereologica (Stockholm)* **63**, 246–249.
Prentice, L.M., Phillips, D.I., Sarsero, D., Beever, K., McLachlan, S.M. & Smith, B.R. (1990) Geographical distribution of subclinical autoimmune thyroid disease in Britain: a study using highly sensitive direct assays for autoantibodies to thyroglobulin and thyroid peroxidase. *Acta Endocrinologica (Copenhagen)* **123**, 493–498.
Ramanathan, M., Abidin, M.N. & Muthukumarappan, M. (1989) The prevalence of skin manifestations in thyrotoxicosis—a retrospective study. *Medical Journal of Malaysia* **44**, 324–328.
Ramasastry, C.V., Dutta, A.K. & Banerjee, B.N. (1978) Serum electrophoretic patterns in vitiligo, psoriasis and discoid lupus erythematosus. *Indian Journal of Dermatology* **24**, 7–12.
Ruzicka, T. (1981) Atypical Kaposi's sarcoma in a patient with vitiligo and pernicious anemia. *Dermatologica* **163**, 199–204.
Saban, J., Rodriguez-Garcia, J.L., Gil, J., Pais, J.R. & Medina, S. (1991) Porphyria cutanea tarda associated with autoimmune hypothyroidism, vitiligo and alopecia universalis. *Netherlands Journal of Medicine* **39**, 350–352.
Saha, K.C., Arya, M. & Saha, A.K. (1979) Neurohistological studies in lichen planus and vitiligo. *Indian Journal of Dermatology* **24**, 51–55.
Sharma, J.B., Tiwari, S., Gulati, N. & Sharma, S. (1990) Schmidt's syndrome: a rare cause of puberty menorrhagia. *International Journal of Gynaecology and Obstetrics* **33**, 373–375.
Shellow, W.V., Edwards, J.E. & Koo, J.Y. (1992) Profile of alopecia areata: a questionnaire analysis of patient and family. *International Journal of Dermatology* **31**, 186–189.
Shong, Y.K. & Kim, J.A. (1991) Vitiligo in autoimmune thyroid disease. *Thyroidology* **3**, 89–91.
Sidi, Y., David, M., Shohat, B., Feuerman, E.J. & Pinkhas, J. (1978) Vitiligo, autoimmune hemolytic anemia and T lymphocyte dysfunction: a mere coincidence or a new entity? *Dermatologica* **157**, 136–137.
Tadzhibaev, T.T. (1971) Some indices of the functional state of the adrenal cortex and copper metabolism in patients with vitiligo. *Vestnik Dermatologii I Venerologii* **45**, 26–29.
Tan, R.S. (1974) Ulcerative colitis, myasthenia gravis, atypical lichen planus, alopecia areata, vitiligo. *Proceedings of the Royal Society of Medicine* **67**, 195–196.

Tham, S.N., Gange, R.W. & Parrish, J.A. (1987) Ultraviolet-B treatment of psoriasis in patients with concomitant vitiligo [letter]. *Archives of Dermatology* **123**, 26–27.

Thompson, D.M., Robinson, T.W. & Lennard-Jones, J. (1974) Alopecia areata, vitiligo, scleroderma and ulcerative colitis. *Proceedings of the Royal Society of Medicine* **67**, 1010–1012.

Todes-Taylor, N., Abel, E.A. & Cox, A.J. (1983) The occurrence of vitiligo after psoralens and ultraviolet A therapy. *Journal of the American Academy of Dermatology* **9**, 526–532.

Torrelo, A., Espana, A., Balsa, J. & Ledo, A. (1992) Vitiligo and polyglandular autoimmune syndrome with selective IgA deficiency. *International Journal of Dermatology* **31**, 343–344.

Valsecchi, R., Pansera, B., Rossi, A. & Cainelli, T. (1989) Pigmentation abnormalities in the course of topical immunotherapy of alopecia areata. *Giornale Italiano Di Dermatologia E Venereologia* **124**, 31–32.

Villaverde, M.M. (1969) Diabetes with vitiligo. *Journal of the Medical Society of New Jersey* **66**, 218–220.

Walker, J., Ober, R.R., Khan, A., Yuen, D. & Rao, N.A. (1993) Intraocular lymphoma developing in a patient with Vogt-Koyanagi–Harada syndrome. *International Ophthalmology* **17**, 331–336.

Walters, T.R., Lerner, A.B. & Nordlund, J.J. (1978) Vitiligo, chronic thrombocytopenia, and autoimmune hemolytic anemia. *Archives of Dermatology* **114**, 1366–1367.

Wang, C. & Crapo, L.M. (1997) The epidemiology of thyroid disease and implications for screening. *Endocrinology and Metabolism Clinics of North America* **26**, 189–218.

Wang, S.J., Shohat, T., Vadheim, C., Shellow, W., Edwards, J. & Rotter, J.I. (1994) Increased risk for type I (insulin-dependent) diabetes in relatives of patients with alopecia areata (AA). *American Journal of Medical Genetics* **51**, 234–239.

Weitzner, J.M. (1990) Alopecia areata. *American Family Physician* **41**, 1197–1201.

Zelissen, P.M., Bast, E.J. & Croughs, R.J. (1995) Associated autoimmunity in Addison's disease. *Journal of Autoimmunity* **8**, 121–130.

13: The Psychological Effects of Vitiligo: Response to Impaired Appearance

JUDITH PORTER

Although many psychosocial studies of the physically handicapped have been conducted in recent years, less attention has been given to the victims of skin disorders. Skin disfigurement, however, may be a barrier to privileges and opportunities because of the profound social significance of appearance and the attitudes and prejudices of society toward one whose appearance is atypical. The cosmetic disfigurement which accompanies skin disease may have profound effects on a patient's self-esteem and social relationships, and vitiligo is no exception.

The social effects of skin diseases may cause more hardship than the physical limitations. Physical disfigurements affect the nature of the impressions we form of individuals, the causes we assign to their behaviour, and whether we choose to affiliate with them (Jones *et al.* 1984). American society places great emphasis on appearance, and people react negatively to those whose appearance is not consonant with cultural standards of beauty. Physically attractive people are believed to have more socially desirable traits than others. Individuals are more likely to attribute traits of kindness and intelligence to good-looking people, and better-looking people are thought to have more self-control, competence, and be better adjusted (Jones *et al.* 1984). Although sometimes traits attributed to those who are physically disfigured may be positive (Comer & Piliavin 1972), for the most part physically disfigured individuals are likely to provoke negative emotions (Goffman 1963).

Physically attractive people are not only evaluated more positively but research has also shown that they are treated better by peers, teachers, friends, strangers, and employers. Visibly disfigured people face special obstacles in efforts to maintain satisfying social relationships. Interactions between the physically disfigured and colleagues are often strained and tension-producing, and marked by stilted and artificial communication, both verbal and nonverbal (Goffman 1963; Jones *et al.* 1984). The physically disfigured are often the victims of discrimination (Kleck & Strenta 1980). In response to these pressures, impaired individuals may exhibit discomfort and strain in social relationships and may anticipate discriminatory interaction with the nonhandicapped (Comer & Piliavin 1972). Because of the social significance of the skin and face, the stigmatization of the cosmetically impaired may equal or exceed that of those with other body afflictions (Nadelson 1978; Cassileth *et al.* 1982).

Beauty presupposes a blemish-free skin. Literature dealing directly with skin disease agrees that the victims of such disorders do indeed experience the same problems in social interaction that are faced by individuals with other types of visible disfigurements (Shuster *et al.* 1978; Porter 1989). There is general consensus that family members are the most supportive and grow accustomed to the appearance of those with skin disorders. The literature is consistent in reporting that comments from strangers are the most unpleasant and difficult to handle. In one study, over half of individuals with vitiligo said that people stare at them, 20% said that they have been the recipients of rude remarks by strangers, and one-third said that interaction with strangers is especially stressful (Porter *et al.* 1979, 1987).

Although skin disease may produce low self-esteem and feelings of inferiority, these psychological reactions are not inevitable. In order to understand why impaired appearance is more stressful to some individuals than to others, we need to direct attention to resources which help people cope with disfigurement. Psychological resources are the personality characteristics people draw upon to help them withstand threats to their self-esteem due to impaired appearance. Those with a positive self-image are better able to cope with the onset of a disfiguring skin condition. Another set of major resources in helping people adjust to disfigurement are social resources, such as the interpersonal networks of which people are a part and which are potential sources of support (Pearlin & Schooler 1978).

Vitiligo patients are no exception to these psychological effects. A questionnaire and interview study by Porter *et al.* (1987) of 326 vitiligo patients treated in two major hospitals illustrates these points about the importance of appearance in psychological adjustment, the impact of the physical disfigurement caused by the depigmentation of vitiligo, and the variation in response to a physically disfiguring condition. Most of these respondents had either moderate or widespread cases of vitiligo which were easily visible. Over two-thirds of these patients described themselves as worried about vitiligo, primarily about its spread, whether their children would inherit the disease, whether new cures would be found, and other general carcinophobic fears. Many patients felt stigmatized by their condition. Over half said that people stared at them, and from 20–25% said that they had been the victim of rude remarks by strangers and that vitiligo interfered with their relationships with the opposite sex. Almost half admitted that they often felt less at ease socially due to vitiligo, with interaction with strangers reported as especially stressful. In order to hide the depigmented areas, approximately half reported using makeup and special clothing to cover the affected body parts (Porter *et al.* 1987). Embarrassment during sexual relationships was especially frequent for men with vitiligo (Porter *et al.* 1990). It is thus not surprising that 7% felt severely depressed by the disease ('I feel like a freak'). Thirty-two per cent reported that they respond to the disease with acute and consistent embarrassment, feeling ill at ease and unsure how to react although not expressing the strong self-hatred of the depressive category. Twenty-seven per cent reported mild embarrassment, and only 34% claimed that vitiligo does not cause them social problems or embarrassment (Porter *et al.* 1986, 1987).

People with more effective coping resources are better able to resist self-stigmatization, regardless of the 'disfigured appearance' label that has been applied to them. Psychological resources are important in adjustment to vitiligo (Wheaton 1983). Self-esteem, or favourable attitude toward the self, is associated with positive reaction to stress, and those with a positive self-image are better able to cope with the effect of physical disabilities. In various studies by Porter and colleagues vitiligo patients with low self-esteem manifested considerably more psychological disturbance due to the disease than did those whose self-esteem was high. Although younger people and working-class individuals tended to show more psychological disturbance due to vitiligo, gender and race did not predict differences in psychological response to this condition (Porter & Beuf 1988, 1991). Social support seemed to help people cope with the disorder, and African-Americans living in predominantly black communities and women received more support from close family and friends (Porter & Beuf 1994). Visibility of vitiligo and discrimination from others also were related to degree of disturbance caused by vitiligo, but severity of the condition was not the most important factor predicting poor adjustment. Someone with low self-esteem may react with depression to even a mild case of vitiligo, while someone with good self-esteem may be relatively unperturbed by more severe manifestations of vitiligo (Porter *et al.* 1984).

Thus, many people with vitiligo are frightened or embarrassed and see themselves discriminated against in many aspects of their lives, although social and psychological resources help to mitigate negative reactions to the disease. The tendency of many doctors to trivialize vitiligo and its consequences was one of the most difficult problems encountered by patients (Porter *et al.* 1978). Being told that vitiligo is 'only a cosmetic disorder' is small comfort to the majority of patients who experience some degree of psychological stress due to the disease. Vitiligo must not be ignored by the physician. The psychosocial effect of skin disease should not be trivialized. Skin conditions are not 'only cosmetic disorders', but may have profound psychological effects on the lives of those whom they afflict because of the importance of appearance in how we evaluate and interact with others.

References

Comer, R. & Piliavin, J. (1972) The effects of physical deviance on face to face interaction: The other side. *Journal of Personality and Social Psychology* **23**, 33–39.

Cassileth, B., Lusk, B. & Tenaglia, A. (1982) A psychological comparison of patients with malignant melanoma and other dermatological disorders. *Journal of the American Academy of Dermatology* **7**, 742–746.

Goffman, E. (1963) *Stigma*. Prentice Hall, Englewood Cliffs, N.J.

Jones, E., Farina, A., Hastorf, A., Markus, H., Miller, D. & Scott, R. (1984) *Social Stigma: the Psychology of Marked Relationships*. W.H. Freeman, New York.

Kleck, R. & Strenta, A. (1980) Perceptions of the impact of negatively valued physical characteristics on social interaction. *Journal of Personality and Social Psychology* **39**, 861–873.

Nadelson, T. (1978) A person's boundaries: a meaning of skin disease. *Cutis* **21**, 90–94.

Pearlin, L. & Schooler, C. (1978) The structure of coping. *Journal of Health and Social Behavior* **19**, 2–21.

Porter, J. (1989) Psychosocial effects of skin disease. In: *Medical and Health Annual: 1989*, pp. 388–390. Encyclopedia Britannica Inc., Chicago, Illinois.

Porter, J. & Beuf, A. (1988) Response of the elderly to impaired appearance: The effect of age on disturbance by vitiligo. *Journal of Aging Studies* **2**, 167–181.

Porter, J. & Beuf, A. (1991) Racial variation in response to physical stigma: a study of degree of disturbance by vitiligo among black and white patients. *Journal of Health and Social Behavior* **32**, 192–204.

Porter, J. & Beuf, A. (1994) The effect of a racially consonant medical context on the adjustment of African American patients to physical disability. *Medical Anthropology* **16**, 1–16.

Porter, J., Beuf, A., Lerner, A. & Nordlund, J. (1978) Personal responses of patients to vitiligo: The importance of physician–patient interaction. *Archives of Dermatology* **114**, 1384–1385.

Porter, J., Beuf, A., Lerner, A. & Nordlund, J. (1979) Psychological reaction to chronic skin disorders: a study of patients with vitiligo. *General Hospital Psychiatry* **1**, 73–77.

Porter, J., Beuf, A., Lerner, A. & Nordlund, J. (1984) Children coping with impaired appearance: Social and psychological influences. *General Hospital Psychiatry* **6**, 294–301.

Porter, J., Beuf, A., Lerner, A. & Nordlund, J. (1986) The psychosocial effect of vitiligo: A comparison of vitiligo patients with 'normal' controls, with psoriasis patients, and with patients with other pigmentary disorders. *Journal of the American Academy of Dermatology* **15** (Part I), 220–225.

Porter, J., Beuf, A., Lerner, A. & Nordlund, J. (1987) Response to cosmetic disfigurement: a study of patients with vitiligo. *Cutis* **39**, 493–494.

Porter, J., Beuf, A., Lerner, A. & Nordlund, J. (1990) The effect of vitiligo on sexual relationships. *Journal of the American Academy of Dermatology* **22**, 221–222.

Shuster, S., Fisher, G., Harris, E. & Binnell, D. (1978) The effects of skin diseases on self image. *British Journal of Dermatology* **99**, 18–19.

Wheaton, B. (1983) Stress, personal coping resources, and psychiatric symptoms: an investigation of interactive models. *Journal of Health and Social Behavior* **24**, 208–229.

14: Differential Diagnosis of Vitiligo Vulgaris

PRANAV B. SHETH

Vitiligo vulgaris is a depigmenting disorder that has as its hallmark a loss of melanocytes. In the clinical setting, with a good history and a thorough full skin examination that often includes the use of a Wood's lamp, the diagnosis of vitiligo vulgaris is usually straightforward. The classical presentation of acquired, well-demarcated, depigmented milk-white patches in which the epidermis is absolutely normal has a very limited differential diagnosis. That is especially true when the macules are distributed in an acral, facial, or generalized symmetrical distribution, or in a segmental or quasi-dermatomal distribution. However, there are presentations of vitiligo that may have a focal or asymmetrical distribution, an atypical age of onset, or a variable amount of hypopigmentation and depigmentation (trichrome or multichrome vitiligo). It is in these cases that additional studies, including histochemical studies and electron microscopy, may be required. The presence of depigmented white hairs in the involved areas or in the scalp may be a helpful clue for the diagnosis of vitiligo. Even then, clues or classical findings may only come with time and observing the course of the disease. For some patients with hypochromic lesions, no definitive diagnosis can be made.

The list of differential diagnoses can be artificially separated into one list for generalized or bilateral, symmetrical leukoderma and another for that of segmental or unilateral, asymmetrical leukoderma. Clearly there can be an overlap between the two.

Those pigmentary disorders that may need to be distinguished from generalized or bilateral vitiligo include: genetic disorders such as piebaldism, hypomelanosis of Ito and tuberous sclerosis; inflammatory disorders such as lupus erythematosus, sarcoidosis, lichen sclerosis et atrophicus; halo naevi and malignancies like mycosis fungoides; infectious disorders such as tinea versicolor, treponemal infections and leprosy; idiopathic disorders such as idiopathic guttate hypomelanosis; and postinflammatory hypopigmentation. Those pigmentary disorders that may need to be distinguished from segmental vitiligo include: naevus anaemicus, steroid-injection-related hypomelanosis, and naevus depigmentosus.

Genetic or congenital disorders

Congenital hypopigmenting disorders, by definition, are present at birth or shortly after birth and typically the lesions are stable. Congenital vitiligo is extremely rare. The lesions of vitiligo first appear usually after 6 months of age or, more commonly, during childhood and tend to progress to involve a segment or large areas of the integument.

Piebaldism

Piebaldism is an uncommon, autosomal dominant, genetic disorder characterized by leukoderma that affects the hair and skin in a distinctive pattern. Often the family is very aware of the abnormality and will point it out to the paediatrician. There are present at birth, or visible soon after, discrete depigmented patches on the ventral surface of the body, most commonly on the mid-frontal scalp, mid-forehead, neck, anterior mid-trunk, flanks, and mid-portion of the extremities. Characteristic in many patients is a white forelock of hair over the mid-frontal scalp with an underlying depigmented patch of epidermis (Fig. 14.1). Unlike vitiligo, the central back, hips, hands and feet are often spared. As in vitiligo, the patches of piebaldism are well-demarcated and milk-white on Wood's lamp examination. However, the patches of piebaldism often have normal or hyperpigmented macules within them or at their periphery (Fig. 14.2) (Pinto & Bolognia 1991), a feature not found in vitiligo. The histological and electron microscopic findings in skin from piebaldism which reveal an absence of melanocytes in the depigmented patches (Breathnach *et al.* 1965; Jimbow *et al.* 1975) are indistinguishable from those of vitiligo by routine and electron microscopy. However, the combination of family history, age of onset, stability of lesions, presence of normal and hyperpigmented macules within the depig-

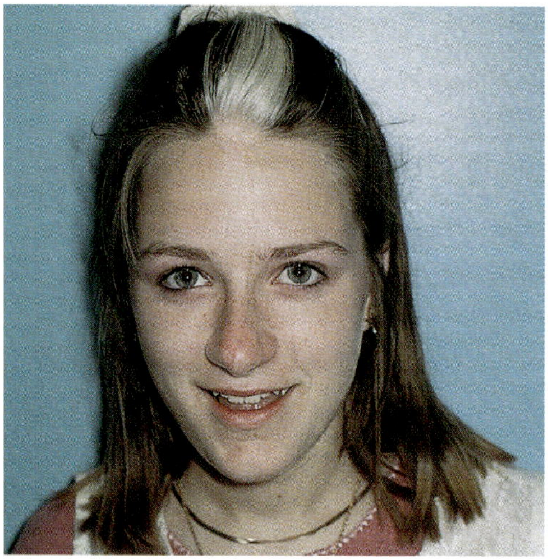

Fig. 14.1 Piebaldism: forelock.

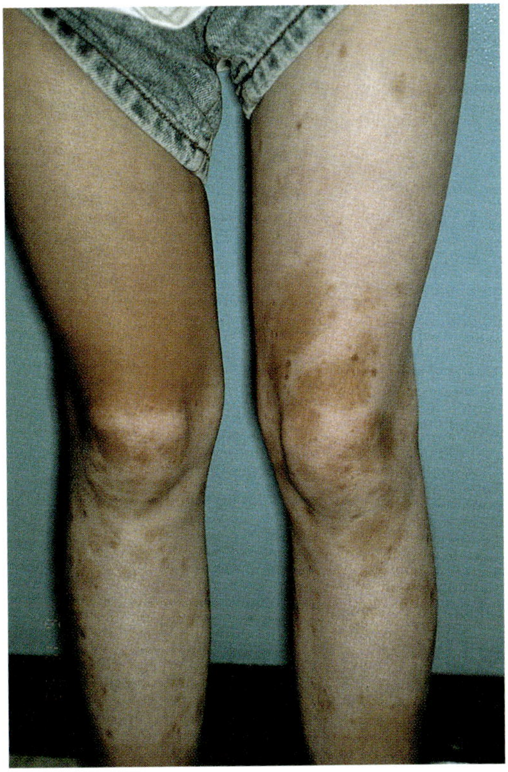

Fig. 14.2 Central lower extremity involvement in piebaldism. Note scattered hyperpigmented macules.

mented lesions and pattern of involvement make it easy to distinguish piebaldism from vitiligo.

Ash leaf macules

The ash leaf macule of tuberous sclerosis complex (TSC) is a hypomelanotic macule that is off-white in colour on Wood's lamp examination. Often well-demarcated, it characteristically is lance ovate or leaf shaped in configuration. The polygonal shape occurs more commonly and confetti shapes can also be seen. Ash leaf macules can be present at birth or often appear within the first year of life. Once present, the hypomelanotic lesions are stable. Distribution is often asymmetrical and random. Other cutaneous stigmata of TSC, including facial angiofibromas, periungual fibromas, and chagrin patch. Forehead plaque or CNS, cardiac or renal involvement, may not be present at time of presentation but may develop over time (Sheth 1998). Unlike mature vitiligo lesions, histology and electron microscopy reveal a normal number of melanocytes with a decrease in the synthesis, melanization and size of melanosomes (Jimbow *et al.* 1975). Early focal hypopigmented vitiligo may be morphologically indistinguishable from the hypomelanotic macule of TSC. However, the constellation of cutaneous and extracutaneous findings of TSC, the random nature of ash leaf macules and the stability of the lesions assist in making the diagnosis.

Hypomelanosis of Ito

Lesions of hypomelanosis of Ito (HI) may be hypopigmented or, rarely, depigmented. The cutaneous lesions of HI are often characteristic in their pattern of distribution in the lines of Blaschko and their different shapes and colours, characteristics now known to be a manifestation of mosaicism. Onset of lesions is most common at birth, but may occur up to the age of three. Characteristically, whorled or linear as well as patchy hypopigmented and depigmented lesions may occur unilaterally or bilaterally. These occur most commonly on two body segments including the trunk and limbs (Fig. 14.3). There may be associated central nervous system, eye, musculoskeletal and/or cardiac defects. Histological and electron microscopic findings are variable, revealing decreased number of melanocytes and melanosomes and increased number of Langerhans cells (Ruiz-Maldonado *et al.* 1992). The characteristic linear and whorled pattern of the lesions and the distribution of the pigmentary lesions in HI allow for easy distinction of this disorder from vitiligo.

Inflammatory/neoplastic disorders

Certain inflammatory disorders more characteristically are associated with hypopigmentation or depigmentation. Whether this is due to a direct role of the melanocyte in the inflammatory process, indirect role of the melanocyte, or the melanocyte as an innocent bystander is not known for many of the disorders (Nordlund & Abdel-Malek 1988). An assumption of direct damage to the melanocyte in disorders such as lupus erythematosus and lichen sclerosus et atrophicus can be made. This is based on the histological finding that there is liquefaction degeneration of the basal cell layer, the site where melanocytes reside. Scarring or sclerotic hypopigmented lesions of these disorders often remain without pigment, probably due to the loss of hair follicle melanocyte reservoir.

Lupus erythematosus

Characteristic lesions of discoid lupus erythematosus are well-demarcated, erythematous, infiltrated plaques with associated epidermal atrophy, telangiectasia, and scaling. The natural progression of the discoid lesion results in hypo/hyperpigmentation and depigmentation and scarring (Laman & Provost 1994). It is these late lesions of cutaneous lupus that may raise the question of vitiligo. The lesions of lupus are frequently distributed on the scalp, ears, and sun-exposed areas of the arms, fingers, chest and upper back. A depigmented lesion of discoid lupus should be easily differentiated from vitiligo by the presence of cutaneous atrophy and scarring (Fig. 14.4) (Hood 1987). The epidermis in a patch of vitiligo is completely normal. If it is not possible to make a clinical diagnosis of lupus, then histological findings of inflammation around the follicles, along the basement

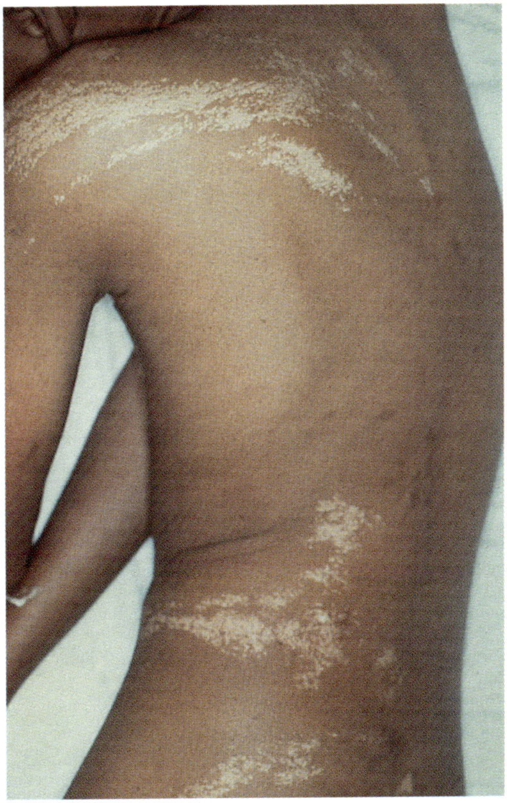

Fig. 14.3 Hypomelanosis of Ito. Unilateral whorled linear depigmented patches.

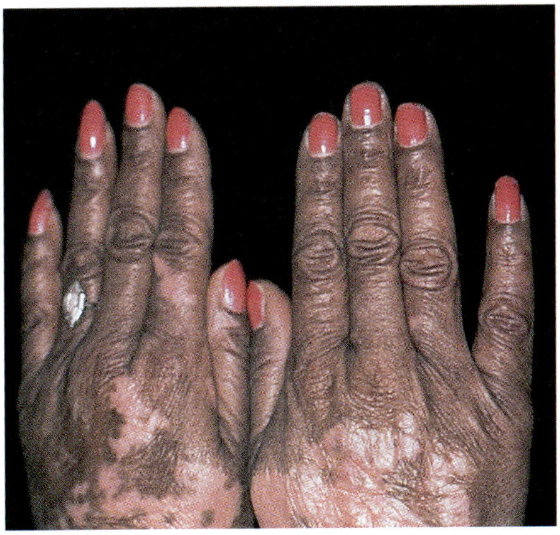

Fig. 14.4 Cutaneous lupus—depigmented atrophic patches.

membrane, epidermal atrophy, pigment incontinence, loss of appendages and fibrosis will assist in the differentiation.

Characteristic lesions of subacute cutaneous lupus and 'acute' lupus may also become hypopigmented or depigmented. The distribution is also in sun-exposed areas and there is often a history of previously inflamed skin

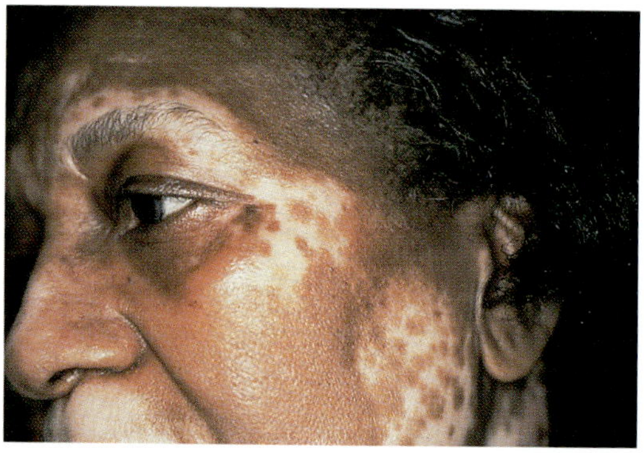

Fig. 14.5 Lupus erythematosus: depigmented lesions on the face.

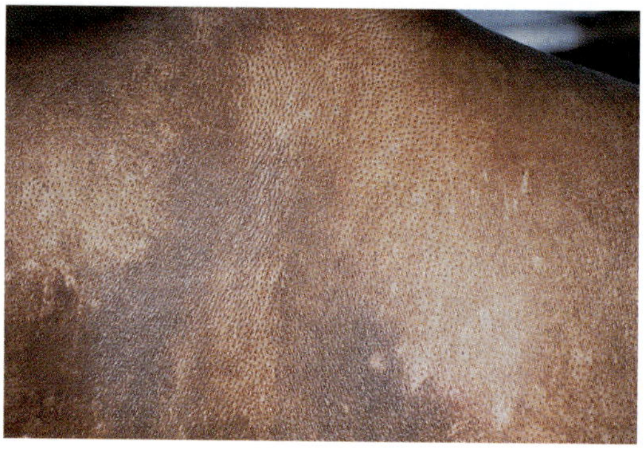

Fig. 14.6 Scleroderma. Hypopigmented and depigmented patches with 'salt and pepper' appearance due to follicular pigmentation.

(Fig. 14.5). Repigmentation is possible. Unlike vitiligo, the lesions are less symmetrical, may show evidence of atrophy and scarring and often have telangiectasias. Irregular fingertip hypopigmentation may occur, however, proximal nail fold capillary loops are often prominent.

Scleroderma

Pigmentary changes in scleroderma may occur in one of three patterns: generalized hyperpigmentation or darkening of exposed regions, focal hyperpigmentation and hypopigmentation in areas of sclerosis, and patches of vitiligo-like depigmentation with follicular repigmentation often in areas of normal skin (Braverman 1998). In this third pattern, patches of perifollicular pigmentation appear on a background of complete pigment loss, which gives a 'salt and pepper' appearance to the skin (Fig. 14.6). These changes are most commonly found on the upper chest and back, although other areas may be involved. These lesions are histologically indistinguishable from vitiligo. Patients will have other changes of scleroderma on examination.

Lichen sclerosis et atrophicus

Genital and extragenital lesions of lichen sclerosis et atrophicus (LSA) may

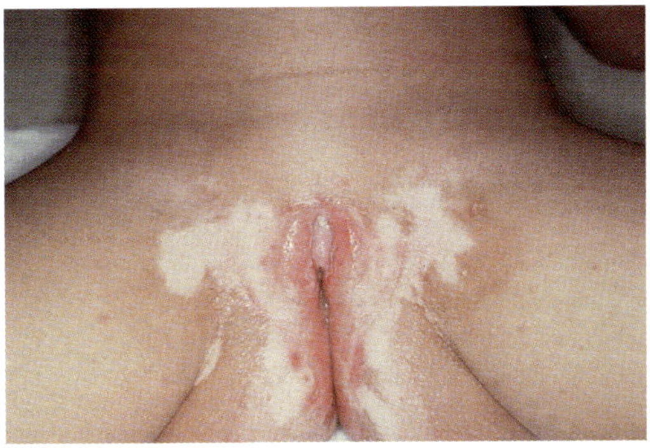

Fig. 14.7 Lichen sclerosis et atrophicus. Atrophic eroded vulvar lesions with depigmentation and peripheral hyperpigmentation.

mimic lesions of vitiligo depending on the age and activity of the lesions. LSA presents in all age groups, greatest in prepubertal children, postmenopausal women and middle-aged men (balanitis xerotica obliterans). Genital lesions in females often involve the inner parts of the vulva (clitoris, vestibule area and the inner part of the labia majora) sometimes extending to the perineum and perianal area (Fig. 14.7). Symptoms of vaginal pruritus, burning and dysaesthesia are common (Leibowitch 1996). In men, the glans penis and/or prepuce are most commonly affected. Phimosis, meatal stenosis and urethral symptoms may occur in men. Genital lesions are often symmetrical, ill-defined, hypo- or depigmented atrophic patches with variable degrees of telangiectasia and occasionally purpura. Early genital LSA in young girls can be most difficult to distinguish from vitiligo.

Extragenital LSA is most common on the neck, shoulders, trunk and extremities. Extragenital lesions begin as white, polygonal papules that coalesce into plaques often with comedo like plugs early on. Later lesions often have an atrophic, porcelain-white appearance.

If needed, histology is distinctive and very useful in distinguishing vitiligo from LSA. It reveals epidermal atrophy, orthohyperkeratosis, vacuolar degeneration of the basal layer, follicular occlusion and a homogenized, oedematous, papillary dermis early on. Histological findings of later lesions reveal a hyalinized and sclerotic dermis. Electron microscopic findings in one report revealed loss of melanocytes in active lesions and decreased number of melanocytes showing degenerative changes in resolving lesions (Meffert *et al.* 1995).

Pityriasis alba

Pityriasis alba is a common, asymptomatic disorder usually seen in children and young adults, often with a personal or family history of atopic diathesis. Characteristically, lesions are ill-defined, hypopigmented macules with slight scaliness and a variable amount of mild erythema at the border. Lesions may be 0.5–5 cm in size. Distribution is commonly on the face, neck, shoulders and extensor surface of the arms (Fig. 14.8). Histology of active

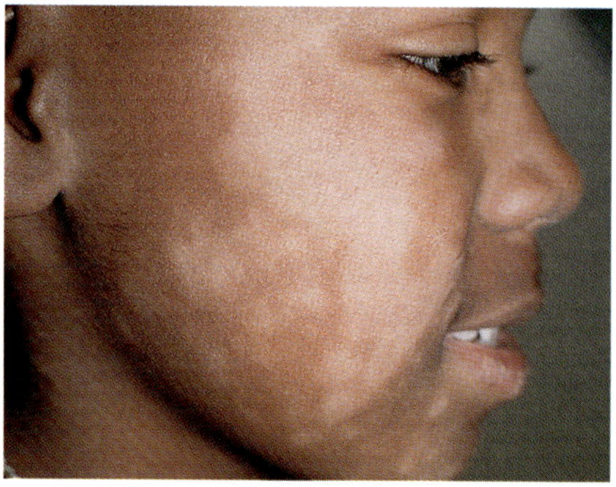

Fig. 14.8 Pityriasis alba. Moderate involvement on the face of an African-American male.

lesions reveals epidermal spongiosis, follicular spongiosis, focal parakeratosis, acanthosis, and a superficial perivascular lymphocytic infiltrate (Martin *et al.* 1990). A histochemical and ultrastructural study on extensive pityriasis alba revealed reduced numbers of active melanocytes and a decrease in number and size of melanosomes in the affected skin (Zaynoun *et al.* 1983). Differentiation from vitiligo in general is not difficult. The ill-defined borders that appear 'air-brushed', the hypopigmentation with mild, fine scaling and the location on the face or extremity of a child are characteristic of pityriasis alba.

Sarcoidosis

Hypomelanotic macules scattered on the trunk and extremities, greatest on the legs, have been described in patients with sarcoidosis (Fig. 14.9). Hypopigmented macules have been more commonly reported in darker skinned patients with sarcoidosis than in those with skin type I or II. The appearance of lesions can vary from ill-defined hypopigmented macules to dermal nodules with surrounding hypopigmentation (Fig. 14.10). Histology of the nonpalpable hypopigmented macules frequently, although not consistently, revealed sarcoidal granulomas (Cornelius *et al.* 1973; Hall *et al.* 1984; Mitchell *et al.* 1986). Ultrastructural evaluation of hypopigmented lesions in one study revealed degenerative changes in the melanocyte resulting in depressed melanogenesis and pigmentary incontinence (Clayton *et al.* 1977). Differentiation from vitiligo is based on the ill-defined, hypopigmented nature of the lesions, other cutaneous or systemic presence of sarcoidosis and histological findings.

Halo naevi

Halo naevi characteristically occur on the trunk, less frequently on the extremities, in the same distribution as melanocytic naevi. Often beginning

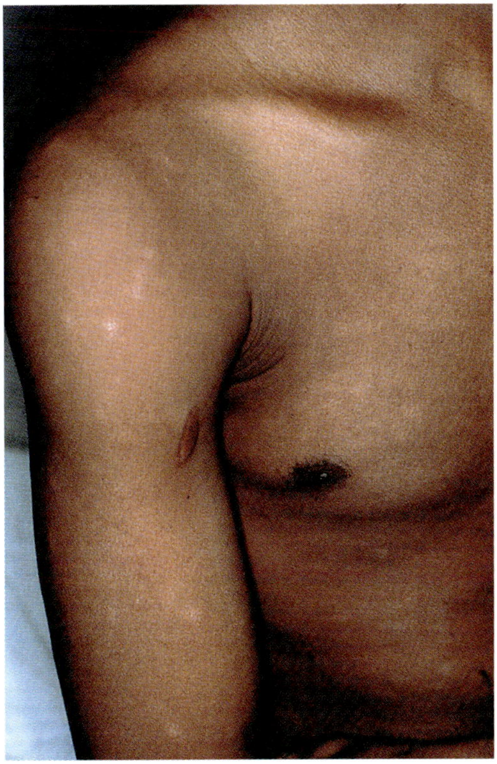

Fig. 14.9 Hypopigmented sarcoidosis. Thirty-three-year-old black female with one month history of hypopigmented macules on trunk and extremities. Has pulmonary sarcoidosis.

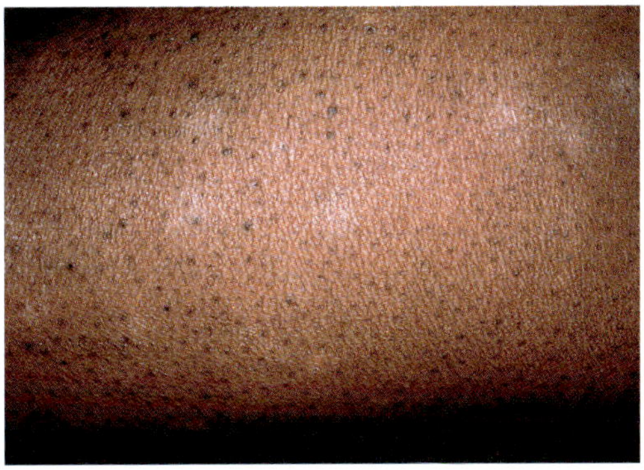

Fig. 14.10 Hypopigmented sarcoidosis, ill-defined macules (same patient as Fig. 14.20).

as a well-defined depigmented macule around a junctional or compound melanocytic naevus, the end stage of a halo naevus is often a depigmented, discrete 0.5–5 cm stable patch (Fig. 14.11). There can be more than one naevus undergoing the halo phenomenon. Histological findings vary with the stage of the lesion, ranging from a junctional or melanocytic naevus with a variable mononuclear infiltrate to a densely lichenoid mononuclear infiltrate and eventual loss of recognizable naevus cells (Frank & Cohen 1964). Differentiation of a late halo naevus that has lost its central pigmented papule from vitiligo can be difficult at times. Often, a history of a previous mole in the area or other hypo- and depigmented

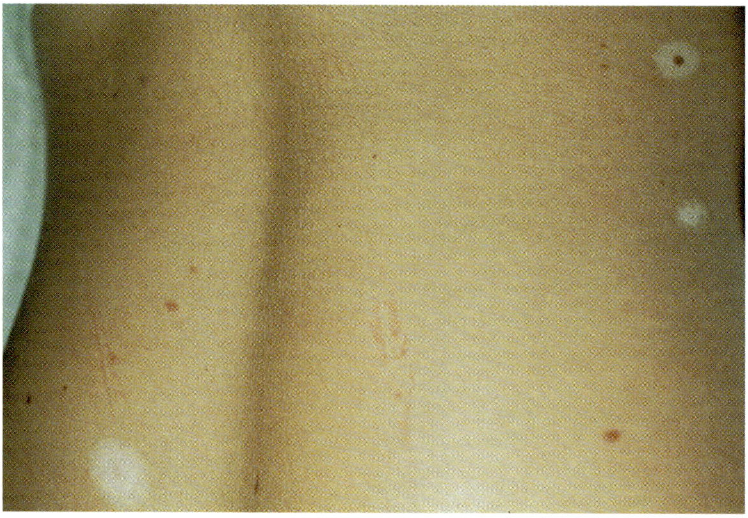

Fig. 14.11 Halo naevi (multiple).

macules with a central naevus on skin examination are helpful in the diagnosis. Histological examination revealing melanocytic naevus cells or dense lymphocytic mononuclear infiltrate differentiates this from vitiligo. Of note, classical vitiligo vulgaris has been reported to occur in conjunction with halo naevi in some patients. Some investigators consider halo naevi a form of vitiligo vulgaris, but most consider them separate pathological entities. The editors of this book favour the latter interpretation.

Mycosis fungoides

Mycosis fungoides is a lymphoma of the skin that may also present with hypomelanotic macules. Often in dark-skinned patients, hypomelanotic macules and diffuse depigmentation have been described. The typical age range of affected patients is 30–40 years, the lesions may have some scale or erythema, are usually located on the trunk and extremities, and are variable in size from less than 1 cm to many centimeters (Figs 14.12 & 14.13). Histology is needed for diagnosis, and this reveals moderate to profound epidermotropism by infiltrating mononuclear cells (Goldberg *et al.* 1986; Lambroza *et al.* 1995). The mechanism of pigment disturbance is unclear and electron microscopic studies have revealed decreased number of melanocytes as well as decreased melanosomes within keratinocytes in some patients (Lambroza *et al.* 1995). Differentiation from vitiligo on a clinical basis should be straightforward, however, a biopsy is needed to confirm the diagnosis of hypopigmented mycosis fungoides.

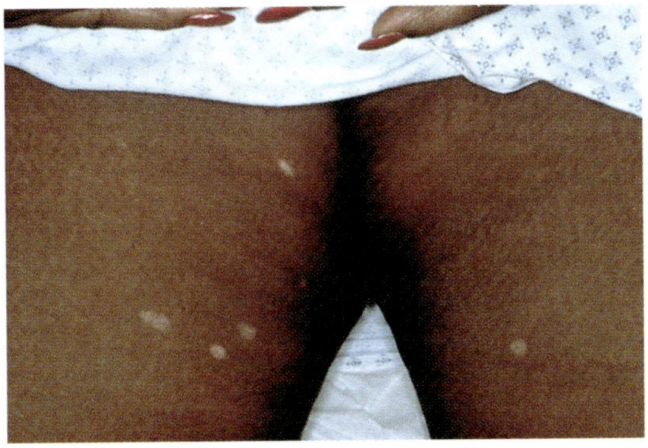

Fig. 14.12 Twenty-six-year-old black female with 2 years history of hypopigmented macules. Biopsy revealed hypopigmented mycosis fungoides.

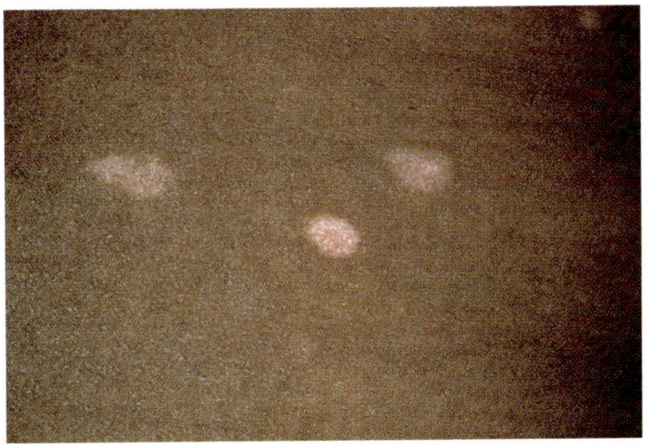

Fig. 14.13 Hypopigmented mycosis fungoides. Close-up of erythematous, scaling, depigmented macules.

Infectious disorders

Tinea versicolor

Tinea versicolor, a mild, chronic, often asymptomatic infection of the epidermis caused by malassezia furfur, may present as hyperpigmented or, more commonly, hypopigmented macules which become confluent and form scaly patches. Hypopigmented lesions typically begin as reddish macules with fine scale upon scraping. They have a seborrheic distribution including the chest, neck, upper arms and back. The face, lower trunk and proximal extremities may be involved in extensive cases (Figs 14.14, 14.15) or in patients with type 4, 5 or 6 skin colour. There is occasional pruritus. Tinea versicolor commonly affects young adults ages 15–35 years. Wood's lamp examination of active lesions reveals yellow or golden fluorescence (Assaf & Weil 1996). Direct microscopy with potassium hydroxide of scale reveals hyphae and spores. Differentiation of vitiligo from active tinea versicolor is straightforward on examination based on the above findings of scaling, Wood's lamp examination and KOH staining. By Wood's lamp, the scale of tinea versicolor has a golden fluorescence. The nonactive hypopigmented lesions of tinea versicolor can last for months and can infrequently be difficult to differentiate from vitiligo. Histochemical and electron micro-

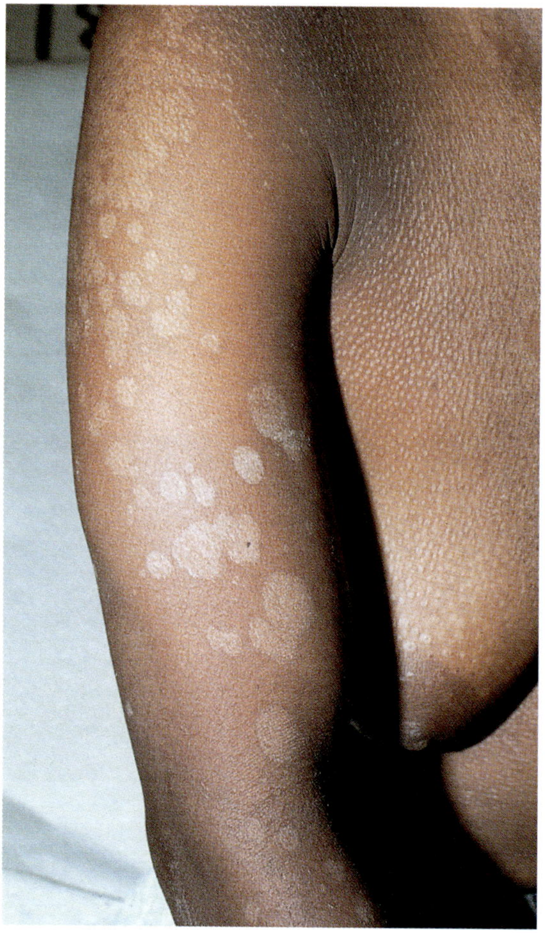

Fig. 14.14 Tinea versicolor. Fine, scaling, discrete and confluent, hypopigmented macules and patches.

scopic findings, however, will confirm the presence of melanocytes in lesional skin.

Pinta

Pinta, a nonvenereal infection caused by the spirochaete *Treponema carateum*, is found in Central and South America. The hallmark of the tertiary or late stage is depigmented lesions over bony prominences, wrists, elbows and ankles. These symmetrical, depigmented lesions develop 3 months to 10 years after the appearance of the secondary lesions (called pintids) which are psoriasiform papules and plaques (Koff & Rosen 1993). Morphologically the lesions may be difficult to distinguish from vitiligo, however, the history of a previous papulosquamous eruption, geographical history and positive serology for treponemal infection distinguishes pinta from vitiligo.

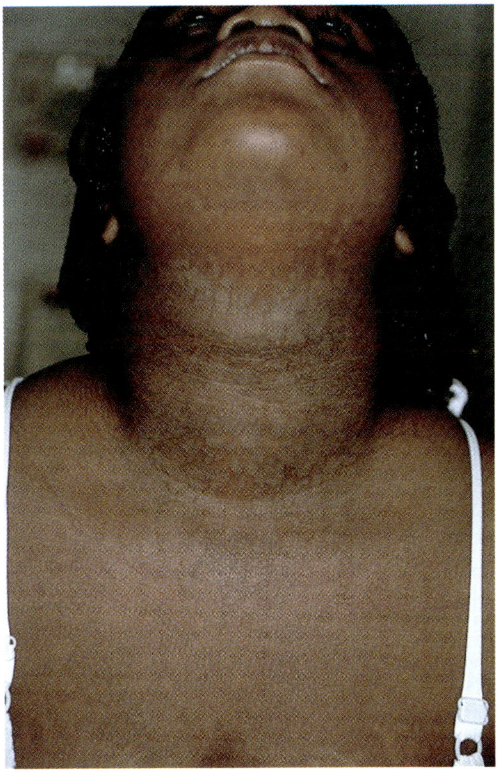

Fig. 14.15 Tinea versicolor. Extensive involvement of neck and trunk.

Syphilis

Leukoderma syphiliticum caused by *Treponema pallidum* is an uncommon presentation of secondary syphilis in which depigmented, round or oval discrete patches measuring 1–2 cm can present around the neck ('necklace of Venus'), trunk, limbs, palms and soles. There have been two variants of leukoderma syphiliticum described. The first type appears to be a form of postinflammatory depigmentation. In this type, 3–6 months after the papulosquamous eruption of secondary syphilis, there are hypomelanotic and depigmented macules and patches occurring in the site of previous syphilitic lesions (Fiumara & Cahn 1982). Treatment of the syphilitic infection allows for repigmentation over a several month period.

The second form is one of depigmented patches with a peripheral reticular hyperpigmentation. There is no preceding history of a skin rash and the leukodermic lesion is felt to be a primary lesion of secondary syphilis. As such, treponemes are found within the lesions (Poulsen *et al.* 1988). Differentiation of leukoderma syphiliticum from vitiligo is based on the history of preceding rash or genital ulcer, supporting sexual history, and positive serological tests for treponemal infection (rapid plasmin reagin (RPR), Venereal Disease Research Laboratory (VDRL) or fluorescent treponemal antibody, absorbed (FTA-ABS)). Yaws, which is caused by the same organism but acquired by nonvenereal routes, can also cause depigmentation. It is most common in Africa and some parts of South America.

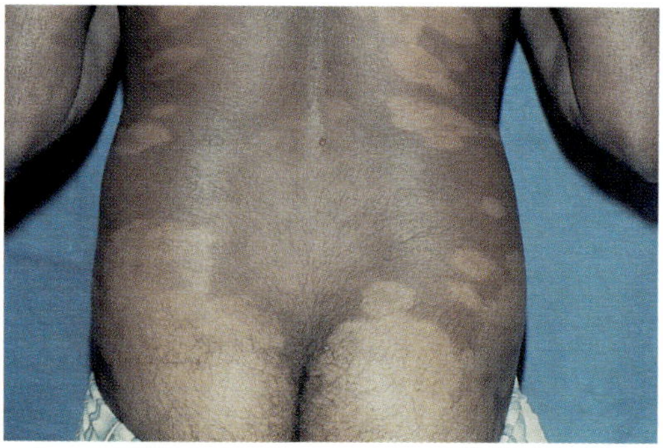

Fig. 14.16 Hypopigmented lesions in borderline leprosy.

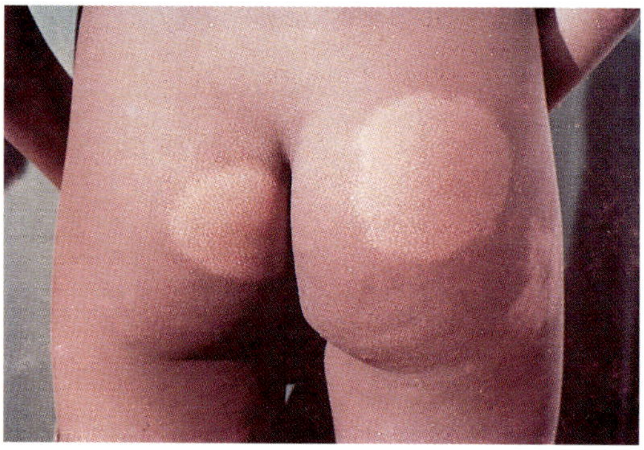

Fig. 14.17 Hypopigmented patches of tuberculoid leprosy.

Leprosy

Hypopigmented patches are one of the cardinal features of leprosy, especially the tuberculoid forms. Caused by *Mycobacterium leprae*, morphology of a hypopigmented lesion varies depending on the type of leprosy. Lesions vary from well-defined to ill-defined, smooth, asymmetrical to symmetrical, variably erythematous patches and variably indurated plaques (Figs 14.16–14.18). Most lesions have a partial to complete loss of sensation of temperature, touch and pain. Histology reveals the spectrum of well-defined, compact granulomas, often around a nerve, in tuberculoid leprosy to diffuse granulomatous inflammation with foamy macrophages in lepromatous leprosy (Sehgal 1973). Differentiation from vitiligo is straightforward if there is anaesthesia of the lesions. In addition, lesions of vitiligo are usually depigmented but those of leprosy are never depigmented, only hypopigmented. However, patients with leprosy who suffer from loss of sensation often get burns on the hands that can depigment as a secondary result of leprosy. If necessary, histochemical and electron microscopic studies can be used to demonstrate the presence of melanocytes and granulomatous inflammation. Repigmentation of hypopigmented lesions of leprosy occurs slowly after appropriate therapy.

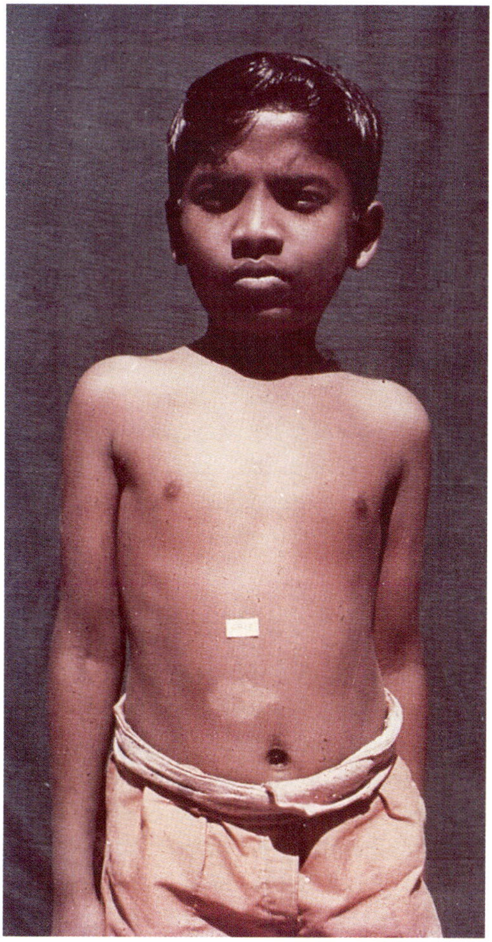

Fig. 14.18 Indeterminate leprosy.

Idiopathic disorders

Idiopathic guttate hypomelanosis

Idiopathic guttate hypomelanosis is a common disorder of adulthood. Lesions are most common on the sun-exposed areas of the arms and legs, but can be found on the trunk as well. They are often hypomelanotic but may appear depigmented. Lesions are well circumscribed, sharply defined, angular or polygonal in shape and small in size (2–5 mm, occasionally up to 1.5 cm) (Fig. 14.19). Histological findings are variable, most commonly revealing a flattening of the dermal–epidermal junction, a moderate to marked reduction in melanin granules, epidermal atrophy and basket weave hyperkeratosis (Falabella 1988). The course of the disease is slowly progressive with age and no spontaneous repigmentation has been reported. Ultrastructural studies reveal both normal number of melanocytes with decreased number of melanosomes and, in one patient, loss of epidermal melanocytes (Ortonne & Perrot 1980). Differentiation from vitiligo is based on the age of onset, the distribution, the persistent small

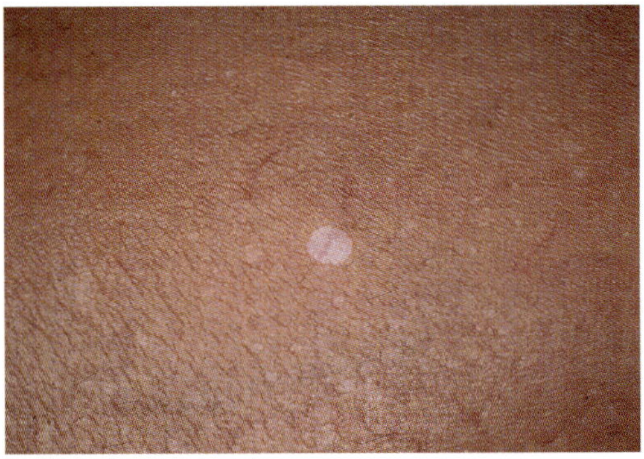

Fig. 14.19 Idiopathic guttate hypomelanosis.

size of the lesions, the slow, progressive nature, the general lack of confluence of lesions and the lack of depigmented hairs in the idiopathic guttate hypomelanosis lesions. If necessary, histological and biochemical studies can be done to differentiate from vitiligo.

Postinflammatory pigment loss

Postinflammatory hypopigmentation and depigmentation can have a variety of presentations based on the preceding inflammatory reaction or insult. Depigmentation from burns often shapes itself in the form of the burn. Repigmentation is possible if there is no scarring or loss of follicles. The depigmentation of discoid lupus has already been discussed. Many inflammatory reactions have the potential of hypopigmenting or depigmenting the skin. More commonly, hypopigmenting inflammatory reactions leave ill-defined, poorly circumscribed lesions. Repigmentation is based on a host of factors including the age of the patient, the type of insult or injury, the location on the skin and presence of hair follicles. Differentiation from vitiligo is based on the history of preceding eruption or injury.

Differential diagnosis of segmental vitiligo

As previously mentioned, there is overlap amongst the differential diagnoses mentioned for generalized vitiligo and segmental vitiligo. As such, in addition to the following disorders, any of the previously mentioned disorders can present with hypopigmenting lesions in a segmental or focal distribution.

Naevus depigmentosus

Naevus depigmentosus can either be a congenital hypopigmenting disorder or, less commonly, form during adolescence or adult life. The macules or patches may not be noticed until later in infancy. Relatively stable in size throughout its life, it is well circumscribed, irregular bordered, hypopigmented, solitary and often unilateral. Its size will vary depending on if it is isolated, segmental or systematized. Hairs within the naevus may be hypopigmented. The lesions are commonly located on the trunk or proximal extremities (Figs 14.20 & 14.21), however, may occur on the head and neck. Histological and electron microscopic studies reveal normal or decreased numbers of melanocytes and few melanosomes, as well as abnormal melanization within the melanocytes (Pinto & Bolognia 1991). Differentiation from segmental vitiligo is based on the age of onset and hypopigmentation vs. depigmentation.

Naevus anaemicus

Naevus anaemicus can also be a congenital or acquired anomaly of hypochromic macules and patches. However, there is no true abnormality in the pigmentary system. The lesion is caused by decreased blood flow through the capillaries in the dermal papillae. A hypochromic or pale lesion of variable size with well defined borders and irregular margins will present at birth but is often missed until later on in life (Fig. 14.22). Usually unilateral and located on the trunk, it is not accentuated by Wood's lamp examination. Pressure at the margin of the lesion obliterates the border making the lesional skin indistinguishable from surrounding skin. This is best demonstrated on diascopy. Histological and electron microscopic

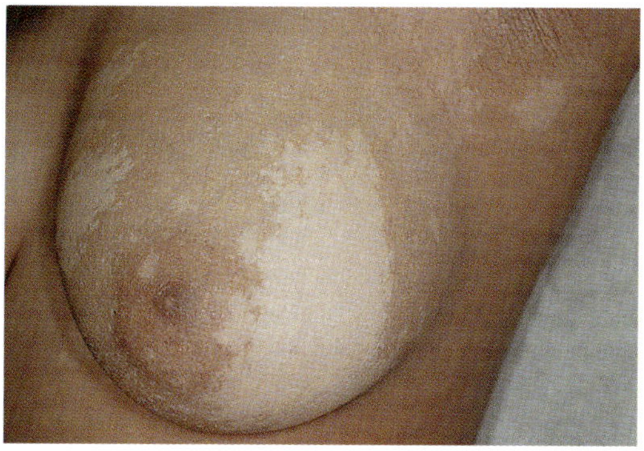

Fig. 14.20 Naevus depigmentosus.

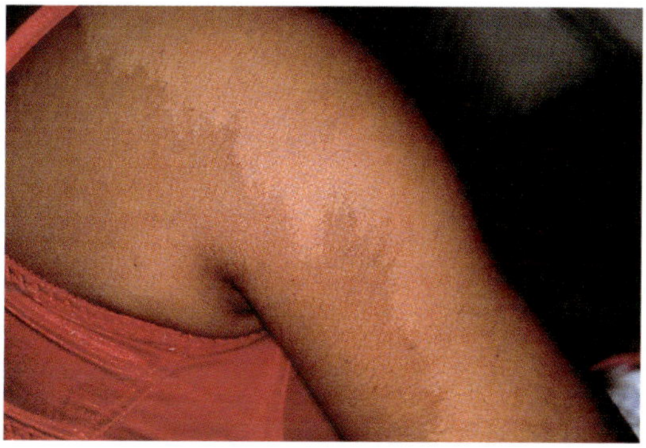

Fig. 14.21 Naevus depigmentosus.

studies reveal no abnormality in melanocytes or melanization. Naevus anaemicus is felt to be due to a localized hypersensitivity of blood vessels within the lesion to catecholamines (Mountcastle *et al.* 1986). Naevus anaemicus is easily distinguished from segmental vitiligo based on clinical and histological findings.

Topical steroids

Although unlikely to be confused with vitiligo, hypopigmentation after intralesional corticosteroid therapy can occur in a focal distribution. The lesion is characterized by linear, irregular and stellate or angulated, ill-defined, hypopigmented streaks often occurring several weeks to months after intralesional or intra-articular injections of steroids (Figs 14.23 & 14.24). The pattern of hypopigmentation is felt to be secondary to lymphogenous spread of the corticosteroid suspension. Histological and electron microscopic findings in one patient revealed decreased numbers of melanocytes in the hypopigmented skin (Friedman *et al.* 1988). Repigmentation is variable. A history of intralesional or intra-articular injection should be obtained. If not, the pattern and ill-defined border of the lesion rule out vitiligo.

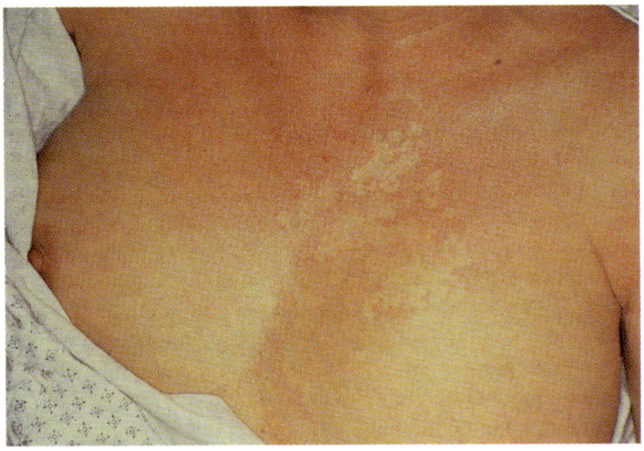

Fig. 14.22 Naevus anaemicus.

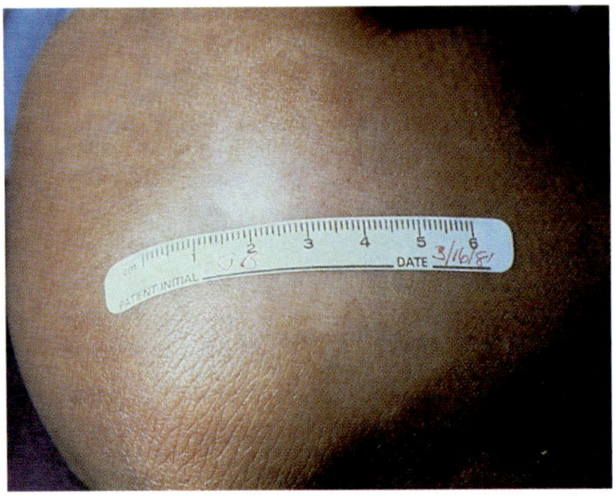

Fig. 14.23 Leukoderma secondary to intra-articular Kenalog.

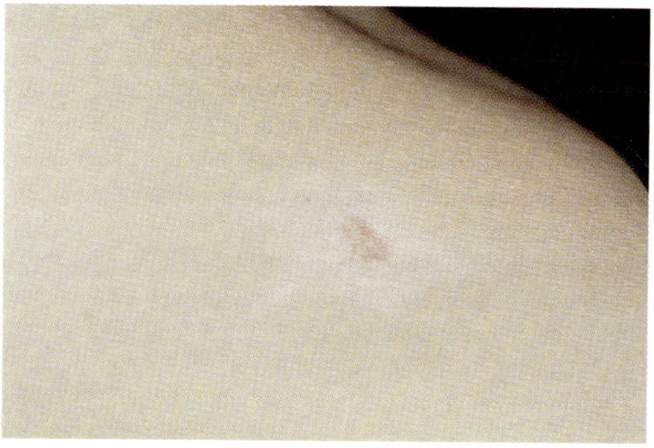

Fig. 14.24 Steroid-induced hypopigmentation.

References

Assaf, R.R. & Weil, M.L. (1996) The superficial mycoses. *Dermatologic Clinics* **14**, 57–67.

Braverman, I.M. (1998) *Skin Signs of Systemic Disease*. 3rd edn., pp. 238–239. W.B. Saunders Company, Philadelphia.

Breathnach, A.S., Fitzpatrick, T.B. & Wyllie, L.M.A. (1965) Electron microscopy of melanocytes in a case of human piebaldism. *Journal of Investigative Dermatology* **45**, 28–37.

Clayton, R., Breathnach, A., Martin, B. & Feiwel, M. (1977) Hypopigmented sarcoidosis in the Negro: Report of eight cases with ultrastructural observations. *British Journal of Dermatology* **96**, 119–125.

Cornelius, C.E., Stein, K.M., Hanshaw, W.J. & Spott, D.A. (1973) Hypopigmentation and sarcoidosis. *Archives of Dermatology* **108**, 249–251.

Falabella, R. (1988) Idiopathic guttate hypomelanosis. *Dermatologic Clinics* **6**, 241–247.

Fiumara, N.J. & Cahn, T. (1982) Leukoderma of secondary syphilis: two case reports. *Sexually Transmitted Diseases* **9**, 140–142.

Frank, S.B. & Cohen, H.J. (1964) The halo nevus. *Archives of Dermatology* **89**, 367–373.

Friedman, S.J., Butler, D.F. & Pittelkow, M.R. (1988) Perilesional linear atrophy and hypopigmentation after intralesional corticosteroid therapy: report of two cases and review of the literature. *Journal of the American Academy of Dermatology* **19**, 537–541.

Goldberg, D.J., Schinella, R.S. & Kechijian, P. (1986) Hypopigmented mycosis fungoides. Speculation about the mechanism of hypopigmentation. *American Journal of Dermatopathology* **8**, 326–330.

Hall, R.S., Floro, J.F. & King, L.E. (1984) Hypopigmented lesions in sarcoidosis. *Journal of the American Academy of Dermatology* **11**, 1163–1164.

Hood, A.F. (1987) Pathology of cutaneous lupus erythematosus. *Advances in Dermatology* **2**, 153–170.

Jimbow, K., Fitzpatrick, T.B., Szabo, G. & Hori, Y. (1975) Congenital circumscribed hypomelanosis: a characterization based on electron microscopic study of tuberous sclerosis, nevus depigmentosus and piebaldism. *Journal of Investigative Dermatology* **64**, 50–62.

Koff, A.B. & Rosen, T. (1993) Nonvenereal treponematoses: yaws, endemic syphilis, and pinta. *Journal of the American Academy of Dermatology* **29**, 519–535.

Laman, S.D. & Provost, T.T. (1994) Cutaneous manifestations of lupus erythematosus. *Rheumatic Disease Clinics of North America* **20**, 195–212.

Lambroza, E., Cohen, S.R., Phelps, R., Lebwohl, M., Braverman, I.M. & DiConstanzo, D. (1995) Hypopigmented variant of mycosis fungoides: demography, histopathology, and treatment of seven cases. *Journal of the American Academy of Dermatology* **32**, 987–993.

Leibowitch, M. (1996) Lichen sclerosus. *Seminars in Dermatology* **15**, 42–46.

Martin, R.F., Lugo-Somolinos, A. & Sánchez, J.L. (1990) Clinicopathologic study on pityriasis alba. *Boletin—Asociacion Medica de Puerto Rico* **82**, 463–465.

Meffert, J.J., Davis, B.M. & Grimwood, R.E. (1995) Lichen sclerosus. *Journal of the American Academy of Dermatology* **39**, 393–416.

Mitchell, I.C., Sweatman, M.C., Rustin, M.H.A. & Wilson, R. (1986) Ulcerative and hypopigmented sarcoidosis. *Journal of the American Academy of Dermatology* **15**, 1062–1065.

Mountcastle, E.A., Diestelmeier, M.R. & Lupton, G.P. (1986) Nevus anemicus. *Journal of the American Academy of Dermatology* **14**, 628–632.

Nordlund, J.J. & Abdel-Malek, Z.A. (1988) Mechanisms for post-inflammatory hyperpigmentation and hypopigmentation. In: *Advances in Pigment Cell Research. Proceedings of the XIII International Pigment Cell Society* (ed. J.Bagnara), pp. 219–236. Alan R. Liss, Inc., New York, NY.

Ortonne, J.P. & Perrot, H. (1980) Idiopathic guttate hypomelanosis. *Archives of Dermatology* **116**, 664–668.

Pinto, F.J. & Bolognia, J.L. (1991) Disorders of hypopigmentation in children. *Pediatric Clinics of North America* **38**, 991–1017.

Poulsen, A., Secher, L., Kobayasi, T. & Weismann, K. (1988) Treponema pallidum in leukoderma syphiliticum demonstrated by electron microscopy. *Acta Dermato-Venereologica (Stockholm)* **68**, 102–106.

Ruiz-Maldonado, R., Toussaint, S., Tamayo, L., Laterza, A. & del Castillo, V. (1992) Hypomelanosis of Ito: diagnostic criteria and report of 41 cases. *Pediatric Dermatology* **9**, 1–10.

Sehgal, V.N. (1973) Hypopigmented lesions in leprosy. *British Journal of Dermatology*. 99–100.

Sheth, P.B. (1998) Tuberous sclerosis complex. In: *The Pigmentary System. Physiology and Pathophysiology* (eds J.J. Nordlund, R.E. Boissy, V.J. Hearing, R.A. King & J.-P. Ortonne), pp. 606–610. Oxford University Press, New York.

Zaynoun, S.T., Aftimos, B.G., Tenekjian, K.K., Bahuth, N. & Kurban, A.K. (1983) Extensive pityriasis alba: a histological histochemical and ultrastructural study. *British Journal of Dermatology* **108**, 83–90.

PART 3
PATHOGENESIS OF VITILIGO: THEORIES FOR DEPIGMENTATION

15: The Intrinsic (Genetic) Theory for the Cause of Vitiligo

RAYMOND E. BOISSY

As has been stated throughout this comprehensive monograph, the aetiology of vitiligo is not clearly understood. At present there have been various causative factors implicated in the depigmentary processes of vitiligo which include cytological, environmental, immunological, and neurological destruction of the melanocytes. However, exposure to these causes may not be unique to individuals who develop vitiligo but may be more globally present throughout the population in general. Therefore, regardless of whether a single or multiple initiating events are responsible for the development of vitiligo, it is probable that an underlying genetic/intrinsic factor predisposes the melanocyte of an individual to be more sensitive to these varied causative factors. This genetic/intrinsic susceptibility would result in only a subset of people exposed to similar environmental or cellular events to develop melanocyte destruction and subsequently vitiligo. This hypothesis of an intrinsic/genetic basis for vitiligo is formulated from the data demonstrating that vitiligo has an inheritable component and that vitiligo melanocytes isolated in culture can selectively express intrinsic defects.

Inheritable component

There is clearly a multifactorial genetic component to vitiligo that appears to predispose individuals to the disease (Merelender & Rywlin 1940; Hafez *et al.* 1983; Majumder *et al.* 1988, 1993; Nath *et al.* 1994). This multifactorial genetic component may be responsible for the complex nature in the presentation of vitiligo by patients.

Vitiligo is not inherited by a simple Mendelian mechanism. Studies on familial inheritance patterns in India and the United States have demonstrated a complex expression for the inheritance of vitiligo (Shah *et al.* 1975, 1977). Mehta demonstrated that in India the incidence of vitiligo in the rural population was 0.47% and in the urban area was 1.78% (Mehta *et al.* 1973). In this study, the investigators stated that there was a grouping of affected individuals within kinships, suggesting a genetic component. Additional descriptions of the familial expression for vitiligo have been subsequently reported (Mayenburg *et al.* 1976; Carnevale *et al.* 1980; Hafez *et al.* 1983; Das *et al.* 1985; Majumder *et al.* 1988; Salamon *et al.* 1989; Bhatia *et al.* 1992; Nath *et al.* 1994).

Ramaiah and colleagues (Ramaiah *et al.* 1988) reported on the Somavamshan Sahasrarjuna Kshatriya (SSK) community of Bangalore, India who were immigrants from the Gujarat-Maharashtra border that originally expressed a high incidence (3.6%) of vitiligo. In the SSK community, the expression of vitiligo was characterized by an earlier age of onset and a very high (90.38%) familial incidence suggesting that continuous inbreeding among the SSK community may have enhanced their genetic predisposition to vitiligo. In a recent epidemiological study of 15685 individuals from 298 families, the investigators found a sevenfold increase of vitiligo in primary family members of individuals with vitiligo (Nath *et al.* 1994). The investigators developed a computer-generated genetic model that postulated a minimum of three unlinked diallelic genes might be coordinately involved with the expression of vitiligo, i.e. as a polygenic disorder (Majumder *et al.* 1993).

Inherent defects

There are data in support of the concept that part of the genetic factors involved in this polygenic disorder may manifest as inherent defects within the melanocyte of patients with vitiligo (Puri *et al.* 1987; Boissy *et al.* 1991b; Chen & Jimbow 1994) as well as animal models for vitiligo (Boissy *et al.* 1986, 1991a; Bowers *et al.* 1992; Cerundolo *et al.* 1993). The morphology and survival of cultured melanocytes, depending on growth factors added to the media, developed from patients with vitiligo have demonstrated selective abnormalities compared to appropriate controls (Puri *et al.* 1987; Boissy *et al.* 1991b; Chen & Jimbow 1994; Im *et al.* 1994). In one of the latter studies (Puri *et al.* 1987), cultured melanocytes derived from uninvolved skin up to 15 cm away from a vitiligo lesion manifested a lag of 8–11 days before the onset of growth. In addition, the initial seeding capacity of the melanocytes from uninvolved and perilesional skin of vitiligo patients were, respectively, 50% and 25% of the normal individuals. Concomitantly, the primary cultures subsequently developed could not be passaged. These abnormal characteristics of cultured vitiligo melanocytes were corrected in patients successfully repigmenting (after PUVA therapy) or when fetal lung fibroblast-derived growth factors were added to the melanocyte cultures (Puri *et al.* 1989). These observations are pivotal because they suggest that an interaction between the melanocyte and environmental regulators of its physiology is important to maintain the survival of the vitiligo melanocyte.

This hypothesis is further strengthened when one considers that Puri *et al.* (Puri *et al.* 1987), in the study described above, had used suboptimal culture conditions in demonstrating survival differences between vitiligo and control melanocytes, i.e. only 12-O-tetradecanolyphorbol-13-acetate (TPA) and a minimal concentration of cholera toxin (CT) was added to basal cell culture media. We (Medrano & Nordlund 1990; Boissy *et al.* 1991b; Swope *et al.* 1995), and colleagues (Halaban 1988; Imokawa *et al.* 1992; Yohn *et al.* 1993), have demonstrated that, in addition to TPA, other factors are required for optimal proliferation of adult-derived human melanocytes in culture. It appears that by using medium optimized for melanocyte proliferation, the inherent survival defect of cultured vitiligo melanocytes can be masked. We have cultured melanocytes, derived from well over three dozen vitiligo patients, in medium containing pituitary extract (or basic fibroblast growth factor), insulin, transferrin and vitamin E, in addition to TPA and have found no significant alteration in growth rate of the vitiligo compared to control melanocytes (Medrano & Nordlund 1990; Boissy *et al.* 1991b). However, under these more permissive culture conditions, we and colleagues have observed dilated rough endoplasmic reticulum and/or autophagocytotic vesicles (resembling similar morphological abnormalities observed *in vivo*) in a majority of the cases (Boissy *et al.* 1991b; Im *et al.* 1994). These observations are consistent with the hypothesis that vitiligo melanocytes are inherently abnormal. Other laboratories culturing vitiligo melanocytes for transplantation have used growth factor enhanced medium containing basic fibroblast growth factor and dibutyryl adenosine monophosphate and demonstrated the *in vitro* proliferation is not compromised (Olsson & Juhlin 1993).

Expression of melanocyte specific proteins has also been shown to be aberrant in vitiligo melanocytes. Recent studies (Chen & Jimbow 1994; Norris *et al.* 1996) have demonstrated that melanocytes cultured from patients with active vitiligo exhibited lack of both c-Kit and stem cell factor (SCF) expression, which are the receptor/ligand system shown to play a role in melanocyte differentiation and thus melanization (Chabot *et al.* 1988; Zsebo *et al.* 1990). In addition, Chen and Jimbow (1994) reported that cultured vitiligo melanocytes demonstrated an elevated expression of tyrosinase related protein-1 (TRP-1) although the size of this TRP-1 product appeared normal.

Cultures of melanocytes developed from the various avian models for vitiligo also demonstrate evidence of genetic/intrinsic melanocyte abnormalities. Melanocytes established in culture from neural tubes isolated from Smyth line chicken embryos selectively demonstrate degenerative events by 90 days in culture that resemble those of the melanocytes in the depigmenting feather follicles (Boissy *et al.* 1986). In contrast, melanocyte cultures developed from feather follicle epithelium of either the White Leghorn (WL) or the Barred Plymouth Rock (BPR) chicken models for vitiligo demonstrate normal growth (Bowers *et al.* 1992). However, if WL and BPR melanocytes are cultured in the presence of the epithelial tissue of origin, or in medium conditioned by WL and BPR melanocytes, they exhibit cell death not seen in control melanocytes (Bowers *et al.* 1992). These investigators hypothesized that the mutant WL and BPR melanocytes are genetically preconditioned to be more sensitive to a precipitating factor present in the feather follicle environment that does not affect normal melanocytes.

A genetic basis may also underlie the development of the occupational/contact form of vitiligo. Both anecdotal and experimental evidence exists demonstrating that certain environmental chemicals (i.e. specific phenolic and catecholic derivatives) may be selectively toxic to melanocytes and thus may instigate the occupational or contact vitiligo (Ortonne & Bose 1993; Cummings & Nordlund 1995). Specifically, these putative environmental toxins are aromatic or aliphatic derivatives of phenols and catechols (i.e. hydroquinone, monobenzyl ether of hydroquinone, 2,4-di-tert-butylphenol (DTBP), p-tert-butylphenol (PTBP), p-methyl-catechol, p-isopropylcatechol, p-chlororesorcinol, p-cresol, diisopropyl fluorophosphate, and physostigmine). These compounds have been shown to be preferentially toxic to melanocytes both in culture and *in vivo* (Bleehen *et al.* 1968; Lerner 1971; Gellin *et al.* 1979). In fact, these compounds have been added to bleaching creams, products used to remove hyperpigmented lesions. Interestingly, these creams are not toxic to all individuals. Even at high dosages only a subset of humans depigment in response to application of these compounds. In contrast, patients with extensive vitiligo readily continue to depigment in response to contact with these compounds. This observation suggests that these agents are not simple poisons for melanocytes but are injurious to only those genetically susceptible (i.e. vitiligo patients).

An important anecdotal clue implicating these environmental agents in melanocyte cytotoxicity is seen in cases where a definitive correlative factor is associated with the onset of vitiligo. Depigmentation develops in a significant number of people who work with or are exposed to phenolic and catecholic derivatives. This includes people working with rubber (Quevedo *et al.* 1986; O'Malley *et al.* 1988) and industrial oils (Gellin *et al.* 1970) containing phenolic antioxidants or plasticizers, phenolic detergent germicides (Kahn 1970), paratertiary-butylphenol containing adhesives (Bajaj *et al.* 1990) and in the general manufacturing of these chemicals. Studies have shown that 1% of individuals who are exposed to these chemicals rapidly develop a vitiligo-like syndrome, while other exposed individuals require years to develop pigment loss (O'Malley *et al.* 1988). These observations suggest that there is a genetic variability in the response to these environmental contaminants. In addition, this suggests that melanocytes in vitiligo patients are genetically susceptible to the cytotoxic action of these phenolic/catecholic agents.

References

Bajaj, A.K., Gupta, S.C. & Chatterjee, A.K. (1990) Contact depigmentation from free paratertiary-butylphenol in bindi adhesive. *Contact Dermatitis* **22**, 99–102.

Bhatia, P.S., Mohan, L., Pandey, O.N., Singh, K.K., Arora, S.K. & Mukhija, R.D. (1992) Genetic nature of vitiligo. *Journal of Dermatological Science* **4**, 180–184.

Bleehen, S.S., Pathak, M.A., Hori, Y. & Fitzpatrick, T.B. (1968) Depigmentation of skin with 4-isopropylcatechol, mercaptoamines and other compounds. *Journal of Investigative Dermatology* **50**, 103–117.

Boissy, R.E., Moellmann, G.E., Trainer, A.A., Smyth, J.R. Jr & Lerner, A.B. (1986) Delayed-amelanotic (DAM-Smyth) chicken: melanocyte dysfunction *in vivo* and *in vitro*. *Journal of Investigative Dermatology* **86**, 149–156.

Boissy, R.E., Beato, K.E. & Nordlund, J.J. (1991a) Dilated rough endoplasmic reticulum and premature cell death in melanocytes cultured from the vitiligo mouse. *American Journal of Pathology* **138**, 1511–1525.

Boissy, R.E., Liu, Y.-Y., Medrano, E.E. & Nordlund, J.J. (1991b) Structural aberration of the rough endoplasmic reticulum and melanosome compartmentalization in long-term cultures of melanocytes from vitiligo patients. *Journal of Investigative Dermatology* **97**, 395–404.

Bowers, R.R., Harmon, J., Prescott, S., Asano, J. & Wynne, S. (1992) Fowl model for vitiligo: Genetic regulation on the fate of the melanocytes. *Pigment Cell Research Supplement* **2**, 242–248.

Carnevale, A., Zavala, C., del Castillo, V., Ruiz Maldonado, R. & Tamayo, L. (1980) [Genetic analysis of 127 families with vitiligo (author's translation)]. *Revista de Investigacion Clinica* **32**, 37–41.

Cerundolo, R., De Caprariis, D., Esposito, L., Maiolino, P., Restucci, B. & Roperto, F. (1993) Vitiligo in two water buffaloes: histological, histochemical, and ultrastructural investigations. *Pigment Cell Research* **6**, 23–28.

Chabot, B., Stephenson, D.A., Chapman, V.M., Besmer, P. & Bernstein, A. (1988) The proto-oncogene c-kit encoding a transmembrane tyrosine kinase receptor maps to the mouse W locus. *Nature* **335**, 88–89.

Chen, H. & Jimbow, K. (1994) Comparison in expression of tyrosinase, TRP-1, and c-kit between normal human melanocytes and 'vitiligo' melanocytes. *Pigment Cell Research Supplement* **3**, 24 (Abstract).

Cummings, M.P. & Nordlund, J.J. (1995) Chemical leukoderma: fact or fancy. *American Journal of Contact Dermatitis* **6**, 122–127.

Das, S.K., Majumder, P.P., Majumder, T.K. & Haldar, B. (1985) Studies on vitiligo II. Familial aggregation and genetics. *Genetic Epidemiology* **2**, 255–262.

Gellin, G.A., Possick, P.A. & Perone, V.B. (1970) Depigmentation from 4-tertiary butyl catechol—an experimental study. *Journal of Investigative Dermatology* **55**, 190–197.

Gellin, G.A., Maibach, H.I. & Misiaszek, M.H. (1979) Detection of environmental depigmenting substances. *Contact Dermatitis* **5**, 201–213.

Hafez, M., Sharaf, L. & El-Nabi, S.M.A. (1983) The genetics of vitiligo. *Acta Dermato-Venereologica (Stockholm)* **63**, 249–251.

Halaban, R. (1988) Responses of cultured melanocytes to defined growth factors. *Pigment Cell Research Supplement* **1**, 18–26.

Im, S., Hann, S.K., Kim, H.I., Kim, N.S. & Park, Y.-K. (1994) Biologic characteristics of cultured human vitiligo melanocytes. *International Journal of Dermatology* **33**, 556–562.

Imokawa, G., Yada, Y. & Miyagishi, M. (1992) Endothelins secreted from human keratinocytes are intrinsic mitogens for human melanocytes. *Journal of Biological Chemistry* **267**, 24675–24680.

Kahn, G. (1970) Depigmentation caused by phenolic detergent germicides. *Archives of Dermatology* **102**, 177–187.

Lerner, A.B. (1971) On the etiology of vitiligo and grey hair. *American Journal of Medicine* **51**, 141–147.

Majumder, P.P., Das, D.K. & Li, C.C. (1988) A genetical model for vitiligo. *American Journal of Human Genetics* **43**, 119–125.

Majumder, P., Nordlund, J.J. & Nath, S.K. (1993) Pattern of familial aggregation of vitiligo. *Archives of Dermatology* **129**, 994–998.

Mayenburg, J.V., Vogt, H.J. & Ziegelmayer, G. (1976) Vitiligo in a pair of enzygotic twins. *Hautarzt* **27**, 426–431.

Medrano, E.E. & Nordlund, J.J. (1990) Successful culture of adult human melanocytes from normal and vitiligo donors. *Journal of Investigative Dermatology* **95**, 441–445.

Mehta, N.R., Shah, K.C., Theodore, C., Vyas, V.P. & Patel, A.B. (1973) Epidemiological study of vitiligo in Surat area, South Gujarat. *Indian Journal of Medical Research* **61**, 145–154.

Merelender, J. & Rywlin, J. (1940) Heredity of aquired vitiligo (vitiligo in 3 generations). *Acta Dermato-Venereologica (Stockholm)* **21**, 583–585.

Nath, S.K., Majumder, P.P. & Nordlund, J.J. (1994) Genetic epidemiology of vitiligo: multilocus recessivity cross validated. *American Journal of Human Genetics* **55**, 981–990.

Norris, A., Todd, C., Graham, A., Quinn, A.G. & Thody, A.J. (1996) The expression of the c-kit receptor by epidermal melanocytes may be reduced in vitiligo. *British Journal of Dermatology* **134**, 299–306.

Olsson, M.J. & Juhlin, L. (1993) Repigmentation of vitiligo by transplantation of cultured autologous melanocytes. *Acta Dermato-Venereologica (Stockholm)* **73**, 49–51.

O'Malley, M.A., Mathias, T., Priddy, M., Molina, D., Grote, A.A. & Halperin, W.E. (1988) Occupational vitiligo due to unsuspected presence of phenolic antioxidant byproducts in commercial bulk rubber. *Journal of Occupational Medicine* **30**, 512–516.

Ortonne, J.-P. & Bose, S.K. (1993) Vitiligo: Where do we stand? *Pigment Cell Research* **6**, 61–72.

Puri, N., Mojamdar, M. & Ramaiah, A. (1987) In vitro growth characteristics of melanocytes obtained from adult normal and vitiligo subjects. *Journal of Investigative Dermatology* **88**, 434–438.

Puri, N., Mojamdar, M. & Ramaiah, A. (1989) Growth defects of melanocytes in culture from vitiligo subjects are spontaneously corrected in vivo in repigmenting subjects and can be partially corrected by the addition of fibroblast-derived growth factors in vitro. *Archives of Dermatological Research—Archiv für dermatologische Forschung* **281**, 178–184.

Quevedo, W.C. Jr, Fitzpatrick, T.B., Szabo, G. & Jimbow, K. (1986) Biology of the melanin pigmentary system. In: *Dermatology in General Medicine* (eds T.B.Fitzpatrick, A.Z.Eisen, K.Wolff, I.M.Freedberg & K.F.Austen), 3rd edn, pp. 224–251. McGraw-Hill, New York.

Ramaiah, A., Mojamdar, M. & Amarnath, V.M. (1988) Vitiligo in the SSK community of Bangalore. *Indian Journal of Dermatology, Venereology and Leprology* **54**, 251–254.

Salamon, T., Hadziselimovic, R. & Halepovic, E. (1989) The heritability of vitiligo. *Hautarzt* **40**, 141–145.

Shah, V.C., Mojamdar, M.V. & Sharma, K.S. (1975) Some genetic, biochemical and physiological aspects of leucoderma vitiligo. *Journal of the Cytologic Genetics Congress (Proceedings of the Second All India Congress on Cytologic Genetics) Supplement* 173–178.

Shah, V.C., Haribhakti, P.B., Mojamdar, M.V. & Sharma, K.S. (1977) Statistical study of 600 vitiligo cases in the city of Ahmedabad. *Gujarat Medical Journal* **42**, 51–59.

Swope, V.B., Medrano, E.E., Smalara, D. & Abdel-Malek, Z. (1995) Long-term proliferation of human melanocytes is supported by the physiologic mitogens a-melanotropin, endothelin-1, and basic fibroblast growth factor. *Experimental Cell Research* **217**, 453–459.

Yohn, J.J., Morelli, J.G., Walchak, S.J., Rundell, K.B., Norris, D.A. & Zamora, M.R. (1993) Cultured human keratinocytes synthesize and secrete endothelin-1. *Journal of Investigative Dermatology* **100**, 23–26.

Zsebo, K.M., Williams, D.A., Geissler, E.N., Broudy, V.C., Martin, F.H., Atkins, H.L *et al* (1990) Stem cell factor is encoded at the Sl locus of the mouse and is the ligand for the c-kit receptor. *Cell* **63**, 213–214.

16: Theories on the Pathogenesis of Depigmentation: Immune Hypothesis

JEAN-CLAUDE BYSTRYN

Introduction

The cause(s) of the localized, spontaneous and complete depigmentation of the skin that occurs in vitiligo and in association with some pigmented naevi and melanomas is (are) not known. The pigment loss in these conditions can occur in otherwise normal skin, around or within a benign or malignant pigmented lesion, or at a site distal to a pigmented lesion. These various forms of leukodermas probably result from different pathophysiological mechanisms as they involve the destruction of different types of pigment cells, i.e. normal or malignant melanocytes, normal or atypical naevi cells. They occur in different locations of the integument, i.e. at the site of, adjacent to, or distal to the cells that initiated the process. And they are associated with different histological abnormalities, i.e. the presence or absence of a dense cellular infiltrate. Whatever their causes, these leukodermas are experiments of nature that demonstrate that there are mechanisms in humans that can selectively kill pigment cells, including melanoma cells.

Pathogenesis of leukoderma in vitiligo

A number of indirect observations suggest vitiligo is an autoimmune disease directed against pigment cells (Bystryn 1997). These include:

1 Vitiligo is a systemic disease. Approximately 25% of patients with vitiligo have destruction of pigment cells in the eye. Choroidal depigmentation associated with panuveitis is common in Sinclair swine and Smyth chickens with a type of leukoderma that resembles human vitiligo.

2 Vitiligo is associated with a variety of nonspecific immune abnormalities.

3 Most treatments for vitiligo, such as PUVA, topical steroids and topical cytotoxic drugs, are immunosuppressive, a point that suggests their benefit could result from suppression of local immune reactions damaging melanocytes.

4 There are relationships between vitiligo and melanoma that suggest that immune reactions targeted to melanoma cells can also destroy normal melanocytes.

Antibodies to melanocytes in vitiligo

The most direct and convincing evidence that vitiligo is an autoimmune disease is that specific autoantibodies to melanocyte cell surface antigens are present in the circulation of most patients with vitiligo. These antibodies were initially demonstrated by immunoprecipitation of melanocyte surface antigens and by indirect immunofluorescence (Naughton *et al.* 1983; Bystryn & Naughton 1985; Bystryn & Xie 1998). Their presence has been confirmed by other techniques including complement-dependent cytotoxicity (Norris *et al.* 1988; Cui *et al.* 1993; Yu *et al.* 1993), antibody-dependent cellular cytotoxicity (Norris *et al.* 1988; Yu *et al.* 1993), immunoblotting by live cell (Harning *et al.* 1991) and conventional enzyme-linked immunosorbent assay (ELISA) (Fishman *et al.* 1993), and passive transfer experiments (Gilhar *et al.* 1995). Antibodies to melanocytes are unusual in persons with nonpigmentary skin diseases.

The incidence and level of vitiligo antibodies correlates with the extent of depigmentation and the activity of the disease. They have been reported in only 50% of persons with minimal vitiligo but in 93% of those with more extensive disease (Naughton *et al.* 1986b). The average level of antibodies increases with increasing extent and activity of the disease (Harning *et al.* 1991; Cui *et al.* 1993). The titre of melanocyte antibodies decreases in vitiligo patients that respond to PUVA therapy (Hann *et al.* 1997), confirming that their level is related to disease activity.

A variety of animals develop vitiligo. All those studied have antibodies to pigment cells. These include Tervuren dogs, Siamese cats, Arabian horses (Naughton *et al.* 1986a), Sinclair miniswine (Cui *et al.* 1995) and Smyth chicken with vitiligo-like depigmentation (Austin *et al.* 1992). The pattern of antigens defined by pigment cell antibodies in these animals is similar to those recognized by vitiligo antibodies in humans. These observations indicate that humans and animals with vitiligo have similar immunological abnormalities.

Vitiligo antibodies have the functional capacity to kill pigment cells *in vitro* and can do so by two different mechanisms—complement-dependent cytotoxicity and antibody-dependent cellular cytotoxicity (Norris *et al.* 1988; Cui *et al.* 1993). They also have the ability to kill melanocytes *in vivo*, when passively administered to nude mice grafted with human skin (Gilhar *et al.* 1995).

Cellular immune responses to pigment cells in vitiligo

Inflammatory cells, a marker for involvement of cellular immune mechanisms, are usually sparse in lesions of vitiligo but not completely absent (Hann *et al.* 1992; Al Badri *et al.* 1993a) (see Chapter 5). When present, they are most prominent at the periphery of active lesions (Al Badri *et al.* 1993b; Le Poole *et al.* 1996). This has variously been interpreted to mean that cellular immunity is not involved in the pathogenesis of vitiligo (because the infiltrate is sparse) or is involved (because the infiltrate is more prominent where the lesions are most active). The infiltrate consists of CD3+ (T cells), CD4+ (helper T cells), and CD8+ (cytolytic T cells) cells and macrophages. The T cells are activated as evidenced by increased expression of class II HLA antigens and intercellular adhesion molecules (ICAM-1) (Al Badri *et al.* 1993b), and are closely associated with zones of melanocyte depletion (Al Badri *et al.* 1993a). The characteristics of the infiltrate do not differ from those seen in other inflammatory skin diseases.

Unfortunately, there are few direct studies of the ability of cellular mechanisms specifically to kill pigment cells in vitiligo. An early study by Mitchell *et al.* (1980) found that lymphocytes from vitiligo patients were unreactive to melanoma cells, though it is unclear whether the melanoma cells used were pigmented. In Smyth chickens with vitiligo-like amelanosis, the infiltrate follows the appearance of morphologically abnormal melanocytes, but actual disappearance of melanocytes does not occur if the infiltrate is prevented by neonatal bursectomy (Boissy *et al.* 1984). This suggests that the infiltrate does not initiate injury to melanocytes but aggravates it. Whether the same is true in humans is not known.

While these observations suggest that cellular mechanisms may play a role in the pathogenesis of vitiligo, the evidence is much weaker than that for antibody responses.

Vitiligo antigens

The pigment cell antigens defined by antibodies in patients with vitiligo called 'vitiligo antigens' play a critical role in the pathogenesis of this disease as they may be both the cause and the target of immune responses that damage melanocytes.

Vitiligo antibodies are predominantly directed to melanocyte antigens of 40–45, 75 and 90 kDa (referred to as VIT40, VIT75, and VIT90, respectively) and occasionally to other antigens of 35 and 150 kDa (Cui *et al.* 1992). All these antigens are expressed on the cell surface. The most interesting is VIT90, because it is selectively expressed on pigment cells, particularly melanocytes. By contrast VIT40 and VIT75 are common tissue antigens expressed on both pigment and unrelated cells, and expressed more strongly on melanoma than on melanocytes. Little is known about the identity of these antigens, apart from VIT40 which shares a cross-reacting epitope with, or is tightly bound to, class I HLA. VIT90 is unrelated to currently known pigment cells antigens of similar size, including gp100, p97, and S100 (Cui *et al.* 1995). VIT75 may be related to tyrosinase or tyrosinase-related protein-1 (TRP-1), as all three molecules have similar molecular weights. However, the available evidence suggests this is unlikely. While antibodies to tyrosinase were initially reported in 61% of 26 patients with vitiligo (Song *et al.* 1994), subsequent studies have not confirmed this association. Some investigators have detected tyrosinase antibodies in only a minority (Baharav *et al.* 1996), 11% (Kemp *et al.* 1997), or none (Xie &

Bystryn 1996) of patients with active vitiligo in three subsequent studies. Thus, antibodies to tyrosinase do not seem to be present often enough in vitiligo to be vitiligo antibodies.

TRP-1 has been suggested to be a vitiligo antigen as passive administration of antibody to this molecule into mice causes loss of pigmentation (Hara *et al.* 1995). However, immunodepletion experiments show that VIT75 and gp75 are immunologically distinct (Cui *et al.* 1995). The protein, gp75, is a cytoplasmic antigen while VIT75 is on the cell surface. Antibodies to gp75 have not been found in patients with vitiligo (Song *et al.* 1994), and the depigmentation caused by anti-gp75 is restricted to regrowing hairs (Hara *et al.* 1995) whereas pigment cells in hair follicles are usually spared in vitiligo. Many molecules on pigment cells have a molecular weight of approximately 75 kDa. Several of these have partial sequence homology with tyrosinase. At this stage VIT75 does not appear to be tyrosinase or TRP-1, but a distinct antigen that may have some homology with these molecules.

That some vitiligo antigens are normal tissue antigens also expressed by nonpigment cells does not exclude their playing a role in the pathogenesis of vitiligo. Melanocytes are unusually susceptible to be damaged by immune mechanisms (Norris *et al.* 1988). The LD50 of melanocytes to peroxide-mediated injury, a major mechanism by which immune cells damage their target, is 10 times greater than that of keratinocytes and 100 times greater than that of fibroblasts. Thus, immune reactions to normal antigens expressed by melanocytes could damage these cells while sparing more resistant unrelated cells expressing the same antigens, resulting in a selective destruction of melanocytes.

The antigenic phenotype of melanocytes derived from hair follicles and from overlying epidermis in the same individual differ from each other (Tobin & Bystryn 1996). Hair follicle melanocytes express more of the antigens recognized by antibodies associated with alopecia areata and less of those recognized by vitiligo antibodies, while the reverse is true for epidermal melanocytes. These differences may account for epidermal but not hair follicle melanocytes being preferentially destroyed in vitiligo, while the reverse is true in alopecia areata; and for the hair follicle serving as the source for melanocytes in lesions of vitiligo that repigment (Cui *et al.* 1991).

Role of immune mechanisms in the pathogenesis of vitiligo

The presence of antibodies to melanocytes in patients with vitiligo, their absence in persons without this disease, and the selective expression of some vitiligo antigens on pigment cells provide the essential framework required for vitiligo to be an autoimmune disease. The key questions, as in other autoimmune diseases, are:

1 Are these abnormal anti-pigment cell immune responses a cause or a result of the disease?

2 Do they actually injure melanocytes *in vivo* or are they simply interesting epiphenomena?

3 If immune mechanisms do injure melanocytes, how do they do so?

These questions remain unresolved.

Are immune abnormalities a cause or a result of vitiligo?

Several observations support the notion that vitiligo antibodies can be involved in pigment cell destruction in vitiligo. They target antigens expressed on the surface of melanocytes where they are available to interact with immune effector mechanisms. The level of vitiligo antibodies parallels the extent of pigment cell destruction and the activity of the disease. Vitiligo antibodies have the functional ability to kill melanocytes *in vitro* and *in vivo*. In both Sinclair swine (Cui *et al.* 1995) and Smyth chickens with vitiligo (Austin *et al.* 1992), the pigment cell antibodies usually appear before the onset of pigment loss. That, together with the observation that neonatal bursectomy in chicken minimizes depigmentation, suggests that the antibodies are involved in causing the disease rather than being a result of it.

If vitiligo antibodies are a primary event in the disease, the stimulus for their appearance remains unknown. One possibility is that they are stimulated by cross-reacting antigens expressed on other cells or microorganisms. This possibility is supported by the frequent association of antibodies to melanocytes in patients with chronic mucocutaneous candidiasis (Bystryn 1997), a finding that suggests that candida and melanocytes share some antigens. Common antigens are also shared by mycobacteria and malignant melanocytes.

Whether the vitiligo antibodies are a cause or a result of vitiligo, they have the potential to aggravate pigment cell destruction. Once melanocytes are damaged, the release of additional pigment cell antigens could amplify whatever immune responses are present, and the immune responses so triggered could further aggravate injury to these cells.

Can immune mechanisms injure melanocytes *in vivo*?

Regardless of whether the immune abnormalities in vitiligo are a primary or secondary, they have the potential to damage melanocytes. This is evident by the ability of vitiligo antibodies to kill melanocytes *in vitro* and *in vivo* (Cui *et al.* 1993; Gilhar *et al.* 1995). Whether immune reactions actually do damage melanocytes in vitiligo is not known. The best evidence that they do is that in Smyth chicken, suppression of humoral immunity by bursectomy or of cellular immunity by cyclosporin A delays the progression of vitiligo.

Possible mechanisms of immune destruction of melanocytes in vitiligo

If vitiligo is an autoimmune disease, how is it mediated? At least two possibilities need to be considered:

1 immune responses specifically directed to antigens preferentially expressed by melanocytes, such as VIT90; and
2 responses to common tissue antigens also expressed by melanocytes, such as VIT40 and VIT75, which could nonetheless selectively destroy melanocytes as these cells are much more sensitive to immune injury than unrelated cells expressing the same antigens (Norris *et al.* 1988).

The actual immune mechanisms responsible for melanocyte killing are likely to be multiple. They probably involve complement-dependent and antibody-dependent cellular cytotoxicity (ADCC), as vitiligo antibodies can kill melanocytes *in vitro* by both mechanisms. Alternatively, vitiligo antibodies may simply be markers of abnormal immunity to melanocytes in vitiligo, and the actual damage may be being mediated by other immune mechanisms such as cellular responses. Injury could also result from alterations in the metabolism of melanocytes triggered by immune reactions occurring on their surface, or from proteolytic enzymes or cytokines released by adjacent immune cells or keratinocytes.

Summary

Though the cause of vitiligo remains unknown, immune mechanisms are clearly involved in some fashion. Abnormal antibodies specifically directed to melanocytes are associated with vitiligo in humans and animals, the presence and level of these antibodies correlates with the extent and activity of the disease, and they can kill melanocytes *in vitro* and *in vivo*. As with most other autoimmune diseases, it is still unknown whether the specific immune abnormalities seen in vitiligo are a cause or an effect of the disease, whether they damage melanocytes or aggravate melanocyte injury initiated by other causes, or are interesting but irrelevant epiphenomena.

Acknowledgements

Supported in part by NIH Research Grant 5R21CA66669, FDA grant FDR-000632, and by grants from the National Vitiligo Foundation and the Rose M. Badgeley Residuary Trust.

References

Al Badri, A.M.T., Foulis, A.K., Todd, P.M. *et al.* (1993a) Abnormal expression of MHC class II and ICAM-1 by melanocytes in vitiligo. *Journal of Pathology* **169**, 203–206.

Al Badri, A.M.T., Todd, P.M., Gariochi, J.J. *et al.* (1993b) An immunohistological study of cutaneous lymphocytes in vitiligo. *Journal of Pathology* **170**, 149–155.

Austin, L.M., Boissy, R.E., Jacobson, B.S. & Smith, J.R. Jr (1992) The detection of melanocyte autoantibodies in the Smyth chicken model for vitiligo. *Clinical Immunology and Immunopathology* **64**, 112–120.

Baharav, E., Merimsli, O., Shoenfeld, Y. *et al.* (1996) Tyrosinase as an autoantigen in patients with vitiligo. *Clinical and Experimental Immunology* **105**, 84–88.

Boissy, R.E., Lamont, S.J. & Smyth, J.R. Jr (1984) Persistence of abnormal melanocytes in immunosuppressed chickens of the autoimmune DAM line. *Cell Tissue Research* **235**, 663–668.

Bystryn, J.-C. (1997) Immune Mechanisms in Vitiligo. *Clinics in Dermatology* **15**, 853–861.

Bystryn, J.-C. & Naughton, G.K. (1985) The significance of vitiligo antibodies. *Journal of Dermatology* **12**, 1–9.

Bystryn, J.-C. & Xie, Z. (1998) Neoplastic hypomelanoses. In: *The Pigmentary System: Physiology and Pathophysiology* (eds J.J.Nordlund, R.E.Boissy, V.J.Hearing, R.A.King & J.P.Ortonne), pp. 647–662, Oxford University Press, New York.

Cui, J., Shen, L. & Wang, G. (1991) Role of hair follicles in the repigmentation of vitiligo. *Journal of Investigative Dermatology* **97**, 410–416.

Cui, J., Harning, R., Henn, M. *et al.* (1992) Identification of pigment cell antigens defined by vitiligo antibodies. *Journal of Investigative Dermatology* **98**, 162–165.

Cui, J., Arita, Y. & Bystryn, J.-C. (1993) Cytolytic antibodies to melanocytes in vitiligo. *Journal of Investigative Dermatology* **100**, 812–815.

Cui, J., Arita, Y. & Bystryn, J.-C. (1995) Characterization of vitiligo antigens. *Pigment Cell Research* **8**, 53–59.

Fishman, P., Azizi, E., Shoenfeld, Y. *et al.* (1993) Vitiligo autoantibodies are effective against melanoma. *Cancer* **72**, 2365–2369.

Gilhar, A., Zelickson, B., Ulman, Y. & Etzioni, A. (1995) *In vivo* destruction of melanocytes by the IgG fraction of serum from patients with vitiligo. *Journal of Investigative Dermatology* **105**, 683–686.

Hann, S.K., Park, Y.-K., Lee, K.-G., Choi, E.H. & Im, S. (1992) Epidermal changes in active vitiligo. *Journal of Dermatology* **19**, 217–222.

Hann, S.-K., Chen, D.L. & Bystryn, J.-C. (1997) Systemic steroids suppress anti-melanocyte antibodies in vitiligo. *Journal of Cutaneous Medicine and Surgery* **1**, 193–195.

Hara, I., Takechi, Y. & Houghton, A.N. (1995) Implicating a role for immune recognition of self in tumor rejection: passive immunization against the brown locus protein. *Journal of Experimental Medicine* **182**, 1609–1614.

Harning, R., Cui, J. & Bystryn, J.-C. (1991) Relation between the incidence and level of pigment cell antibodies and disease activity in vitiligo. *Journal of Investigative Dermatology* **97**, 1078–1080.

Kemp, E.H., Gawkrodger, D.J., MacNeil, S., Watson, P.F. & Weetman, A. (1997) Detection of tyrosinase autoantibodies in patients with vitiligo using ^{35}S-labeled recombinant human tyrosinase in a radioimmunoassay. *Journal of Investigative Dermatology* **109**, 69–73.

Le Poole, I.C., van den Wijngaard, R.M., Westerhof, W. & Das, P.K. (1996) Presence of T cells and macrophages in inflammatory vitiligo skin parallels melanocyte disappearance. *American Journal of Pathology* **148**, 1219–1228.

Mitchell, M.S., Nordlund, J.J. & Lerner, A.B. (1980) Comparison of cell-mediated immunity to melanoma cells in patients with vitiligo, halo nevi, or melanoma. *Journal of Investigative Dermatology* **75**, 144.

Naughton, G.K., Eisinger, M. & Bystryn, J.-C. (1983) Antibodies to normal human melanocytes in vitiligo. *Journal of Experimental Medicine* **158**, 246–251.

Naughton, G.K., Mahaffey, M. & Bystryn, J.-C. (1986a) Antibodies to surface antigens of pigmented cells in animals with vitiligo. *Proceedings of the Society for Experimental Biology and Medicine* **181**, 423–426.

Naughton, G.K., Reggiardo, M.D. & Bystryn, J.-C. (1986b) Correlation between vitiligo antibodies and extent of depigmentation in vitiligo. *Journal of the American Academy of Dermatology* **15**, 978–981.

Norris, D.A., Capin, L., Muglia, J.J. *et al.* (1988) Enhanced susceptibility of melanocytes of different immunologic effector mechanisms *in vitro*: potential mechanisms for postinflammatory hypopigmentation and vitiligo. *Pigment Cell Research Supplement* **1**, 113–123.

Song, Y.H., Connor, E., Li, Y. *et al.* (1994) The role of tyrosinase in autoimmune vitiligo. *Lancet* **344**, 1049–1052.

Tobin, D.J. & Bystryn, J.-C. (1996) Different populations of melanocytes are present in hair follicles and epidermis. *Pigment Cell Research* **9**, 304–310.

Yu, H.-S., Kao, C.-H. & Yu, C.-L. (1993) Co-existence and relationship of antikeratinocyte and antimelanocyte antibodies in patients with non-segmental-type vitiligo. *Journal of Investigative Dermatology* **100**, 823–828.

Xie, Z. & Bystryn, J.-C. (1996) Anti-tyrosinase antibodies in vitiligo. *Journal of Investigative Dermatology* **106**, 938.

17: Autocytotoxic Hypothesis for the Destruction of Melanocytes as the Cause of Vitiligo

SEUNG-KYUNG HANN AND WOO-HYUNG CHUN

The autocytotoxic theory for the destruction of melanocytes

Vitiligo is a disorder or group of disorders characterized by the destruction of some, or more commonly all, epidermal melanocytes. In the skin or hair, melanocytes are the sole source of the pigment melanin. Thus their disappearance results in a complete absence of melanin and the skin appears white. The mechanisms for the destruction of melanocytes are likely to be multiple and complex, possibly a composite of several normal processes influencing melanocyte function, proliferation and/or survival. The various theories extant to explain the disappearance of melanocytes from the epidermis are not all inclusive nor mutually exclusive. One theory is the autocytotoxic theory.

The autocytotoxic hypothesis is based on the observation that phenol and some of its derivatives are capable of preferentially killing pigment cells (Lerner & Nordlund 1978). Tyrosine, the substrate for the enzyme tyrosinase, is itself a derivative of phenol and has an alkyl-carboxylic acid chain attached in the position para to the hydroxy group. The tyrosine molecule is oxidized into melanin via a complex series of oxidative reactions, often accompanied by electronic rearrangements within molecules. Some of these products are unstable and capable of forming radicals that react with other molecules in the cell. It is thought that melanin synthesis is confined within the melanosome to prevent these melanin precursors from diffusing into the cell where they might disrupt essential metabolic pathways.

A large number of melanin precursors, derivatives of phenol or hydroquinone with aromatic (monobenzyl ether of hydroquinone) or aliphatic side chains in this particular position (such as para tert butyl phenol, 4 isopropyl catechol) have been identified, which are known to be capable of destroying pigment cells both *in vitro* and also in the skin of some individuals exposed to these chemicals. There are a number of ways in which phenolic derivatives might destroy a melanocyte.

Phenols and free radicals

Bleehen *et al.* (1968) suggested destruction of melanocytes resulted from free radical formation from or by exogenous phenolic compounds. Riley (1970) suggested that an enhanced phenol production is more likely in individuals with certain genes that he labelled vitiligo genes, that is, susceptibility genes. Excessive quantities of toxic by-products generated either in the epidermis or upper dermis damaged the melanocyte that seems to have a limited ability to proliferate and replace dying or dead cells.

Genetic protective mechanisms

Lerner (1971) postulated that melanocytes have a genetically based protective mechanism that eliminates any toxic precursors or by-products (such as dopa, DOPAchrome, 5,6-dihydroxyindole) produced during the synthesis of melanin. In individuals of kinships sharing certain genes, these genetic protective mechanisms are deficient. There is an accumulation of melanocytotoxic products causing the death of pigment cells. The end result clinically is depigmentation.

Membrane permeability

Wick (1977) noted that the outer membranes of melanosomes are normally responsible for retarding or blocking the diffusion of the toxic intermediary products of melanin synthesis into the cytoplasm and nucleus where they might cause irreversible damage and death to the cell. Defects either inherited or acquired in the membranes of melanosomes probably would result in the demise of the melanocytes.

Peroxidation of membrane lipids

Riley (1970) suggested that depigmentation produced by infusions of hydroxyanisole is brought about by the formation of semiquinone free radicals. He suggested the hydroxyanisole is taken up like tyrosine into the melanosome where it is oxidized by the enzyme tyrosinase. It can only be partially oxidized and forms a semiquinone. These compounds diffuse out of the melanosomes to initiate the chain of peroxidation of lipids in the membranes of mitochondria or the cell itself. The peroxidation causes damage to critical cellular organelles and ultimately the selective destruction of melanocytes. However, neither semiquinone free radicals nor increased levels of the two tyrosine derivatives described by Brun (1972) have been found in vitiliginous skin. These four ways by which phenolic derivatives might kill melanocytes are not mutually incompatible nor all inclusive.

Chemical leukoderma

There are many *in vitro* observations that suggest or confirm a toxic role for tyrosine-like molecules, melanin precursors or by-products. Chemicals with structures similar to melanin intermediates have been added to cultures of melanocytes or melanoma cells. The cells undergo cytolysis (Wick 1987; Prezioso *et al.* 1990). Most of the chemicals that have a cytotoxic potential are phenols and quinones. Brun (1972) suggested that vitiligo might be due to the inhibitory action on the tyrosine-tyrosinase system by a phenolic derivative which may be a degradative product of a normally occurring component in melanin synthesis. Such a chemical disrupts melanogenesis, possibly by competitive inhibition for tyrosinase and leads to melanocyte death. Graham *et al.* (1978) have shown that dopachrome produced during melanin synthesis is a highly toxic metabolite specifically for melanocytes.

Derivatives of hydroquinone (monobenzyl ether of hydroquinone), catechols or phenol applied to the skin of humans, or some animals, may induce vitiligo-like cutaneous depigmentation. Frenk (1969) reported the ultrastructure of chemically induced depigmentation to be similar to that of vitiligo. (See Chapter 32 for a detailed presentation about topical melanocytotoxic chemicals.) Many depigmenting agents show striking structural similarity to tyrosine or dopa. Brun (1972) observed two tyrosine derivatives, p-hydroxycinnamic acid and p-hydroxyphenylpyruvic acid to be strong inhibitors of melanogenesis. Tyrosine, dopa, and tryptophan (a second amino acid that also can be incorporated into the synthesis of melanin) show a selective cytotoxicity towards melanin-producing cells. Treatment of cells with phenylthiourea, a selective inhibitor of tyrosinase activity and melanin formation, completely protects the cells from the toxicity of the melanin precursors.

Melatonin and the melatonin receptor

Other investigators have suggested that melanin synthesis is disrupted by abnormalities of the melatonin receptor. Melatonin is derived from the pineal gland, the retina, cells in the gastrointestinal tract and, perhaps, other extrapineal sites. In amphibians and some mammals it is responsible for rapid decrease in colour and down-regulation of melanin formation (Slominski *et al.* 1989). That is, melatonin is a naturally occurring inhibitor and modulator of melanin synthesis (Logan & Weatherhead 1980). It exerts its regulatory role by an interaction with a specific receptor and is a product of the multistep conversion of L-tryptophan to serotonin and subsequently melatonin. The synthesis and secretion of melatonin are stimulated by catecholamines (Ebadi & Govitrapong 1986). Melatonin exhibits a host of activities including immunomodulatory and antitumour activities.

A defective receptor might result in the uncontrolled production of melanin with the release of free radicals and toxic products of melanogenesis. This process damages melanocytes by a build up of toxic products and free radicals generated during melanogenesis without a parallel increase in the production of the scavenger melanin. In addition, keratinocytes are damaged by toxic products released from melanocytes or by transport of metabolically active melanosomes into keratinocytes. Release of cellular proteins could provoke a secondary autoimmune response against intracellular or altered cell surface antigens on the melanocytes and increase the propensity of melanocytes to undergo malignant transformation. Other scavenger systems may also be defective and render the patient more vulnerable to toxic products generated. As a consequence, the melanocyte damage is magnified by a vicious cycle: decrease or loss of melanocyte support by keratinocytes within a functional pigmentary unit (Nordlund 1985).

Melatonin and the autoimmune hypothesis

A secondary autoimmune response to altered cell surface proteins on the damaged melanocytes and keratinocytes, as well as to intracellular antigens sharing homology with surface antigens, leads to an irreversible loss of melanocytes ('point of no return').

The melatonin receptor could be subject to abnormal activation by several mechanisms that include:

1 an increased concentration of melatonin in the skin caused by excessive production of melatonin in the pineal gland or in peripheral production sites (perhaps the skin) initiated by an increased release of catecholamines and other neurotransmitters;

2 a hereditary tendency toward expression of an increased number of melatonin receptors; and

3 a dysfunction of the melatonin receptor caused by an intrinsic activation without binding of ligand, activation by binding of a ligand other than melatonin or via stimulating autoantibodies against the melatonin receptor.

The latter speculation is suggested by the association of vitiligo with Grave's disease, which displays stimulatory autoantibodies against thyroid-stimulating hormone (TSH) receptors. The immunomodulatory properties of melatonin could further contribute to the autoimmune phenomena associated with vitiligo.

The melatonin hypothesis emphasizes the pivotal role of a hyperactive melatonin receptor in the initial phase of vitiligo pathogenesis, and stresses the interdependence of the different systems affected. All the experimental and clinical findings about vitiligo and depigmentation can be explained within the confines of the melatonin hypothesis, including the association with other autoimmune diseases, neurologic/psychiatric disorders and stress, melanoma, hereditary factors and Koebner's phenomenon. Spontaneous or therapeutically induced repigmentation of vitiligo skin lesions would be possible before the 'point of no return' has been reached. It has been suggested (but there are no data yet to confirm) that there is a higher incidence of vitiligo in patients with Addison's disease. If this supposition were true, the phenomenon could be explained by the stimulatory effect of melanocyte-stimulating hormone (MSH) and ACTH on the generation of toxic products and free radicals of melanogenesis.

Although the melatonin hypothesis is consistent with the many clinical observations about vitiligo, the theory is without any substantial experimental basis. For example, it is still necessary to establish that human melanocytes actually have functional melatonin receptors and that activation of these receptors can lead to a build up of toxic products of melanogenesis. There is no clinical evidence that melatonin has any role in the regulation of melanin production in humans. The recently reported finding that 5-methoxypsoralen actually increased melatonin serum levels in 11 normal volunteers awaits explanation (Souetre *et al.* 1987). In vitiligo, serum melatonin levels may be of minor relevance, as opposed to melatonin concentration in the skin and degree of receptor activation of the target cells.

Conclusion

The clinical and laboratory observations noted here provide some basis for the autocytotoxic theory for melanocyte destruction but much more work needs to be done before this hypothesis is confirmed. In the meantime, the pathogenesis of vitiligo remains a mystery.

References

Bleehen, S.S., Pathak, M.A., Hori, Y. & Fitzpatrick, T.B. (1968) Depigmentation of skin with 4-isopropylcatechol, mercaptoamines, and other compounds. *Journal of Investigative Dermatology* **50**, 103–117.

Brun, R. (1972) A propos de l'etiologie du vitiligo. *Dermatologica* **145**, 169–174.

Ebadi, M. & Govitrapong, P. (1986) Neural pathways and neurotransmitters affecting melatonin synthesis. *Journal of Neural Transmission* **21** (Suppl.), 125–155.

Frenk, E. (1969) Experimentelle Depigmentierung der Meerschweinchenhaut durch selektiv toxische Wirkung von Hydrochinon-monoathylather auf die Melanocyten. *Archiv Klinische und Experimentelle Dermatologie* **235**, 16–24.

Graham, D.G., Tiffany, S.M. & Vogel, F.S. (1978) The toxicity of melanin precursors. *Journal of Investigative Dermatology* **70**, 113–116.

Lerner, A.B. (1971) On the etiology of vitiligo and gray hair. *American Journal of Medicine* **51**, 141–147.

Lerner, A.B. & Nordlund, J.J. (1978) Vitiligo: loss of pigment in skin, hair and eyes. *Japanese Journal of Dermatology* **5**, 1–8.

Logan, A. & Weatherhead, B. (1980) Post-tyrosinase inhibition of eumelanogenesis by melatonin in hair follicles *in vitro*. *Journal of Investigative Dermatology* **74**, 47–50.

Nordlund, J.J. (1985) The pigmentary system: new interpretations of old data. *Journal of Dermatology* **12**, 105–116.

Prezioso, J.A., Fitzgerald, G.B. & Wick, M.M. (1990) Effects of tyrosinase activity on the cytotoxicity of 3,4-dihydroxybenzylamine and buthionine sulfoximine in human melanoma cells. *Pigment Cell Research* **3**, 49–54.

Riley, P.A. (1970) Mechanism of pigment cell toxicity produced by hydroxyanisole. *Journal of Pathology* **101**, 163–169.

Slominski, A., Paus, R. & Bomirski, A. (1989) Hypothesis: Possible role for the melatonin receptor in vitiligo: Discussion paper. *Journal of the Royal Society of Medicine* **82**, 539–541.

Souetre, E., Salvati, E., Belugou, J.L. *et al.* (1987) 5-Methoxypsolaren increases the plasma melatonin levels in humans. *Journal of Investigative Dermatology* **89**, 152–155.

Weatherhead, B. & Logan, A. (1981) Interaction of α-melanocyte stimulating hormone, melatonin, cyclic AMP and cyclic GMP in the control of melanogenesis in hair follicle melanocytes *in vitro*. *Journal of Endocrinology* **90**, 89–96.

Wick, M.M. (1977) 1-Dopa methyl ester as a new antitumour agent. *Nature* **269**, 512–513.

Wick, M.M. (1987) Inhibition of transformation by levodopa-carbodopa in lymphocytes derived from patients with melanoma. *Journal of Investigative Dermatology* **88**, 532–534.

18: Neural Pathogenesis

GIOVANNI E. ORECCHIA

Dedication: To my wife Laura

One commonly accepted theory for the pathogenesis of vitiligo is the neural hypothesis. The neural theory is supported by clinical, physiological, microscopic, ultrastructural, immunohistochemical and biochemical findings.

Clinical evidence for the neural hypothesis

Melanocytes are neural crest derived cells giving them an embryological link to the nervous system (Reedy *et al.* 1998). It is not surprising that an association between neurological disorders and skin pigmentation changes has been observed. Furthermore, melanocytes are known to be present in other areas besides the skin such as the retinal pigment epithelium, the uveal tract, the inner ear and the leptomeninges. Therefore it is plausible to think that whatever process destroys the melanocyte in the skin can also affect melanocytes and related cells in the central nervous system (Barnes 1988).

In lower vertebrate species, movement of melanosomes within pigment cells leading to skin colour change is regulated by autonomic nerve fibres (Fujii & Novales 1969). In humans, increased numbers of nerve fibres have been found in benign melanocyte skin lesions such as acquired and congenital naevi.

Disorders of the central nervous system like neurofibromatosis and tuberous sclerosis (epiloia) can present with hyperpigmentation and hypopigmentation of the skin (Koplon & Shapiro 1968; Zvulunov & Esterly 1995). Abnormal myelination of the brain has been demonstrated by magnetic resonance imaging scan in a young woman with vitiligo who also had segmental spinal muscular atrophy and a deletion of a portion of the long arm of chromosome 18 (Weiss *et al.* 1991).

The bacteria causing diseases like syphilis, leprosy and pinta characteristically infect both the nervous system and the skin producing pigmentary abnormalities (Mosher *et al.* 1993). In tuberculoid leprosy, depigmentation and anaesthesia coexist in areas innervated by the affected peripheral nerves (McDougall & Ulrich 1993).

Some cutaneous disorders have a dermatomal distribution such as herpes zoster. On occasion vitiligo appears to be dermatomal, such as in the area of the trigeminal nerve (Lerner 1959; Nordlund 1986). In fact, vitiligo has been described to follow peripheral nerve damage (Arnozan 1922). Vitiligo has developed in the area supplied by nerves damaged after a brachial plexus injury, suggesting that 'sympathetic repercussion' ended in depigmentation (Costea 1961).

Vitiligo has been associated with viral encephalitis (Nellhaus 1970) and with multiple sclerosis (Jonesco-Siseti *et al.* 1973).

One patient with a transverse myelitis, paralysed from the waist down, had vitiligo only in the upper part of the body and preservation of pigmentation in the areas below the level of cord damage (Lerner *et al.* 1966). Spontaneous repigmentation of extensive vitiligo was described in the areas made anaesthetic by diabetic neuropathy (Lerner 1972).

Physiological evidence for the neural hypothesis

Denervation modifies skin pigmentation in guinea pigs (Fabian 1951). Injections of acetylcholine, noradrenaline, adrenaline and melatonin into a frog cause lightening of the dermal melanocytes (Lerner 1959). In fish, electrical stimulation of cutaneous nerves induces blanching and sectioning of them or induces darkening (McBurney 1979). α-adrenergic stimulation lightens skin colour by dispersing melanosomes or darkens the skin by aggregating melanosomes (Zvulunov & Esterly 1995). These observations suggest that the peripheral nerves produce some factors that affect melanocytes (Lerner 1959). A dysfunction of some nervous function or structure (Panja 1977) might be involved in the pathogenesis of vitiligo.

In patients with the generalized form of vitiligo, studies conducted on sweating, skin temperature and bleeding times in depigmented and normal skin, revealed that surface temperature and sweat production were increased in vitiliginous skin and that the bleeding was prolonged compared to the normal skin. Injections of or iontophoresis with acetylcholine, epinephrine and histamine did not produce differences in sweating between depigmented and normal areas (Chanco-Turner & Lerner 1965). These findings are consistent either with cholinergic hyperactivity or a depressed adrenergic function in vitiliginous skin. In contrast, Gokhale found a decreased perspiration rate in generalized vitiligo (Gokhale *et al.* 1977).

In patients suffering from segmental vitiligo, Dutta observed abnormalities in vitiliginous skin. He tested blister resorption time, bleeding time and epinephrine vasoconstrictor effect (Dutta & Dermat 1972). However Gopinathan did not note any differences of cutaneous sensation and perspiration between normal and vitiliginous skin (Gopinathan 1965). The local nerve tonus was regarded by Dutta as a 'conditioning factor' of the longer blanch reaction after intradermal injection of epinephrine solution (Dutta & Mandal 1972).

Koga reported that the inhibitor of cholinesterase, physostigmine, induced an abnormal response of sweating much more frequently in patients with segmental vitiligo than in those with the generalized form

(Dutta & Mandal 1972). In segmental vitiligo the skin is likely to show adrenergic hypotonia in the early phases, whereas in later phases hyperactive adrenergic responses are observed (Koga 1977).

Sudomotor dysfunction has also been recently evidenced as an abnormal sympathetic response (Merello *et al.* 1993). Moreover, the importance of innervation is evidenced by surgical transplant studies. The grafted skin acquires the characteristics of the area where it is transplanted only after the local innervation has taken place (Haxthausen 1947; Spencer & Tolmach 1952; Eriksson *et al.* 1968).

A numerical decrease of active melanocytes in the inner ear, which results in an impairment of the ion exchange between the endolymph and perilymph, has been suggested to explain the abnormalities of the auditory brainstem response on vitiligo (Nikiforidis *et al.* 1993).

Microscopic and ultrastructural findings

Skin is innervated primarily by sensory nerves and by postganglionic parasympathetic and sympathetic fibres. Sensory nerves function as an afferent and as an efferent system able to stimulate target tissues by secreting several neuropeptides (Maggi & Meli 1988). Alteration of the neuroreceptor apparatus and dystrophic changes of nerve trunks and terminals have been previously reported in vitiligo (Chan-Gen 1959). Degenerative and regenerative changes in terminal regions of cutaneous nerves supplying central and marginal areas of vitiliginous lesions have been described (Mori 1964; Breathnach *et al.* 1966; Nozaky 1976).

There is a close overlap between the distribution of nerve fibres and some dermatological diseases. This seems true in vitiligo in which it has been demonstrated (Morohashi *et al.* 1977) that there is direct contact between cutaneous free nerve endings and epidermal melanocytes, as is observed in guinea pigs (Mihara *et al.* 1982). In vitiliginous skin, subtle, ultrastructural changes, including degeneration and regeneration, were consistently found in dermal nerves, with increased thickness of the basement membrane of Schwann cells. Regeneration was more prominent than degeneration in both marginal and central maculae, as evidenced by the great metabolic activity of both nerves and Schwann cells demonstrated by higher mitochondrial density, by increased rough endoplasmic reticulum and by small pockets of collagen entrapped in Schwann cells. The findings are consistent with remodelling and reorganization of Schwann cells (Al'Abadie *et al.* 1994).

Very recently an intimate physical connection of intra-epidermal axon terminals with melanocytes has been shown (Hara *et al.* 1996). There is thickening of pre- and postsynaptic membranes and vesicle aggregation, analogous to a nervous system synapse.

Immunohistochemical findings

The immunoreactivity of neuropeptide and neuronal markers was studied in lesional and marginal areas of vitiligo. The results support the concept of neuronal or neuropeptide involvement in vitiligo and, in particular, confirm a role for neuropeptide Y (NPY) in the pathogenesis of disease (Al'Abadie *et al.* 1994). An increased immunoreactivity for NPY was found around the vessels and in the dermis, the marginal areas and, to a lesser extent, in the lesional areas. The NPY is released by either exogenous stimuli (e.g. trauma, like in Koebner's phenomenon) or by endogenous stimuli (e.g. stress) (Al'Abadie *et al.* 1994).

An altered balance of neuropeptides in vitiliginous skin supports a role for the nervous system in the pathogenesis of vitiligo (Liu *et al.* 1996). In fact, a reduction in the number and intensity of low affinity (p75) immunoreactive nerve growth factor receptors (NGFr-IR) was demonstrated in vitiligo skin. The number of NGFr-IR nerve fibres was significantly increased. Moreover the number of immunoreactive calcitonin gene-related peptide (CGRP-IR) nerve fibres in the epidermis and in papillary dermis was greatly increased in vitiliginous skin (Cheng *et al.* 1995).

Neuropeptides are able to induce melanocyte dendricity and participate in the regulation of cell substrate adhesion and, ultimately, cell motility and shape (Rozengurt 1995). Neuropeptides may regulate melanin synthesis or affect melanosomal transfer to surrounding keratinocytes. NPY has been reported to regulate the secretory activity of melanin containing cells in *Xenopus laevis* (Scheenen *et al.* 1994).

Some neuropeptides are known to have immunoregulatory effects (Covelli & Jirillo 1988; Rameshwar *et al.* 1992), a potential link between the autoimmune hypothesis and the neural pathogenic theory of vitiligo. Moreover, neuropeptides can mediate alteration of sweating reported in vitiligo skin (Chanco-Turner & Lerner 1965) and vasoconstriction (Lerner 1972). Vasoconstriction might be an indirect cause of damage to melanocytes (Morrone *et al.* 1992).

Merkel cells seem to be absent from vitiliginous skin although normal in the surrounding epidermis (Bose 1994).

Biochemical evidence for the neural hypothesis

An increased release of catecholamines from the autonomic nerve endings in the microenvironment of melanocytes in the affected skin areas has been suggested, since changes in the content of epinephrine and norepinephrine in the blood of patients with vitiligo have been measured (Durneva 1973). More recently, the urine levels of homovanillic acid (HVA) and vanillmandelic acid (VMA) from dopamine and from norepinephrine and epinephrine, appeared to be elevated in subjects affected either with the early active phase or with the progression of vitiligo. A higher, although not significant, concentration of these neurotransmitters was found also in the plasma of patients with generalized and acrofacial vitiligo (Orecchia *et al.* 1994).

These neurotransmitters are known for having toxic properties by:

1 interacting with cellular sulphydryl groups,

2 inhibiting enzyme activities,

3 impairing some mitochondrial energy processes such as calcium uptake and

4 forming cytotoxic products such as free radicals, orthoquinones and hydroxylated indoles (Bindoli *et al.* 1992).

Besides a direct cytotoxicity, they could have an indirect action by activating α-receptors of skin arterioles causing a severe vasoconstriction. Hypoxia produces toxic oxygen radicals (Morrone *et al.* 1992).

An enormously high concentration of norepinephrine and its metabolites in vitiligo has been recently related to a decrease of phenylethanolamine-N-methyl transferase activity (PNMT) and an increased activity of tyrosine hydroxylase (TH), the key enzyme in the catecholamine pathway, producing L-dopa from L-tyrosine (Schallreuter *et al.* 1994b). The rate-limiting cofactor/electron donor for TH is (6R)-5,6,7,8-tetrahydrobiopterin (6-BH_4), which is increased due to a decreased 4a-hydroxy-6-BH_4 dehydratase (DH) activity (Schallreuter *et al.* 1994a). The presence of this nonenzymatic by-product in epidermis is supposed to initiate the process of depigmentation in the vitiligo, by blocking the supply of L-tyrosine either directly in the melanocytes or from the surrounding basal keratinocytes. These alterations are said to produce melanocyte dysfunction or injury (see Chapter 19).

A derangement of the enzymes dealing with catabolism of adrenergic transmitters has been reported, namely, catechol-o-methyltransferase (COMT) and monoamino oxidase (MAO-A). COMT normally prevents the formation of toxic orthoquinones during melanin synthesis. Epidermal homogenates from vitiligo patients express a higher COMT activity, probably induced in the tissues by elevated levels of catecholamines secreted by keratinocytes or by nerve endings. Toxic products may be damaging to the melanocytes because of their slow turnover rate (Le Poole *et al.* 1994). COMT activity is also related to decreased Ca^{2+} concentrations in vitiligo for a defective calcium uptake in keratinocytes (Schallreuter & Pittelkow 1988) and may contribute to depigmentation by decreasing the amount of precursor molecules available for melanin formation. This effect can be further aggravated by an increased expression of β_2-adrenoreceptors (Schallreuter *et al.* 1993), which regulate intracellular calcium concentrations (Koizumi *et al.* 1991) and are increased in numbers at low calcium levels (Schallreuter *et al.* 1993).

An alteration of calcium metabolism in vitiligo has been recently confirmed by a study on defective calcium transport in vitiliginous melanocytes (Schallreuter-Wood *et al.* 1996) correlating with reduced thioredoxin reductase/thioredoxin. Thioredoxin functions as an allosteric inhibitor of tyrosinase through an increase of the concentration of hydrogen peroxide in the epidermis of vitiligo patients (Schallreuter *et al.* 1991).

A consequence of increased norepinephrine appears to be the induction of another catecholamine degrading enzyme, the monoamino oxidase (MAO-A) (Bindoli *et al.* 1992). The increased MAO-A activity favours the formation of toxic levels of hydrogen peroxide (Schallreuter *et al.* 1996). The damage to the melanocytes is not buffered by the low catalase activity (Schallreuter *et al.* 1996).

Since stress also influences the catecholamine secretion, a trial correlating their levels with the personality structure of vitiligo patients has been made (Salzer & Schallreuter 1995), correlating the neurotransmitter patterns with the diagnosis, treatment, and pathophysiology of several neurogenetic disorders (Goldstein *et al.* 1996).

The effect of acetylcholine, another neurotransmitter, was studied. The acetylcholine esterase activity is lowered in vitiliginous skin during depigmentation, giving further support to the neural influences on the pathogenesis of vitiligo (Iyengar 1989).

References

Al'Abadie, M.S., Senior, H.J., Bleehen, S.S. & Gawkrodger, D.J. (1994) Neuropeptide and neuronal marker studies in vitiligo. *British Journal of Dermatology* **131**, 160–165.

Arnozan, L. (1922) Vitiligo avec troubles nerveus sensitifs et sympathetiques: l'origine sympathique du vitiligo. *Bulletin de la Societe Francaise de Dermatologie et de Syphiligraphie* **29**, 338–342.

Barnes, L. (1988) Vitiligo and the Vogt-Koyanagi–Harada syndrome. *Dermatologic Clinics* **6**, 229–239.

Bindoli, A., Rigobello, M.P. & Deeble, D.J. (1992) Biochemical and toxicological properties of the oxidation products of catecholamines. *Free Radical Biology and Medicine* **13**, 391–405.

Bose, S.K. (1994) Probable mechanisms of loss of Merkel cells in completely depigmented skin of stable vitiligo. *Journal of Dermatology* **21**, 725–728.

Breathnach, A.S., Bor, S. & Wyllie, L.M. (1966) Electron microscopy of peripheral nerve terminals and marginal melanocytes in vitiligo. *Journal of Investigative Dermatology* **47**, 125–140.

Chanco-Turner, M.L. & Lerner, A.B. (1965) Physiologic changes in vitiligo. *Archives of Dermatology* **91**, 390–396.

Chan-Gen, S. (1959) Changes of the neuroreceptor apparatus in vitiligo. *Vestnik Dermatologii I Venerologii* **33**, 20–24.

Cheng, L., Khan, M. & Mudge, A.W. (1995) Calcitonin gene-related peptide promotes Schwann cell proliferation. *Journal of Cell Biology* **129**, 789–796.

Costea, V. (1961) Leukoderma patches in the course of traumatic paralysis of the brachial plexus in a subject with insular cavities. *Dermatovenerologica* **2**, 161–166.

Covelli, V. & Jirillo, E. (1988) Neuropeptides with immunoregulatory function: current status of investigations. *Functional Neurology* **3**, 253–261.

Durneva, S.G. (1973) Changes in the content of epinephrine and norepinephrine in the blood of patients with vitiligo. *Vestnik Dermatologii I Venerologii* **47**, 33–36.

Dutta, A.K. & Dermat, D. (1972) Non-nervous vascular reactions in vitiligo patches (an experimental study). *Indian Journal of Dermatology* **17**, 29–36.

Dutta, A.K. & Mandal, S.B. (1972) A study of non-nervous vasoconstrictor responses. *International Journal of Dermatology* **11**, 177–180.

Eriksson, G.P., Klingenstroem, B., Nylen, B. & Wersaell, J. (1968) Electron microscopic studies on the epidermis in human split-skin auto-graft. *Scandinavian Journal of Plastic and Reconstructive Surgery and Hand Surgery* **2**, 83–90.

Fabian, G. (1951) The spread of black pigment of the denervated skin of the guinea pig. *Acta Biologica Academiae Scientiarum Hungaricae* **4**, 471–480.

Fujii, R. & Novales, R.R. (1969) Cellular aspects of the control of physiological color changes in fish. *American Zoologist* **9**, 453–463.

Gokhale, B.B., Mebta, L.N. & Damle, P.S. (1977) Skin resistance to electric current and its correlation with sweat gland histology in vitiligo. *Indian Journal of Medical Research* **66**, 859–864.

Goldstein, D.S., Lenders, J.W., Kaler, S.G. & Eisenhofer, G. (1996) Catecholamine phenotyping: clues to the diagnosis, treatment and pathophysiology of neurogenetic disorders. *Journal of Neurochemistry* **67**, 1781–1790.

Gopinathan, T. (1965) A study of the lesion of vitiligo. *Archives of Dermatology* **91**, 397–404.

Hara, M., Toyoda, M., Yaar, M., Bahawan, J., Avila, E.M., Penner, I.R. & Gilchrest, B.A. (1996) Innervation of melanocytes in human skin. *Journal of Experimental Medicine* **184**, 1385–1395.

Haxthausen, H. (1947) Studies on the pathogenesis of morphea, vitiligo and acrodermatitis atrophicans by means of transplantation experiments. *Acta Dermato-Venereologica (Stockholm)* **27**, 352.

Iyengar, B. (1989) Modulation of melanocytic activity by acetylcholine. *Acta Anatomica* **136**, 139–141.

Jonesco-Siseti, M.M., Vasilesco, N. & Palade, G. (1973) Sclerose en plaques avec syndrome of Claude Bernard-Homer et vitiligo. *Bulletins et Memoires de la Societe Medicale de Hopitaux de Paris* **53**, 941–944.

Koga, M. (1977) Vitiligo: a new classification and therapy. *British Journal of Dermatology* **97**, 255–261.

Koizumi, H., Yasui, C., Fukaya, T., Ohkawara, A. & Ueda, T. (1991) Beta-adrenergic stimulation induces intracellular calcium increase in human epidermal keratinocytes. *Journal of Investigative Dermatology* **96**, 234–237.

Koplon, B.S. & Shapiro, L. (1968) Poliosis overlying a neurofibroma. *Archives of Dermatology* **98**, 631–633.

Le Poole, I.C., van den Wijngaard, R.M., Smit, N.P., Oosting, J., Westerhof, W. & Pavel, S. (1994) Catechol-O-methyltransferase in vitiligo. *Archives of Dermatological Research—Archiv für dermatologische Forschung* **286**, 81–86.

Lerner, A.B. (1959) Vitiligo. *Journal of Investigative Dermatology* **32**, 285–310.

Lerner, A.B. (1972) Vitiligo. *Progress in Dermatology* **6**, 1–6.

Lerner, A.B., Snell, R.S., Chanco-Turner, M.L. & McGuire, J.S. (1966) Vitiligo and sympathectomy. The effect of sympathectomy and alpha-melanocyte stimulating hormone. *Archives of Dermatology* **94**, 269–278.

Liu, P.Y., Bondesson, L., Loentz, W. & Tohansson, O. (1996) The occurrence of cutaneous nerve endings and neuropeptides in vitiligo vulgaris: a case-control study. *Archives of Dermatological Research—Archiv für dermatologische Forschung* **288**, 670–675.

Maggi, C.A. & Meli, A. (1988) The sensory-efferent function of capsaicinsensitive sensory neurons. *General Pharmacology* **19**, 1–43.

McBurney, E.I. (1979) Vitiligo. Clinical picture and pathogenesis. *Archives of Internal Medicine* **139**, 1295–1297.

McDougall, A.C. & Ulrich, M.I. (1993) Mycobacterial disease: leprosy. In: *Dermatology in General Medicine*, Vol. 1 (eds T.B.Fitzpatrick, A.Z.Eisen, K.Wolff, I.M.Freedberg & K.F.Austen), 4th edn, pp. 2395–2410. McGraw-Hill, New York.

Merello, M., Nogues, M., Leiguarda, R., Lopez Saubidet, C. & Florin, A. (1993) Abnormal sympathetic skin response in patients with autoimmune vitiligo and primary autoimmune hypothyroidism. *Journal of Neurology* **240**, 72–74.

Mihara, M., Hashimoto, K. & Kumakiri, M. (1982) Intraepidermal free nerve endings relating to epidermal melanocytes in spotted guinea pigs. A statistical and electron microscopic study. *Journal of Dermatology* **9**, 63–72.

Mori, H. (1964) Neurohistological studies on vitiligo vulgaris skin with special reference to vegetative nerves. *Japanese Journal of Dermatology* **74**, 411–431.

Morohashi, M., Hashimoto, K., Goodman, T.F. Jr, Newton, D.E. & Rist, T. (1977) Ultrastructural studies of vitiligo, Vogt–Koyanagi syndrome, and incontinentia pigmenti achromians. *Archives of Dermatology* **113**, 755–766.

Morrone, A., de Picardo, M., Luca, C., Terminali, O., Passi, S. & Ippolito, F. (1992) Catecholamines and vitiligo. *Pigment Cell Research* **5**, 65–69.

Mosher, D., Fitzpatrick, T., Hori, H. & Ortonne, J.-P. (1993) Disorders of pigmentation. In: *Dermatology in General Medicine* (eds T.Fitzpatrick, A.Eisen, K.Wolff, I.Freedberg & K.Austen), 4th edn, pp. 903–995. McGraw-Hill, New York.

Nellhaus, G. (1970) Acquired unilateral vitiligo and poliosis of the head and subacute encephalitis with partial recovery. *Neurology* **20**, 961–974.

Nikiforidis, G.C., Tsambaos, D.G., Karamitsos, D.S., Koutsojannis, C.C. & Georgiou, S.V. (1993) Abnormalities of the auditory brainstem response in vitiligo. *Scandinavian Audiology* **22**, 97–100.

Nordlund, J.J. (1986) Vitiligo. In: *Pathogenesis of Skin Diseases* (eds B.H.Thiers & R.L.Dobson), pp. 99–127. Churchill Livingston, New York.

Nozaky, T. (1976) Histochemical and electronmicroscopic studies of peripheral nerve terminals and clinical studies in vitiligo vulgaris. *Japanese Journal of Dermatology* **86**, 1–19.

Orecchia, G., Frattini, P., Cucchi, M.L. & Santagostino, G. (1994) Normal-range plasma catecholamines in patients with generalized and acrofacial vitiligo: preliminary report. *Dermatology* **189**, 350–353.

Panja, R.K. (1977) Etiology of vitiligo—a problem. *Indian Journal of Dermatology, Venereology and Leprology* **43**, 185–189.

Rameshwar, P., Gascon, P. & Ganea, D. (1992) Immunoregulatory effects of neuropeptides: Stimulation of interleukin-2 production by substance P. *Journal of Neuroimmunology* **37**, 65–74.

Reedy, M.V., Parichy, D.M., Erickson, C.A., Mason, K.A. & Frost-Mason, S.K. (1998) Regulation of melanoblast migration and differentiation. In: *The Pigmentary System. Physiology and Pathophysiology* (eds J.J.Nordlund, R.E.Boissy, V.J.Hearing, R.A.King & J.-P.Ortonne), pp. 75–95. Oxford University Press, New York.

Rozengurt, E. (1995) Convergent signalling in the action of integrins, neuropeptides, growth factors and oncogenes. *Cancer Surveys* **24**, 81–96.

Salzer, B.A. & Schallreuter, K.U. (1995) Investigation of the personality structure in patients with vitiligo and a possible association with impaired catecholamine metabolism. *Dermatology* **190**, 109–115.

Schallreuter, K.U. & Pittelkow, M.R. (1988) Defective calcium uptake system in vitiligo. *Archives of Dermatological Research—Archiv für dermatologische Forschung* **280**, 137–139.

Schallreuter, K.U., Wood, J.M. & Berger, J. (1991) Low catalase levels in the epidermis of patients with vitiligo. *Journal of Investigative Dermatology* **97**, 1081–1085.

Schallreuter, K.U., Wood, J.M., Pittelkow, M.R., Swanson, N.N. & Steinkraus, V. (1993) Increased *in vitro* expression of beta 2-adrenoceptors in differentiating lesional keratinocytes of vitiligo patients. *Archives of Dermatological Research—Archiv für dermatologische Forschung* **285**, 216–220.

Schallreuter, K.U., Wood, J.M., Pittelkow, M.R., Gutlich, M., Lemke, K.R., Rodl, W., Swanson, N.N., Hitzemann, K. & Ziegler, I. (1994a) Regulation of melanin biosynthesis in the human epidermis by tetrahydrobiopterin. *Science* **263**, 1444–1446.

Schallreuter, K.U., Wood, J.M., Ziegler, I., Lemke, R., Pittelkow, M.R., Lindsey, N.J. & Gutlich, M. (1994b) Defective tetrahydrobiopterin and catecholamine biosynthesis in the depigmentation disorder vitiligo. *Biochimica et Biophysica Acta* **1226**, 181–192.

Schallreuter, K.U., Wood, J.M., Pittelkow, M.R., Buttner, G., Swanson, N., Korner, C. & Ehrke, C. (1996) Increased monoamine oxidase A activity in the epidermis of patients with vitiligo. *Archives of Dermatological Research—Archiv für dermatologische Forschung* **288**, 14–18.

Schallreuter-Wood, K.U., Pittelkow, M.R. & Swanson, N.N. (1996) Defective calcium transport in vitiliginous melanocytes. *Archives of Dermatological Research—Archiv für dermatologische Forschung* **288**, 12–13.

Scheenen, W.J., Jenks, B.G., Willems, P.H. & Roubos, E.W. (1994) Action of stimulatory and inhibitory α-MSH secretagogues on spontaneous calcium oscillations in melanotrope cells of Xenopus laevis. *European Journal of Physiology* **427**, 244–251.

Spencer, G.A. & Tolmach, J.A. (1952) Exchange grafts in vitiligo. *Journal of Investigative Dermatology* **19**, 1–5.

Weiss, B.J., Kamholz, J., Ritter, A., Zackai, E.H., McDonald-McGinn, D.M., Emanuel, B. & Fischbeck, K.H. (1991) Segmental spinal muscular atrophy and dermatological findings in a patient with chromosome 18q deletion. *Annals of Neurology* **30**, 419–423.

Zvulunov, A. & Esterly, N.B. (1995) Neurocutaneous syndromes associated with pigmentary skin lesions. (Review). *Journal of the American Academy of Dermatology* **32**, 915–935.

19: Biochemical Theory of Vitiligo: a Role of Pteridines in Pigmentation

KARIN U. SCHALLREUTER, WAYNE D. BEAZLEY AND JOHN M. WOOD

Introduction

Vitiligo is an acquired idiopathic depigmentation disorder affecting 0.5–4% of the world population (Ortonne & Bose 1993). A significant decrease in the numbers of functioning epidermal melanocytes or their complete absence in the white skin of affected individuals has been described (Gokhale & Mehta 1983; Le Poole *et al.* 1993a, Chapters 1 and 2). There have been several hypotheses proposed in the past but none of them seems to cover the entire spectrum of this enigmatic disorder.

The clinical hallmarks of vitiligo are white patches together with normal pigmented skin in the same individual (Fitzpatrick *et al.* 1979). The diagnosis is usually made by eye because the distribution and localization is, in the majority, characterized by symmetrical appearance. However, there are also clinical forms of the disease which can mimic other clinical leukodermas (Ortonne & Bose 1993). A very simple clinical observation has been useful to overcome this difficulty. We suggest that, upon Wood's light examination at 351 nm the clinically white skin of vitiligo shows a characteristic yellow/green or bluish fluorescence, whereas we propose that other leukodermas lack this phenomenon (Schallreuter *et al.* 1994b, c) (Fig. 19.1). We attribute this fluorescence originates in the accumulation of two different oxidized pteridines, 6-biopterin with a bluish fluorescence and 7-biopterin, its isomer, with yellow/green fluorescence (Schallreuter *et al.* 1994b, c).

What are these pteridines and what is their physiological role/function?

More than a hundred years ago, Frederick Gowland Hopkins isolated a yellow pigment from the English Brimstone butterfly and the white pigment from the Cabbage White butterfly (Hopkins 1889). In 1925 Wieland and Schöpf introduced these pigments as pteridines and named them according to their colours, xanthopterin and leucopterin. The discovery of the natural pteridines opened the field of pteridine chemistry.

(6R)-L-erythro 5,6,7,8 tetrahydrobiopterin ($6BH_4$) is the essential cofactor/electron donor for various intracellular metabolic steps including the hydroxylation of the aromatic amino acids L-phenylalanine, L-tyrosine and L-tryptophan (Ziegler 1990). In addition, nitric oxide synthase requires $6BH_4$

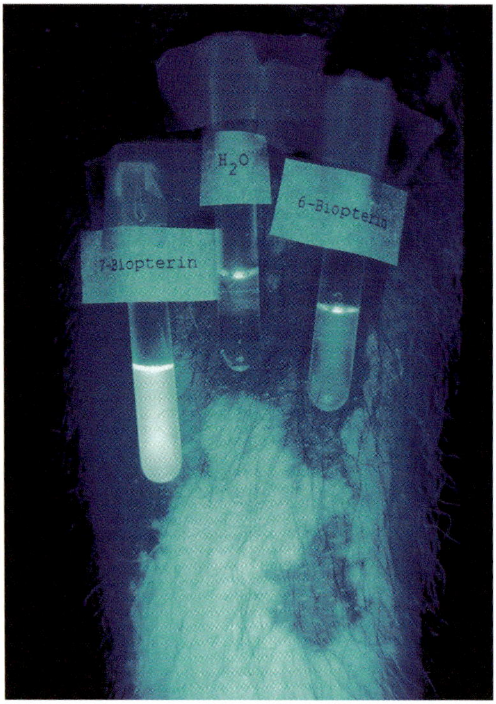

Fig. 19.1 The fluorescence of involved skin in vitiligo. Typical fluorescence of involved skin on the leg of a patient with vitiligo upon Wood's light examination. This patient expresses a more yellow/green colour in accordance with the presence of 7-biopterin, while in the surrounding pigmented areas melanins quench the fluorescence.

for activity, and there is accumulating evidence that pteridines are synthesized during activation of cell-mediated immunity and haematopoiesis (Ziegler 1990). $6BH_4$ is synthesized *de novo* from guanosine triphosphate (GTP) via the rate limiting enzyme GTP-cyclohydrolase I, followed by two steps involving 6-pyruvoyl tetrahydropterin synthase and sepiapterin reductase. The cofactor serves for phenylalanine hydroxylase in the presence of oxygen (O_2) to convert the essential amino acid L-phenylalanine to L-tyrosine, and the metabolic intermediate 4a-carbinolamine. This reaction starts the recycling of the cofactor. Additionally, a nonenzymatic by-product (7R)-L-erythro 5,6,7,8 tetrahydrobiopterin ($7BH_4$), is formed (Curtius *et al.* 1990). Under physiological conditions $7BH_4$ production appears to be negligible. The function and purpose of $7BH_4$ at these low concentrations has escaped definition so far. The next step in the cycling process involves the important enzyme/transcription factor 4a-OH-tetrahydrobiopterin dehydratase (synonyms: phenylalanine hydroxylase stimulating factor; 4a-carbinolamine dehydratase) for dehydration of 4a-carbinolamine to produce quinonoid dihydropterin (qBH_2), which is further reduced by dihydropteridine reductase to $6BH_4$. The pathway for $6BH_4$ *de novo* synthesis/recycling is presented in Fig. 19.2.

Pteridines in the human epidermis

The presence of the entire $6BH_4$ *de novo* synthesis/recycling mechanism has been recognized in human epidermal cell extracts, as well as in cell extracts

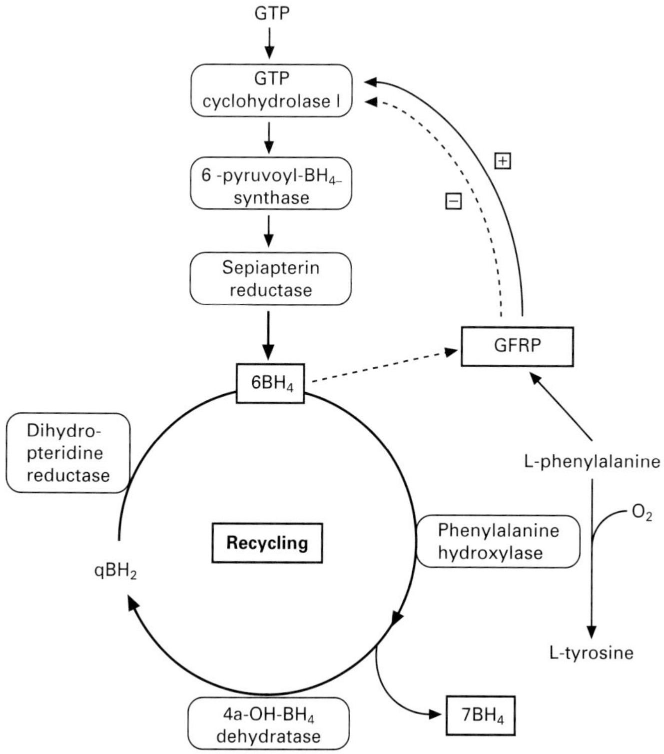

Fig. 19.2 Scheme for the *de novo* synthesis and recycling of $6BH_4$. GTP-cyclohydrolase I is the rate-limiting enzyme for *de novo* synthesis of $6BH_4$ from GTP, involving two other steps. This cofactor serves phenylalanine hydroxylase in the presence of O_2 for the conversion of the essential amino acid L-phenylalanine to L-tyrosine. During this metabolic step $7BH_4$ is nonenzymatically produced from the intermediate 4a-carbinolamine. The latter is the substrate for 4a-OH-tetrahydrobiopterin dehydratase forming qBH_2, which is further reduced to $6BH_4$. The growth factor regulatory protein (GFRP) may be bound by phenylalanine, up-regulating GTP-cyclohydrolase I, or by $6BH_4$, down-regulating this key enzyme.

from cultured melanocytes and keratinocytes (Schallreuter *et al.* 1994b,c). Enzyme activities and expression of specific mRNA for all of the enzymes involved in this biosynthetic pathway have been demonstrated. Only very recently the presence of 4a-OH-tetrahydrobiopterin dehydratase in epidermal keratinocytes has been confirmed by Lei *et al.* (1997). Taking these results into consideration, they would imply that under physiological conditions the cofactor $6BH_4$ is crucial, in both melanocytes and keratinocytes, to drive phenylalanine hydroxylase enzyme activity for synthesis of L-tyrosine from the essential amino acid L-phenylalanine. L-tyrosine represents the central substrate for catecholamine synthesis in keratinocytes and for melanogenesis in melanocytes (Prota 1992; Naoi & Parvez 1993). Moreover, $6BH_4$ is also the rate limiting step for catecholamine synthesis via tyrosine hydroxylase and controls tyrosinase activity in melanocytes by uncompetitive inhibition of a specific tetrahydrobiopterin binding domain on this enzyme (Wood *et al.* 1995).

The importance of epidermal pteridine redox status

The redox status of the pteridines controls $6BH_4$-dependent enzyme activities where the oxidized pterins are inactive (Schallreuter-Wood & Wood 1995; Wood *et al.* 1995). However, it has been demonstrated that 2×10^{-7} M 6-biopterin is cytotoxic to human melanocytes under *in vitro* conditions (Schallreuter *et al.* 1994a). The ubiquitous antioxidant system thioredoxin/thioredoxin reductase (T/TR) has the capacity to reduce the oxidized biopterin back to qBH_2 (Wood *et al.* 1995) (Fig. 19.2). The presence of specific mRNA as well as activities for the T/TR system in epidermal melanocytes and keratinocytes has been identified earlier. Since the T/TR system is under allosteric regulation by calcium via a single EF-hands binding site on TR, it can be concluded that the redox status of the pteridines is under control of this important ion (Schallreuter & Wood 1991). Furthermore, it has also been recognized that the levels of the cofactor $6BH_4$ are controlled by a GTP-cyclohydrolase I feedback regulatory protein (GFRP). L-phenylalanine binds to GFRP causing an up-regulation of the rate-limiting enzyme GTP-cyclohydrolase I (positive feedback), whereas $6BH_4$ exerts the opposite effect (Harada *et al.* 1993; Milstien *et al.* 1996). The presence of specific mRNA for GFRP has only recently been identified in melanocytes and keratinocytes for the first time (Schallreuter *et al.* 1998).

Overproduction of 6- and 7-tetrahydrobiopterins in vitiligo

In vitiligo an overproduction of $6BH_4$, in association with a micromolar accumulation of the isomer $7BH_4$, indicates a metabolic defect in tetrahydrobiopterin homeostasis in these patients (Schallreuter *et al.* 1994b, c). How can these observations be reconciled in the depigmentation process of this disorder?

So far two major causes for the overproduction of the tetrahydrobiopterins have been identified:

1 there is increased activity of GTP-cyclohydrolase I, the key enzyme in *de novo* synthesis of $6BH_4$;

2 there is defective recycling of $6BH_4$ in association with significantly impaired 4a-OH-tetrahydrobiopterin dehydratase activities. This low enzyme activity leads to increased nonenzymatic production of $7BH_4$, concomitant with an increased production of hydrogen peroxide (H_2O_2), via an enhanced short circuit in the recycling process.

Earlier it was established by several groups that $7BH_4$ can competitively inhibit $6BH_4$, binding on phenylalanine hydroxylase (Adler *et al.* 1992; Davis *et al.* 1992). This specific enzyme inhibition was also demonstrated in epidermal cell extracts from patients with vitiligo. As a consequence, a build up of epidermal L-phenylalanine followed by a shortage of L-tyrosine can be predicted (Fig. 19.3).

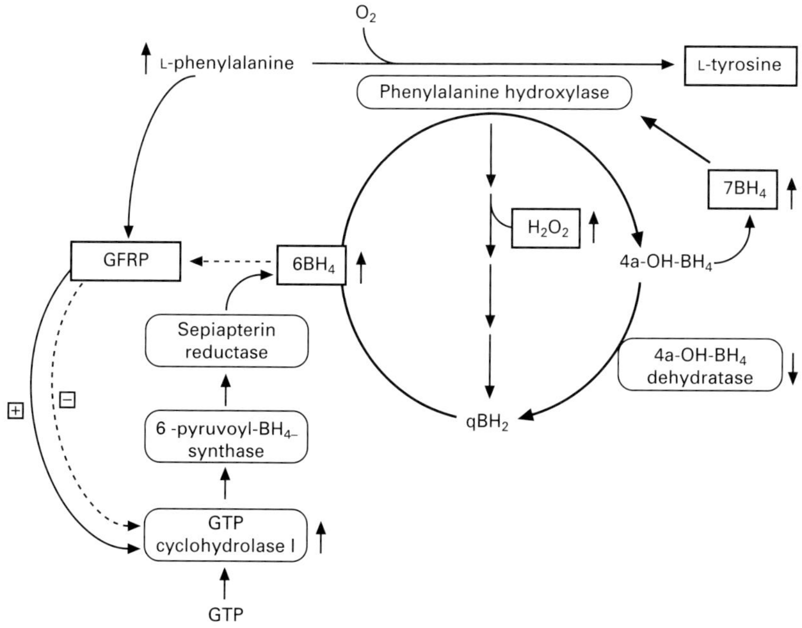

Fig. 19.3 Scheme for overproduction of $6BH_4$ in vitiligo. An increase in epidermal L-phenylalanine levels would lead to increased activity of GTP-cyclohydrolase I and an accumulation of $6BH_4$ via the regulatory protein GFRP. Decreased 4a-OH-tetrahydrobiopterin dehydratase activities result in defective $6BH_4$ recycling and subsequent H_2O_2 production. There is a concomitant build-up of $7BH_4$, which competitively inhibits $6BH_4$ binding to phenylalanine hydroxylase, reducing epidermal conversion of L-phenylalanine to L-tyrosine. The feedback mechanism of $6BH_4$ on its rate-limiting enzyme GTP-cyclohydrolase I via GFRP appears to be defective in vitiligo.

Impaired L-phenylalanine turnover in vitiligo

This hypothesis has been tested very recently using noninvasive Fourier Transform Raman spectroscopy directly *in vivo* on patients ($n = 23$) and on age and sex matched control skin ($n = 10$). The results demonstrated unambiguously that all patients had higher levels of phenylalanine in their white skin compared to their normal skin (Fig. 19.4a). This observation was further substantiated with *in vivo* studies, where the individual phenylalanine hydroxylase activities were followed in patients ($n = 32$) and in controls ($n = 10$) over 4 hours after a single oral loading with L-phenylalanine. The results showed that all patients had a slower turnover from L-phenylalanine to L-tyrosine, but 41% of the patients were significantly slower ($P = 0.0001$). However, all patients returned to normal levels after 4 hours, underlining that these patients do not express a peripheral hyperphenylalaninemia under normal conditions (Schallreuter *et al.* 1998) (Fig. 19.4b). These results also confirmed earlier studies, where patients with vitiligo never displayed any evidence for a peripheral accumulation of this essential amino acid (Cormane *et al.* 1985).

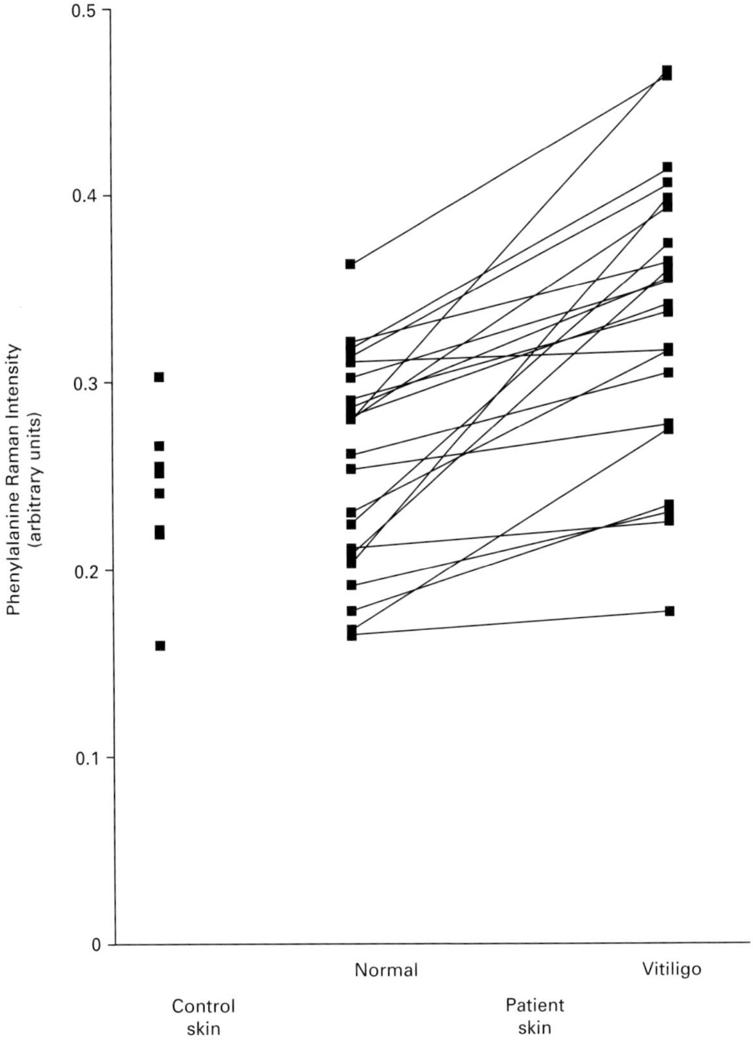

(a)

Fig. 19.4 (a) Epidermal phenylalanine levels. FT-Raman spectroscopy was utilized *in vivo* to determine epidermal phenylalanine concentrations. All patients ($n = 23$) showed higher levels in their involved skin compared to their uninvolved skin. Levels between healthy controls and uninvolved skin did not differ significantly. (b) L-phenylalanine turnover in vitiligo patients and controls. After a single oral loading with L-phenylalanine (100 mg/kg), the turnover of this essential amino acid to L-tyrosine was followed over four hours in 32 patients and 10 healthy controls. In all vitiligo patients, L-phenylalanine clearance was significantly slower than in controls, returning almost back to normal after four hours. The patient group could be divided into two subsets with 13 patients yielding phenylalanine to tyrosine ratios between 4.0 and 7.0 (■–■), and the remaining 19 patients revealing a normal phenylalanine to tyrosine ratio, <4.0. This second subset had a less hindered L-phenylalanine clearance (Δ–Δ) compared to controls (o–o).

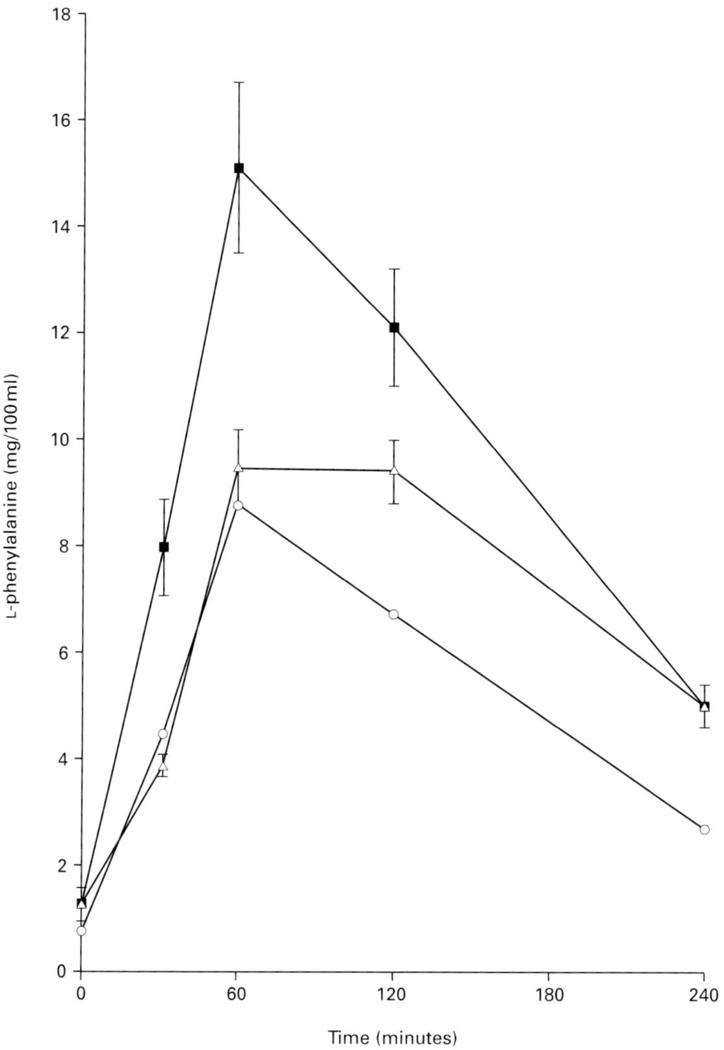

(b)

Fig. 19.4 *Continued.*

One consequence of increased epidermal L-phenylalanine levels would be the positive feedback on the *de novo* synthesis of $6BH_4$, via the regulatory protein GFRP (Harada *et al.* 1993). This would lead to increased activity of GTP-cyclohydrolase I, and therefore enhance the production of $6BH_4$. This cascade of events has been observed in vitiligo. Under physiological conditions, once there is sufficient amount of cofactor, enzyme activities should be down-regulated via the regulatory protein GFRP. However, this step does not appear to function properly in vitiligo because concentrations of $6BH_4$ accumulate to approximately 10^{-6} M. In addition the defective recycling of $6BH_4$ leads to the formation of micromolar levels of $7BH_4$ and H_2O_2 in the epidermis of these patients (Schallreuter *et al.* 1994b, c). The oxidative stress in vitiligo caused by H_2O_2 will be discussed in more detail in our chapter on pseudocatalase (Chapter 23). However, there is increasing evidence that epidermal $7BH_4$-inhibited phenylalanine hydroxylase considerably hampers the epidermal homeostasis for L-phenylalanine conversion to L-tyrosine in vitiligo (see Fig. 19.3).

One intriguing question remains. Are there still melanocytes present in the white skin of patients with vitiligo? Le Poole *et al.* (1993b) re-examined this issue using extensive histochemical and immunohistochemical methodology. Based on their results, this group concluded that there is no evidence for melanocytes in the white skin of these patients. Our own results contradict this conclusion. Recently we have found that decreased numbers of melanocytes are still present in the white skin, and that these cells can produce pigment under *in vivo* and *in vitro* conditions after correction of the impaired homeostasis in patients skin or under culture conditions (Tobin & Schallreuter 1997). Our examination was conducted on 14 randomly selected patients with vitiligo, where the duration of the disease ranged from three to 20 years.

Summary

In summary, the above observations shed some new light on the aetiology of this disease. At the present time at least four possible consequences arise from altered tetrahydrobiopterin homeostasis in vitiligo:

1 the GFRP/$6BH_4$ binding is defective,

2 $7BH_4$ competes with $6BH_4$ for binding on GFRP,

3 $7BH_4$ inhibited phenylalanine hydroxylase is the target, or

4 inefficient recycling of $6BH_4$ due to very low 4a-OH-tetrahydrobiopterin dehydratase activities leads to the enhanced production of $7BH_4$.

Whether each or all of these metabolic aberrations are cause or consequence for the phenomenon vitiligo still remains to be identified.

References

Adler, C., Ghisla, S., Rebrin, I., Haavik, J., Heizmann, C.W., Blau, N., Kuster, T. & Curtius, H.C. (1992) 7-Substituted pterins in humans with suspected pterin-4a-carbinolamine dehydratase deficiency—mechanism of formation via non-enzymatic transformation from 6-substituted pterins. *European Journal of Biochemistry* **208**, 139–144.

Cormane, R.H., Siddiqui, A.H. & Schutgens, R.B.H. (1985) Phenylalanine and UVA light for the treatment of vitiligo. *Archives for Dermatological Research* **277**, 126–130.

Curtius, H.C., Adler, C., Rebrin, I., Heizmann, C. & Ghisla, S. (1990) 7-substituted pterins: formation during phenylalanine hydroxylation in the absence of dehydratase. *Biochemical and Biophysical Research Communications* **172**, 1060–1066.

Davis, M.D., Ribeiro, P., Tipper, J. & Kaufman, S. (1992) '7-Tetrahydrobiopterin', a naturally occurring analogue of tetrahydrobiopterin is a cofactor for, and a potential inhibitor of, the aromatic amino acid hydroxylases. *Proceedings of the National Academy of Sciences, USA* **89**, 10108–10113.

Fitzpatrick, T.B., Eisen, A.Z., Wolff, K., Freedberg, I.M. & Austen, K.F. (1979). *Dermatology in General Medicine*, 2nd edn. McGraw-Hill International Book Co, New York.

Gokhale, B.B. & Mehta, L.H. (1983) Histopathology of vitiliginous skin. *International Journal of Dermatology* **22**, 447.

Harada, T., Kagamiyama, H. & Hatakeyama, K. (1993) Feedback regulatory mechanisms for the control of GTP cyclohydrolase I activity. *Science* **260**, 1507–1510.

Hopkins, F.G. (1889) Note on a yellow pigment in butterflies. *Proceedings of the Chemical Society* 5, 117. &. *Nature (London)* **40**, 335.

Lei, X.-D., Woodworth, C.D., Johnen, G. & Kaufman, S. (1997) Expression of 4a-carbinolamine dehydratase in human epidermal keratinocytes. *Biochemical and Biophysical Research Communications* **238**, 556–559.

Le Poole, I.C., Das, P.K., van den Wijngaard, R.M., Bos, J.D. & Westerhof, W. (1993a) Review of the etiopathomechanism of vitiligo: a convergence theory. *Experimental Dermatology* **2**, 146–153.

Le Poole, I.C., van den Wijngaard, R.M., Westerhof, W., Dutrieux, R.P. & Das, P.K. (1993b) Presence or absence of melanocytes in vitiligo lesions: an immunohistochemical investigation. *Journal of Investigative Dermatology* **100**, 816–822.

Milstien, S., Jaffe, H., Kowlessur, D. & Bonner, T.I. (1996) Purification and cloning of the GTP Cyclohydrolase I Feedback Regulatory Protein, GFRP. *Journal of Biological Chemistry* **271**, 19743–19751.

Naoi, M. & Parvez, S.-H. (1993). *Tyrosine Hydroxylase*. VSP, Utrecht, The Netherlands.

Ortonne, J.P. & Bose, S.K. (1993) Vitiligo: Where do we stand? *Pigment Cell Research* **8**, 61–72.

Prota, G. (1992). *Melanins and Melanogenesis*. Academic Press, New York.

Schallreuter, K.U. & Wood, J.M. (1991) EF-hands calcium-binding regulates the thioredoxin reductase/thioredoxin electron transfer in human keratinocytes and melanocytes. In: *Novel Calcium-Binding Proteins* (ed. C. Heizmann), pp. 339–360. Springer Verlag, Berlin.

Schallreuter, K.U., Büttner, G., Pittelkow, M.R., Wood, J.M., Swanson, N.N. & Körner, C. (1994a) The cytotoxicity of 6-biopterin to human melanocytes. *Biochemical and Biophysical Research Communications* **204**, 43–48.

Schallreuter, K.U., Wood, J.M., Pittelkow, M.R., Gütlich, M., Lemke, K.R., Rödl, W., Swanson, N.N., Hitzemann, K. & Ziegler, I. (1994b) Regulation of melanin biosynthesis in the human epidermis by tetrahydrobiopterin. *Science* **263**, 1444–1446.

Schallreuter, K.U., Wood, J.M., Lemke, K.R., Pittelkow, M.R., Lindsey, N.J., Gütlich, M. & Ziegler, I. (1994c) Defective tetrahydrobiopterin and catecholamine biosynthesis in the depigmentation disorder vitiligo. *Biochimica et Biophysica Acta* **1226**, 181–192.

Schallreuter, K.U., Zschiesche, M., Moore, J., Panske, A., Hibberts, N.A., Herrmann, F.H., Metelmann, H.R. & Sawatzki, J. (1998) *In vivo* evidence for compromised phenylalanine metabolism in vitiligo. *Biochemical and Biophysical Research Communications* **243**, 395–399.

Schallreuter-Wood, K.U. & Wood, J.M. (1995) Control of melanogenesis in the human epidermis by the redox-status of tetrahydrobiopterins. *Pteridines* **6**, 104–107.

Tobin, D.J. & Schallreuter, K.U. (1997) Low numbers of melanocytes and abnormal melanocyte/keratinocyte interaction in vitiligo. *Pigment Cell Research* **10**, 357.

Wieland, H. & Schöpf, C. (1925) Über den gelben Flügelforbstoff des Citronen-falters (Gonepteryx rhemni) *Berichte der Deutschen Chemischen Gesellschaft* **58**, 2178.

Wood, J.M., Schallreuter-Wood, K.U., Lindsey, N.J. *et al.* (1995) A specific tetrahydrobiopterin binding domain on tyrosinase controls melanogenesis. *Biochemical and Biophysical Research Communications* **206**, 480–485.

Ziegler, I. (1990) Production of pteridines during hematopoiesis and T-lymphocyte proliferation — potential participation in the control of cytokine signal transmission. *Medicinal Research Reviews* **10**, 95–114.

PART 4
TREATMENT OF VITILIGO

20: The Melanocyte Reservoir and its Necessity

JIAN CUI

There are no identifiable melanocytes in the epidermis and the matrices of hair follicles of vitiliginous lesions. However, new melanocytes are readily identified in the repigmented skin. Therefore, it is necessary to have a preserved melanocyte reservoir in the depigmented areas. The clinical observation that early repigmentation usually appears at the orifice of hair follicle indicates that a melanocyte reservoir may reside in the hair follicle. In fact, on the palm, sole and mucosal surface, where hair follicles are absent, vitiligo is very difficult to repigment further supporting the melanocyte reservoir theory.

Melanocyte reservoir of hair follicle

In the late 1950s, Staricco (1959) found that there were some DOPA-negative, amelanotic melanocytes in the outer root sheaths (ORS) of normal hair follicles which showed light cytoplasm and dark blue nuclei by DOPA-Toluidine Blue stain. These melanocytes did not synthesize melanin under normal circumstances but became active to produce melanin when stimulated by ultraviolet light (UVL) or by the removal of the epidermis and the upper part of follicles by dermabrasion (Staricco 1960, 1961, 1962). The author concluded that these amelanotic melanocytes could move up along with the regenerated epidermis and mature morphologically and functionally. Ortonne *et al.* (1980) used DOPA stain and scanning electron microscopy (SEM) to examine the repigmented skin after treatment with PUVA and found that the pigment islands had follicular cores and that there were some large melanocytes in the ORS of hair follicles. They postulated that there was a melanocyte reservoir in the human hair follicles and that the melanocytes in the repigmented vitiligo skin might be derived from this reservoir, although there were no mitoses of melanocytes in the repigmented epidermis examined by multiple section ultrastructural study (Ortonne *et al.* 1979). Cui *et al.* (1991) studied the different stages of repigmentation of vitiligo and confirmed the existence of a melanocyte reservoir in the ORS of hair follicles. Vitiligo is a process in which only active (melanin-producing) melanocytes are destroyed and the inactive melanocytes in the ORS are preserved and serve as the only source for repigmentation. Recovery of vitiligo is initiated by the proliferation of these inactive melanocytes, followed by the upward migrating to the nearby

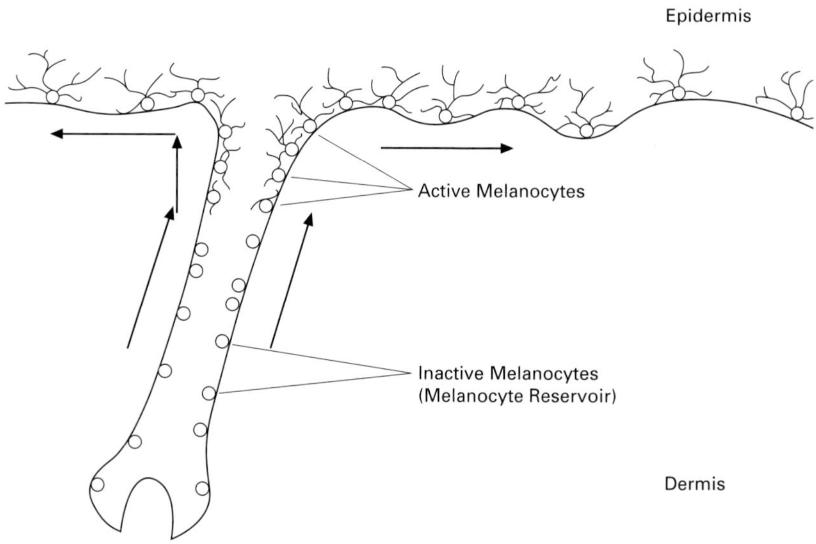

Fig. 20.1 Schematic diagram of repigmentation of vitiligo. Inactive melanocytes divide, proliferate and migrate upward along the surface of hair follicle to the nearby epidermis where they continue to move radially, and downward to the hair matrix. During the migration, the melanocytes mature gradually in function and morphology.

epidermis to form perifollicular pigment islands and the downward migration to the hair matrices to produce melanin (Fig 20.1). During this process, the melanocytes mature morphologically and functionally (Cui *et al.* 1991). Further characterization of these melanocytes by immunohistochemistry and immunoelectron microscopy revealed that the majority of the inactive melanocytes in the ORS were found in the mid- to upper portion of the hair follicles and were readily identified by using MoAb NKI/beteb and A4F11, which recognize premelanosome-related antigens (Horikawa *et al.* 1996; Narisawa *et al.* 1997). The melanocytes in the mid-portion were smaller in size and showed less dendricity. These inactive melanocytes could not be identified by antibodies to tyrosinase, TRP-1, TRP-2, and melanosome-associated antigen, respectively, and they may contain early structural proteins but not any enzymatic proteins necessary for melanogenesis.

Proliferation of follicular melanocytes

What triggers the proliferation of the ORS-inactive melanocytes in vitiligo is not known. Identification of the stimuli, however, will be the key to the development of any specific new treatment for vitiligo. Melanocytes have the ability to proliferate under certain circumstances, such as UVL exposure or injury to the epidermis (Starrico 1961; Bessou *et al.* 1995). But the effects of different stimuli on melanocytes are usually mediated by the production of some molecules that can modify the behaviour of melanocytes.

Many factors are shown to stimulate melanocytes to proliferate and to migrate under different conditions. UVL exposure, endothelins, granulocyte/macrophage colony-stimulating factor (GM-CSF), and stem cell factor (SCF) are just a few of the molecules that enhance the growth of melanocytes. Endothelins are a powerful stimulus to melanocytes and are found to enhance the proliferation and melanogenesis of human melanocytes *in vitro* (Hara *et al.* 1995; Lahav *et al.* 1996; Reid *et al.* 1996). After ultraviolet irradiation, synthesis and secretion of endothelin-1 by keratinocytes are up-regulated, which, along with several other growth factors, produced by keratinocytes, stimulate melanocyte to proliferate, to migrate, and to form dendrites (Hara *et al.* 1995). It is believed that the effects of endothelins on melanocytes are mediated by protein kinase C and tyrosine kinase pathways (Imokawa *et al.* 1996a). GM-CSF, another intrinsic keratinocyte-derived growth factor after UVL irradiation, binds to the specific binding sites on human melanocytes and stimulates DNA synthesis and melanization (Imokawa *et al.* 1996b), which may play an essential role in the maintenance of melanocyte proliferation and UVL-induced pigmentation in the epidermis. SCF, also known as mast cell growth factor and kit ligand, has been shown markedly to promote human melanocytes to proliferate and to melanize *in vivo* (Costa *et al.* 1996). SCF, acting through the tyrosine kinase receptor c-kit on melanocytes, regulates integrin protein expression *in vitro* and induces a rapid increase in actin stress fibre formation, thereby enhances melanocyte adhesion and migration on fibronectin (Scott *et al.* 1996). Interestingly, the expression of the c-kit receptor by epidermal melanocytes was found to be reduced in vitiligo, which may contribute to the defective growth and survival of melanocytes in vitiligo (Norris *et al.* 1996). However, it may also be a consequence of melanocyte damage of unknown aetiology.

When proliferating, melanocytes undergo dramatic morphological changes to speed the process: dendrites are drawn back into the cell body; cells become spherical and detach from their support; and cell division takes place while the cell is suspended (Kippenberger *et al.* 1997). These changes are mediated by the selective expression of adhesion molecules, such as integrins, ICAM-1, E-cadherin, and CD44, etc. Danen *et al.* (1996) demonstrated that nonproliferating melanocytes have an increased surface expression of alpha 2 beta 1 and alpha 6 beta 1 integrins which induce cell adhesion to basement membrane collagen and laminin. On the other hand, focal contact proteins, the transmembrane proteins that link the extracellular matrix to the actin cytoskeleton of cells and play a key role in the control of melanocyte migration (Scott *et al.* 1995), may also be modified to enhance the mobility of melanocytes. After exposure to therapeutic agents, especially UVL exposure, it is believed that keratinocytes as well as other inflammatory cells in vitiligo lesions may release different melanocyte growth factors to stimulate the inactive melanocyte reservoir in the ORS of hair follicles. Some of the factors may be able to modify the expression of adhesion molecules and focal contact proteins on the surface of melanocytes and keratinocytes and to prepare the melanocytes for proliferation and migration. The newly proliferated melanocyte population, attracted by higher concentrations of growth factors in the epidermis, gradually migrates into the nearby epidermis and further differentiates to produce melanin.

References

Bessou, S., Surleve-Bazeille, J.E., Sorbier, E. & Taieb, A. (1995) *Ex vivo* reconstruction of the epidermis with melanocytes and the influence of UVB. *Pigment Cell Research* **8**, 241–249.

Costa, J.J., Demetri, G.D., Harrist, T.J. *et al.* (1996) Recombinant human stem cell factor (kit ligand) promotes human mast cell and melanocyte hyperplasia and functional activation *in vivo*. *Journal of Experimental Medicine* **183**, 2681–2686.

Cui, J., Shen, L.Y. & Wang, G.C. (1991) Role of hair follicles in the repigmentation of vitiligo. *Journal of Investigative Dermatology* **97**, 410–416.

Danen, E.H., Jansen, K.F., Klein, C.E. *et al.* (1996) Loss of adhesion to basement membrane components but not to keratinocytes in proliferating melanocytes. *European Journal of Cell Biology* **70**, 69–75.

Hara, M., Yaar, M. & Gilchrest, B.A. (1995) Endothelin-1 of keratinocyte origin is a mediator of melanocyte dendricity. *Journal of Investigative Dermatology* **105**, 744–748.

Horikawa, T., Norris, D.A., Johnson, T.W. *et al.* (1996) DOPA-negative melanocytes in the outer root sheath of human hair follicles express premelanosomal antigens but not melanosomal antigens or the melanosome-associated glycoproteins tyrosinase, TRP-1, and TRP-2. *Journal of Investigative Dermatology* **106**, 28–35.

Imokawa, G., Yada, Y., Kimura, M. & Morisaki, N. (1996a) Granulocyte/macrophage colony-stimulating factor is an intrinsic keratinocyte-derived growth factor for human melanocytes in UVA-induced melanosis. *Biochemical Journal* **313** (2), 625–631.

Imokawa, G., Yada, Y. & Kimura, M. (1996b) Signaling mechanisms of endothelininduced mitogenesis and melanogenesis in human melanocytes. *Biochemical Journal* **314** (1), 305–312.

Kippenberger, S., Bernd, A., Bereiter-Hahn, J., Ramirez-Bosca, A. & Kaufmann, R. (1997) Melanocytes *in vitro*: how do they undergo mitosis? *Pigment Cell Research* **10**, 85–87.

Lahav, R., Ziller, C., Dupin, E. & Le Douarin, N.M. (1996) Endothelin 3 promotes neural crest cell proliferation and mediates a vast increase in melanocyte number in culture. *Proceedings of the National Academy of Sciences of the United States of America* 93, 3892–3897.

Narisawa, Y., Kohda, H. & Tanaka, T. (1997) Three-dimensional demonstration of melanocyte distribution of human hair follicles: special reference to the bulge area. *Acta Dermato-Venereologica (Stockholm)* **77**, 97–101.

Norris, A., Todd, C., Grahamm, A., Quinn, A.G. & Thody, A.J. (1996) the expression of the c-kit receptor by epidermal melanocytes may be reduced in vitiligo. *British Journal of Dermatology* **134**, 299–306.

Ortonne, J.P., MacDonald, D.M., Micoud, A. & Thivolet, J. (1979) PUVA-induced repigmentation of vitiligo: a histochemical (spli-DOPA) and ultrastructural study. *British Journal of Dermatology* **101**, 1–12.

Ortonne, J.P., Schmitt, D. & Thivolet, J. (1980) PUVA-induced repigmentation of vitiligo: scanning electron microscopy of hair follicles. *Journal of Investigative Dermatology* **74**, 40–42.

Reid, K., Turnley, A.M., Maxwell, G.D. *et al.* (1996) Multiple roles for endothelin in melanocyte development: regulation of progenitor number and stimulation of differentiation. *Development* **122**, 3911–3919.

Scott, G.A., Liang, H. & Cassidy, L.L. (1995) Developmental regulation of focal contact protein expression in human melanocytes. *Pigment Cell Research* **8**, 221–228.

Scott, G., Liang, H. & Luthra, D. (1996) Stem cell factor regulates the melanocyte cytoskeleton. *Pigment Cell Research* **9**, 134–141.

Staricco, R.G. (1959) Amelanotic melanocytes in the outer sheath of the hair follicles. *Journal of Investigative Dermatology* **33**, 295–297.
Staricco, R.G. (1960) The melanocytes and the hair follicle. *Journal of Investigative Dermatology* **35**, 185–194.
Staricco, R.G. (1961) Mechanism of migration of the melanocytes from the hair follicle into the epidermis following dermabrasion. *Journal of Investigative Dermatology* **36**, 99–104.
Staricco, R.G. (1962) Activation of amelanotic melanocytes in the outer root sheath of the hair follicle following ultraviolet exposure. *Journal of Investigative Dermatology* **39**, 163–164.

21: PUVA Therapy

WARWICK L. MORISON

Photochemotherapy with psoralen compounds and subsequent exposure to UVA (320–400 nm) radiation is commonly termed PUVA therapy. This treatment has been used in the management of vitiligo for over 2500 years and is still the main treatment available for achieving repigmentation in this condition. PUVA therapy for vitiligo is tedious and prolonged, usually requiring 100–300 exposures to achieve maximal repigmentation and even then only a few patients achieve total repigmentation. These features deter many physicians from offering the treatment to their patients but this is unfortunate since careful selection of patients can produce quite satisfactory results. Furthermore, use of combination treatments can considerably improve results.

Selection of patients

There are three important issues to consider before suggesting use of PUVA therapy for vitiligo (Ortonne *et al.* 1983).

The disease

Several characteristics of the disease require evaluation.

1 Type. Segmental vitiligo sometimes does not respond as readily to PUVA therapy as generalized vitiligo (Halder *et al.* 1987). Segmental vitiligo commonly causes leukotrichia, an indication that the reservoir for repigmentation located in the hair bulb is missing (see Chapters 7 and 20). These patients cannot respond to PUVA alone, because the reservoir from which the melanocytes migrate is missing. Epidermal grafting followed by PUVA therapy can be used in patients with this type of disease (Chapter 24).

2 Site. Response to PUVA therapy varies with anatomical regions. The face is the most responsive area. The distal parts of the extremities are less responsive and about equal. The tips of the fingers, the dorsum of the feet and genitalia rarely respond to PUVA. All of these areas are glabrous, i.e. do not have hair follicles in which the reservoir resides. For these areas, PUVA therapy alone should not be used.

3 Hair colour. Loss of pigmentation of hair in any patch of vitiligo usually indicates that patch will not respond. This is not absolute and sometimes such a patch will pigment but the chances are low.

4 Progress. Rapidly spreading vitiligo is often unresponsive to treatment. Occasionally PUVA, UVB or sunlight alone seem to retard or stop the progression of the vitiligo. Whether this is an effect of the therapy or the natural history of the vitiligo is not known.
5 Duration and extent. Long duration and widespread disease are often mentioned as negative features but this is not well documented. Some patients with extensive disease or disease present for many years can repigment.

Motivation of patient

PUVA therapy for vitiligo is not a quick-fix treatment and therefore it is important to establish initially how much concern the disease is causing the patient and how easily a prolonged and inconvenient therapy will fit their lifestyle. People with dark skin and young people are more likely to adhere to treatment than are fair-skinned and elderly patients. In addition, treatment heightens the contrast between normal and vitiliginous skin by causing a maximal pigmentation response in normal skin so the vitiligo is much more evident until repigmentation occurs. This should be explained to the patient before commencing treatment.

Age of patient

This consideration mainly applies to young children with concerned parents. Children should only be treated when they are sufficiently disturbed by the vitiligo that they want to engage in a prolonged treatment. Girls usually want treatment at a younger age than boys but there is considerable variation.

Investigations

The only mandatory investigation is a complete eye examination about the time of commencing PUVA therapy to establish a baseline for any ocular pathology. Any history of connective tissue disease or photosensitivity should be investigated by a full history, examination and a lupus package including a test for Ro antibody.

Treatment protocols

Several different protocols are used but they can be broadly divided into oral, topical and combination therapy.

Oral PUVA therapy

This form of treatment gives the most consistent results with the lowest risk of adverse effects (Parrish *et al.* 1976). The psoralen of choice is methoxsalen in a dose of 0.4 mg/kg body weight (Table 21.1) taken one or two hours prior to exposure to radiation. In this dose nausea is a very uncommon problem but if it occurs the patient should be asked to eat a sandwich or light meal at the time of ingestion of the medication. The exposure to UVA radiation is given in a whole-body or area radiator equipped with UVA fluorescent bulbs starting at a dose of 1 J/cm^2. The dose is increased with each treatment until a light pink colour is produced in the patches of vitiligo. Subsequent increases are given to maintain this pink, which is a mild, asymptomatic manifestation of phototoxicity. Treatments should be given twice or three times weekly and must always be at least 48 hours apart. Patients must avoid exposure to sunlight from the time of ingestion of psoralen until sunset and eye protection is essential for the same time period. Patients who are unable to attend a treatment centre may use sunlight as the source of UVA radiation. Trioxsalen in these circumstances is the psoralen of choice because due to poor absorption it is much less phototoxic than methoxsalen (Wennersten & Hagermark 1984). The dose is 0.6 mg/kg body weight taken two hours before exposure to sunlight. The initial exposure is five minutes and the dose is increased by five minutes each time up to a maximum of about an hour. Treatments should be taken on alternate days or at least twice weekly. Eye protection is essential using UV-opaque glasses from the time of ingestion of psoralen until sunset.

Topical PUVA therapy

Methoxsalen in a concentration of 0.1% is the most frequently used psoralen for this therapy (Grimes *et al.* 1982). The 1% methoxsalen lotion available commercially is diluted in 5% propylene glycol and 95% ethanol to give a solution or in white petrolatum to give an ointment. This is applied to the areas of vitiligo 30–60 minutes before exposure to radiation. The initial UVA radiation dose is 0.25 J/cm^2 with increments of 0.12 to 0.25 J/cm^2 until pink erythema is reached; further increments are given to maintain a faint erythema. Following the exposure the area is washed and a sunscreen containing a benzophenone is applied. Exposure to sunlight should be avoided for the remainder of the day of treatment. Treatments must be at least 72 hours apart and a weekly schedule can be effective. Methoxsalen should never be used with sunlight as a source of UVA radiation.

Table 21.1 Dose schedule for methoxsalen ultra.

Patient weight		
lb	kg	Drug dose (mg)
<66	<30	10
66–143	30–65	20
144–200	65–90	30
>200	>90	40

Topical PUVA therapy intuitively is preferable when treating limited disease since it avoids systemic exposure to the medication. Thus it is often advised as the treatment of choice for young children and patients with <20% body surface involvement. The main problem with this treatment is that many patients experience unexpected bullous phototoxic reactions sometimes on more than one occasion. There is evidence this is due to incidental sun exposure causing crosslinking of psoralen monoadducts that remain for days in DNA of skin (Gange *et al.* 1984).

Combination therapy

Epidermal grafting using a suction-induced blister as the source of the grafts is a very useful adjunct to PUVA therapy (Skouge *et al.* 1992, Chapter 24). It can be used initially for areas that are not expected to respond to PUVA therapy or later in the course of treatment for nonresponding areas. Topical corticosteroids (Chapter 22) are also a useful adjunctive treatment but should be used with caution because of a risk of atrophy occurring (Bleehen 1976).

Response to treatment

Repigmentation can occur in several ways. The borders of patches may gradually move inwards often with preliminary hyperpigmentation of the border and perifollicular repigmentation (Fig. 21.1) is also common with gradual expansion of the pigment. When topical corticosteroids are used an even repigmentation may gradually occur across the patches of vitiligo (Fig. 21.2). About 20% of patients will achieve very significant repigmentation and another 50% will achieve partial but satisfactory repigmentation. These results will take 100–300 treatments. A good rule-of-thumb is that if significant repigmentation has not occurred within 30 treatments it will

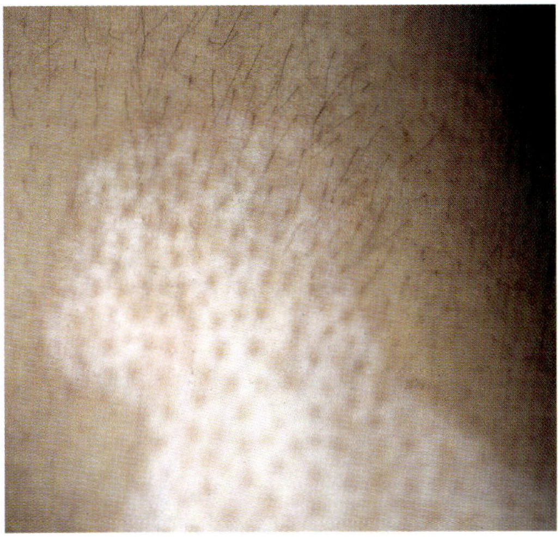

Fig. 21.1 Perifollicular repigmentation plus hyperpigmentation of border of patch of vitiligo.

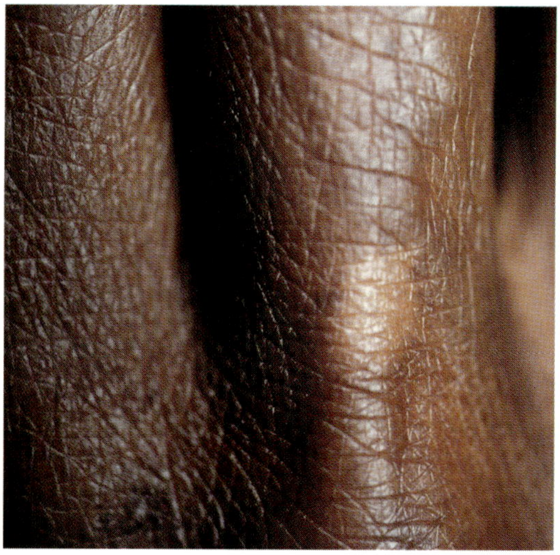

Fig. 21.2 Even repigmentation of vitiligo macule treated with PUVA therapy and topical corticosteroids.

probably never occur. After treatment is completed, pigmentation that completely fills a patch of vitiligo is seldom lost again but partial repigmentation of a patch is frequently lost within a few months (Kenney 1971).

References

Bleehen, S.S. (1976) The treatment of vitiligo with topical corticosteroids. Light and electron-microscopic studies. *British Journal of Dermatology* **94** (Suppl. 12), 43–50.

Gange, R.W., Levins, P. *et al.* (1984) Prolonged skin photosensitization induced by methoxsalen and subphototoxic UVA irradiation. *Journal of Investigations Dermatology* **82**, 219–222.

Grimes, P.E., Minus, H.R., *et al.* (1982) Determination of optimal topical photochemotherapy for vitiligo. *Journal of the American Academy of Dermatology* **7** (6), 771–778.

Halder, R.M., Grimes, P.E., *et al.* (1987) Childhood Vitiligo *Journal of the American Academy of Dermatology* **16** (5 Part 1), 948–954.

Kenney, J.A. Jr (1971) Vitiligo treated by psoralens. A long-term follow-up study of the permanency of repigmentation. *Archives of Dermatology* **103** (5), 475–480.

Ortonne, J.P., Mosher, D.V., *et al.* (1983) *Vitiligo and Other Hypomelanoses.* Plenum Publishing Co., New York.

Parrish, J.A., Fitzpatrick, T.B., *et al.* (1976) Photochemotherapy of vitiligo. Use of orally administered psoralens and a high-intensity long-wave ultraviolet light system. *Archives of Dermatology* **112** (11), 1531–1534.

Skouge, J.W., Morison, W.L., *et al.* (1992) Autografting and PUVA. A combination therapy for vitiligo. *Journal of Dermatologic Surgery and Oncology* **18** (5), 357–360.

Wennersten, G. & Hagermark, O. (1984) Outdoor and office photochemotherapy of vitiligo: a comparison. *Photodermatology* **1** (2), 91–93.

22: Steroid Treatment for Vitiligo

SEUNG-KYUNG HANN

Introduction

Vitiligo involves 0.5–4% of the world's population (see Chapter 4) and causes alterations in the physiology of the epidermis (see Chapter 31) as well as cosmetic and psychological problems (see Chapter 13 and 27). A large variety of therapeutic agents are used for the treatment of vitiligo, but none is clearly a definitive cure. Some therapies do stimulate repigmentation, occasionally completely, more often partially.

PUVA (psoralen plus ultraviolet A) is widely used as the main treatment for vitiligo. However, PUVA therapy is expensive and time consuming. Approximately 1/3 of patients achieve excellent results from PUVA therapy (Hann *et al.* 1991, Chapter 21). It can have side-effects such as fatigue, headache, dizziness, stomach discomfort and rarely hepatitis (Hann *et al.* 1992). More importantly, patients with vitiligo who are receiving PUVA may develop new lesions while the other old lesions are repigmenting (Nordlund & Ortonne 1992). For patients who have either failed or who are unsuitable for PUVA therapy it is necessary to use other types of therapies. Non-PUVA treatment modalities include topical and systemic corticosteroids, levamisole, melagenina, prostaglandin inhibitors, 5-fluorouracil, topical pseudocatalase, autologous minigrafting, and autologous epidermal grafting (Nordlund & Ortonne 1992; Hann *et al.* 1995, Chapter 24), but even with this multiplicity of treatments, the results are limited (see Chapter 29).

Topical steroids

Topical steroid preparations are often the first treatment of choice for patients with vitiligo because they are easy and convenient for both doctors and patients to maintain the treatment. Results of therapy have been reported as moderately successful, particularly in patients who have localized vitiligo and/or who have an inflammatory component to their vitiligo, even if the inflammation is subclinical. However, relatively few studies have reported results obtained from studies that have generated data in the most rigorous manner.

Kandil (1970b) studied the efficacy of topical steroid treatment in vitiligo. Lesions on the face responded best and those on the extremities responded favourably as well. They commented on the pattern of repigmentation, noting that the patches on the neck, trunk and extremities showed follicular repigmentation. On the face, a diffuse increase of pigmentation occurred until normal skin colour was attained. From this author's experience, it is difficult to get repigmentation on the lesions on the distal parts of the fingers, although the dorsum of the hand responds favourably (see Chapter 20). On the face, patches of the eyelid and lateral sides of the orbit are satisfactorily repigmented by topical steroids. The reason why repigmentation occurs easily on the face is unknown. High permeability of steroids into the facial skin, large numbers of residual melanocytes in unaffected facial skin and a high incidence of reversible melanocyte damage in facial lesions may be possible explanations. However, great caution must be exercised when using topical steroids on the eyelid area. There have been reports of topical steroids leading to increased intraocular pressure, as well as complicating congenital glaucoma in infants, aggravating developmental glaucoma and worsening of adult glaucoma (Spiers 1965; Morman 1981).

Skin colour could be a factor affecting repigmentation in topical steroid treatment. Kumari (1984) showed that facial lesions of vitiligo in dark skinned patients responded better than in light skinned patients. A higher success rate in dark skinned patients may be due to higher prevalence of reversible melanocyte damage.

The type of vitiligo was reported to affect the efficacy of topical steroid treatment. Koga (1977) concluded that segmental vitiligo did not respond to 0.12% betamethasone-17-valerate, 0.01% fluocinolone acetonide or 0.1% triamcinolone acetonide, but partial or complete response was found in 82.5% of patients with bilateral localized or generalized vitiligo. Lesions on the face responded more completely than other areas. However, Koga's study (1977) has some deficiencies. He tested only five patients with segmental vitiligo and did not mention the sites of the lesions. From Moon *et al.*'s study (1995), segmental vitiligo which occurs on the face or which is of short duration responds well to topical steroids (Fig. 22.1).

Duration of disease can also affect repigmentation of vitiligo induced by applications of topical steroids. Geraldez and Gutierrez (1987) studied 25 Filipino patients with vitiligo who had no more than 20% of the body surface involved. Clobetasol propionate cream was applied twice daily for 2 weeks and thereafter once daily. Patients were followed for 4 months after the therapeutic trial was completed. They found that 23 of 25 (92%) patients experienced at least 90% repigmentation; two patients (8%) failed to respond. Younger lesions tended to respond better; lesions on the face responded more quickly; and only two relapses were reported. Vitiligo often responds better to topical steroids in darker skinned individuals.

Contrary to previous reports, in Goldstein *et al.*'s experience (1992), only a small percentage of patients responded to topical steroids, and of those, many soon became refractory to therapy and/or relapsed. About 40% of patients with vitiligo referred to their centre had tried a 3–4 month course of

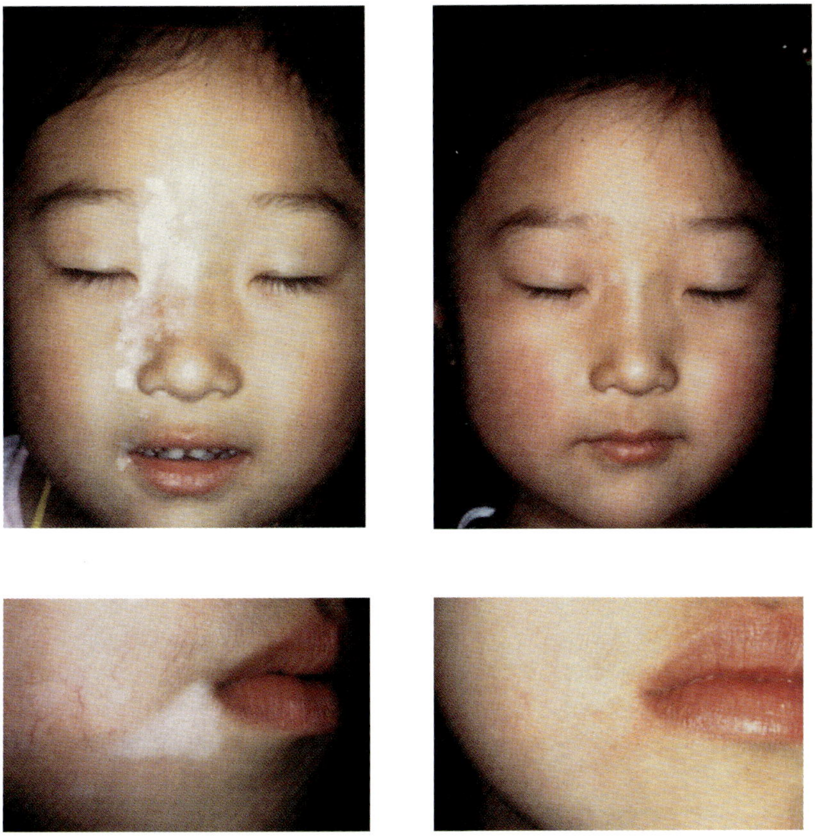

Fig. 22.1 Repigmentation appeared in a segmental vitiligo patient after topical steroid treatment. (a) Before treatment, (b) after treatment.

topical steroids. Of these, about 70% failed to respond to hydrocortisone 1%, hydrocortisone butyrate 1%, desonide 0.05%, or other low potency steroids. The remaining 30% failed with medium potency to high potency fluorinated steroids. The potency of the steroid seems to a important factor in their study.

The efficacy of topical steroids in repigmenting vitiliginous skin varies with the investigators. However, it is difficult to compare the results of various studies objectively. Some patients received therapy to small isolated patches; whereas other patients received therapy to large areas or all affected areas. Often the duration of disease and sites of lesions were not specified in the evaluation of treatment efficacy. Several studies were conducted using the patients as their own controls. Other studies had no controls. End points varied from improvement in single patches to improvement in all patches. Side-effect profiles varied from none to all patients experiencing side-effects. Different steroid preparations with different potencies and vehicles were used, factors that might influence penetration and therapeutic efficacy. Although topical corticosteroids are a suitable first line therapy for many patients, there are a significant number

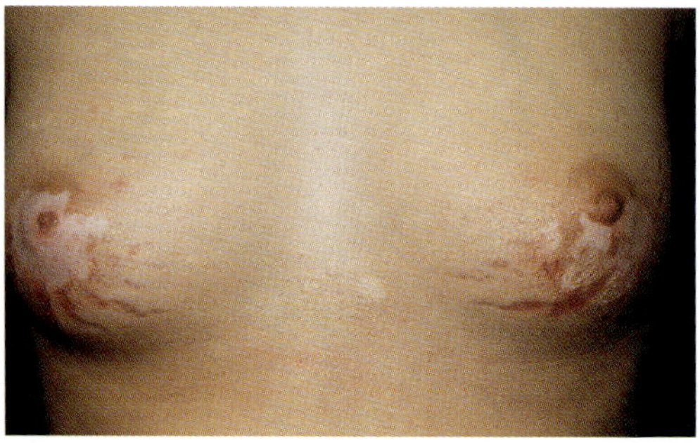

Fig. 22.2 Striae distensae appeared on the breast after intralesional injection of triamcinolone acetonide.

of patients who do not respond to topical steroids and for whom another form of therapy is needed.

Intralesional corticosteroids

The problem of penetration of topical medications and their delivery to deeper target structures in the epidermis and dermis can be obviated by intralesional injections of a steroid preparation. Kandil (1970a) treated 26 patients with vitiligo by injecting triamcinolone acetonide 10 mg/mL. Of 52 patches treated in 26 patients, 30 (58%) were 'completely or almost completely cured'; 15 (29%) had 'satisfactory repigmentation'. Of those treated, four out of 52 (8%) still exhibited atrophy 10 months after the last injection. Mild to no improvement was seen in three patients. It is difficult to draw any conclusions from this study because there was no control group, the end points were only loosely defined and side-effects were not fully explained.

Contrary to Kandil's report (1970a), Vasistha and Singh (1979) reported that there was no significant difference in the amount of repigmentation induced by steroid injections compared to that produced by injections of water to a control group. They observed numerous types of side-effects from steroid injections such as atrophy, telangiectasia and intradermal haemorrhage. They did not recommend intralesional steroids for the treatment of vitiligo.

Goldstein *et al.* (1992) reported that triamcinolone acetonide administered by intralesional injection was ineffective and left slight dermal atrophy and telangiectasia. Striae distensae is one of the more severe complications of intralesional corticosteroids (Fig. 22.2). A decrease in the mobility of finger joints from atrophy of the skin has also been observed following intralesional injection sites of hands. Previous reports have not mentioned the intense pain experienced by some patients during intralesional injections. Severe pain and discomfort can be a reason for patients to abandon intralesional treatments. Leukotrichia on the scalp can be treated with triamcinolone acetonide injection, since topical steroid application on the scalp is troublesome. If there is no repigmentation of hair or skin with triamcinolone acetonide injections, topical PUVA after shaving hair can be initiated.

Systemic steroids

Although topical application of steroids is sometimes effective for vitiligo, application of steroid creams to widespread and extensive lesions is difficult and side-effects are common. Therefore systemic steroid treatment has been used to manage extensive and actively spreading vitiligo. Some investigators have considered vitiligo to be a result of an autoimmune attack against melanocytes (see Chapter 16). Thus it has been proposed that systemic corticosteroids which suppress immunity, may arrest the progression of vitiligo and lead to repigmentation. Several studies supporting steroid treatment in vitiligo have been reported. A decrease of complement-mediated cytotoxicity by autoantibodies to melanocytes and reduced antibody titres to surface antigens of melanocytes were noticed in the serum of vitiligo patients who received oral corticosteroid treatment with clinical improvement (Hann *et al.* 1993, 1997).

There are several clinical studies from which the results of systemic steroid therapy for the treatment of vitiligo have been reported. One group of investigators reported the results of administering 25–40 IU of long acting adrenocorticotropin hormone (ACTH) twice weekly for a period of 5–6 weeks to the patients who previously failed PUVA therapy. A break of 2–4 weeks was followed by repeat treatments as needed to effect satisfactory results, or until a maximum of four courses were given. After 6 months, 80% repigmentation occurred in 16 (59%) of those treated; 50% repigmentation in six (22%); and 20% repigmentation or less in four (15%). There was no improvement in one case (Gokhale & Gokhale 1976).

Contrary to this report, other investigators observed poor results with the use of ACTH gel. In this latter study, 40 mg of ACTH gel was given twice a week for 5 weeks; and after a 5-week rest period, a second 5-week series was administered. Fourteen of 20 patients (70%) showed poor results defined as less than 20% repigmentation. Six (30%) of 20 patients showed more than 80% repigmentation (Hermandez-Perez 1979). However depigmentation occurred rapidly after discontinuation of therapy. It should be noted that ACTH might have a direct effect on epidermal melanocytes via one of the MSH receptors located on the surface of the melanocytes. The medication might stimulate proliferation without intervention in the immune system.

Imamura and Tagami (1976) reported their results from the use of oral corticosteroid therapy (a mixture of prednisolone, betamethasone, paramethasone acetate and methylprednisolone) for vitiligo. The therapy gave satisfactory results in 6 (35%)of 22 patients within 6 months with temporary and minimal side-effects. They noticed that a better response was seen in exposed areas, that generalized lesions responded better than localized lesions and that lesions of more than 10 years duration or those resistant to PUVA therapy responded less well.

Treatment with systemic steroids may produce unacceptable side-effects such as gastrointestinal distress, facial swelling, an increase of body weight, striae distensae, acneiform eruptions, insomnia, urinary frequency, menstrual disturbance, osteoporosis and, rarely, avascular necrosis of bone. To minimize the side-effects, oral mini pulse therapy with betamethasone or dexamethasone in patients with extensive or fast-spreading vitiligo have been tried.

Pasricha and Khaitan (1993) tried oral mini pulse therapy with betamethasone. Forty patients were given betamethasone/dexamethasone 5 mg as a single oral dose after breakfast on 2 consecutive days. This dose was repeated every week. Within 1–3 months of starting the treatment, the progression of vitiligo was arrested in 32 of the 36 patients (89%). Two patients needed an increase in dose of steroids to 7.5 mg per day to achieve complete arrest of lesions. Within 2–4 months, areas of repigmentation in the existing vitiligo lesions were visible in 32 of the patients (80%). The extent of repigmentation varied in different patients and in different lesions in the same patient. Repigmentation was less than 10% in 14 patients (35%), 10–25% repigmentation in seven patients (17.5%), 26–50% repigmentation in 10 patients (25%), 51–75% repigmentation in three patients (7.5%), and 76–99% repigmentation in six patients (15%). Seventeen patients experienced one or more of the following side-effects: weight gain, bad taste, headache, transient mild weakness for 2 days, acne, mild puffiness of the face, perioral dermatitis, herpes zoster, glaucoma or amenorrhoea.

Kanwar *et al.* (1995) also studied the effectiveness of oral mini pulse therapy for vitiligo. Thirty-seven patients with rapidly spreading vitiligo were treated with dexamethasone. Adult patients received dexamethasone 5 mg given on 2 consecutive days a week after breakfast. In children (<16-year-old) the dose was halved. A minimum of five doses and a maximum of 25 doses were tried. The result of this study was not as encouraging as those reported by the previous authors. In only 14 (43.8%) of 32 patients who completed the trial, there was also a mild to moderate repigmentation without appearance of new lesions. In 18 (56.2%) there was no response. The pigmentation appeared mostly within the first 15 weeks (doses) of treatment. It has to be noted that only four children out of nine who completed the trial had mild to moderate repigmentation. No side-effects were reported.

Kim *et al.* (1999) tried low dose steroid therapy (0.3 mg prednisolone/kg) for actively spreading vitiligo in order to avoid or minimize the side-effects of therapy. After 4 months of treatment, 57 of the 81 patients' (70.4%) vitiligo showed some repigmentation. Arrest of progression of vitiligo was noted in 71 of 81 patients (87.7%). The effect of treatment was better in the younger group. Those patients who had vitiligo for 2 years or less showed a better response, repigmentation occurring in 38 of 49 patients (77.6%). However, for those with vitiligo over 2 years repigmentation was noted in only 20 (62.5%) and spreading occurred in nine (28.1%) of 32 patients.

The results differed for those with segmental compared to bilateral vitiligo. Repigmentation was noticed in 23 of 30 patients (76.7%) with segmental vitiligo and in seven of the eight patients (87.5%) with localized depigmentation. In the generalized type, repigmentation occurred in 27 (62.8%) of 43 patients but spreading of vitiligo also developed in 10 (23.2%) of those treated.

The site of vitiligo seemed to have an effect on outcome. Facial lesions proved to be most amenable to therapy (69.8% of 63 patients). Segmental and localized legions were mostly commonly located on the face, a factor that might be important in interpreting the results. Thirty-five patients had no side-effects with this treatment schedule, while 46 patients complained of one or more of the following: facial oedema was the most common side-effect and was noticed in 17 (21%) of the 81 patients; weight gain and acneiform eruption occurred in 14 (17.3%) and eight (9.9%) patients, respectively. Increased appetite, gastrointestinal distress, frequent urination, abdominal pain, hypertrichosis, insomnia, dizziness, diarrhoea, striae distensae, and irregularity of menstruation were also noticed. Some complications of systemic steroids were severe enough to force patients to cease taking the medication. A newly developed methyloxazolin derivative of prednisolone called deflazacort, which is known to have the same therapeutic effects of prednisolone but fewer side-effects was used successfully for those patients with complications.

Other steroids

Muto *et al.* (1995) reported successful treatment of vitiligo with a sex steroid-thyroid hormone mixture which was developed for modulating hormonal imbalances associated with menopausal syndrome. Mixture of a sex steroid-thyroid hormone was administered daily to four patients with generalized vitiligo. Some perifollicular repigmentation was noticed with no significant side-effects after treatment.

Conclusion

Steroid therapy can be an effective therapy for patients with vitiligo. The outcome seems to depend on clinical manifestations. The method of steroid administration should be chosen cautiously to get maximal treatment effects. Considering the frequency of side-effects from systemic steroids, all patients should be screened for any contraindication of systemic steroids, such as diabetes mellitus, tuberculosis, gastrointestinal disease, glaucoma, hypertension and osteoporosis. Serial routine laboratory tests in addition to X-ray studies should be done to detect any side-effects early.

References

Geraldez, C.B. & Gutierrez, G.T. (1987) A clinical trial of Clobetasol propionate in Filipino vitiligo patients. *Clinical Therapeutics* **9**, 474–482.

Gokhale, B.B. & Gokhale, T.B. (1976) Corticotropin and vitiligo (preliminary observations). *British Journal of Dermatology* **95**, 329.

Goldstein, E., Haberman, H.F., Menon, I.A. & Pawlowski, D. (1992) Non-psoralen treatment of vitiligo. Part II. Less commonly used and experimental therapies. *International Journal of Dermatology* **31**, 314–319.

Hann, S.K., Im, S., Cho, M.Y. & Park, Y.K. (1991) Treatment of vitiligo with oral 5-methoxypsoralen. *Journal of Dermatology* **18**, 324–329.

Hann, S.K., Park, Y.K., Im, S., Koo, S.W. & Haam, I.B. (1992) The effect of liver transaminase of phototoxic drugs used in systemic photochemotherapy. *Journal of the American Academy of Dermatology* **26**, 646–648.

Hann, S.K., Kim, H.I., Im, S. *et al.* (1993) The change of melanocyte cytotoxicity after systemic steroid treatment in vitiligo patients. *Journal of Dermatological Science* **6**, 201–205.

Hann, S.K., Im, S., Bong, H.W. & Park, Y.K. (1995) Treatment of stable vitiligo with autologus epidermal grafting and psoralen plus UVA (PUVA). *Journal of the American Academy of Dermatology* **32**, 943–948.

Hann, S.K., Chen, L. & Bystryn, J.C. (1997) Systemic steroids suppress anti-melanocyte antibodies in vitiligo. *Journal of Cutaneous Medicine and Surgery* **1**, 193–195.

Hermandez-Perez, E. (1979) Vitiligo treated with ACTH. *International Journal of Dermatology* **18**, 587–589.

Imamura, S. & Tagami, H. (1976) Treatment of vitiligo with oral corticosteroids. *Dermatologica* **153**, 179–185.

Kandil, E. (1970a) Treatment of localized vitiligo with intradermal injection of triamcinolone acetonide. *Dermatologica* **140**, 195–206.

Kandil, E. (1970b) Vitiligo-response to 0.2% betamethasone 17-valerate in flexible collodion. *Dermatologica* **141**, 277–281.

Kanwar, A.J., Dhar, S. & Dawn, G. (1995) Oral minipulse therapy in vitiligo. *Dermatology* **190**, 251–252.

Kim, S.M., Lee, H.S. & Hann, S.K. (1999) The efficacy of low-dose oral corticosteroids in the treatment of vitiligo patients. *International Journal of Dermatology* **38**, 546–550.

Koga, M. (1999) Vitiligo: A new classification and therapy. *British Journal of Dermatology* **97**, 255–261.

Kumari, J. (1984) Vitiligo treated with topical clobetasol propiomate. *Archives of Dermatology* **120**, 631–635.

Park, Y.K. (1995) The effect of small doses of oral corticosteroids in vitiligo patients. *Korean Journal of Dermatology* **33**, 880–885.

Morman, M.R. (1981) Possible side effects of topical steroids. *American Family Physician* **23**, 171–174.

Muto, M., Furumoto, H., Ohamura, A. *et al.* (1995) Successful treatment of vitiligo with a sex-steroid-thyroid hormone mixture. *Journal of Dermatology* **22**, 770–772.

Nordlund, J.J. & Ortonne, J.-P. (1992) Vitiligo and depigmentation. *Current Problems in Dermatology* **4**, 1–18.

Pasricha, J.S. & Khaitan, B.K. (1993) Oral mini-pulse therapy with betamethasone in vitiligo patients having extensive or fast-spreading disease. *International Journal of Dermatology* **31**, 753–757.

Song, M.S., Hann, S.K., Ahn, P.S., Im, S. & Park, Y.K. (1994) Clinical study of vitiligo. *Annals of Dermatology* **6**, 22–30.

Spiers, F. (1965) A case of irreversible steroid-induced rise in intra-ocular pressure. *Acta Ophthalmology (Copenhagen)* **43**, 735–745.
Visistha, L.K. & Singh, G. (1979) Vitiligo and intralesional steroids. *Indian Journal of Medical Research* **69**, 308–311.

23: Pseudocatalase in the Treatment of Vitiligo

KARIN U. SCHALLREUTER, JEREMY MOORE AND JOHN M. WOOD

The aetiology of vitiligo is still not completely understood (Nordlund & Ortonne 1992; Ortonne & Bose 1993). Nowadays there is accumulating evidence for increased oxidative stress in the entire epidermis of these patients. Several reports have shown earlier peroxidative damage in melanocytes as well as in keratinocytes, where vacuolar degeneration and granular deposits have been described in both involved/depigmented and uninvolved/normal pigmented epidermis (Moellman *et al.* 1982; Bhawan & Bhutani 1983; Boissy *et al.* 1991). Increased sensitivity to hydrogen peroxide (H_2O_2) has been documented in normal human melanocytes under *in vitro* conditions (Yohn *et al.* 1991). Other authors were able to protect melanocytes established from individuals with vitiligo against H_2O_2 cytotoxicity upon the addition of catalase to the culture medium (Medrano & Nordlund 1990). We have been able to demonstrate oxidative stress/vacuolation in freshly established cell cultures of melanocytes and keratinocytes from involved and uninvolved skin of these patients (Schallreuter *et al.* 1999). In addition, functionally altered Langerhans cells have been found.

Low catalase levels in vitiligo

The discovery of low epidermal catalase levels in involved and uninvolved skin of patients with vitiligo suggested a major stress arising from increased epidermal H_2O_2 generation (Schallreuter *et al.* 1991) (Fig. 23.1). Recently these data were supported by Maresca *et al.* (1997), who were able to show decreased catalase activities in melanocytes from uninvolved vitiligo epidermis. However, the expression of catalase mRNA in melanocytes and keratinocytes from this patient group is normal compared to healthy controls. Very recently the presence of high epidermal H_2O_2 levels in vitiligo was confirmed by utilizing *in vivo* noninvasive Fourier Transform Raman spectroscopy (FT-Raman). This method allows the precise assignment of H_2O_2 at 875 cm^{-1} based on the well separated O-O stretch. Figure 23.2 presents an example of the *in vivo* FT-Raman spectra of a patient with vitiligo compared to healthy control skin, indicating the presence of higher levels of H_2O_2 in this disorder. One consequence of H_2O_2 accumulation is the oxidative degradation of the porphyrin active site of catalase, which has been confirmed earlier by detailed kinetic analysis where

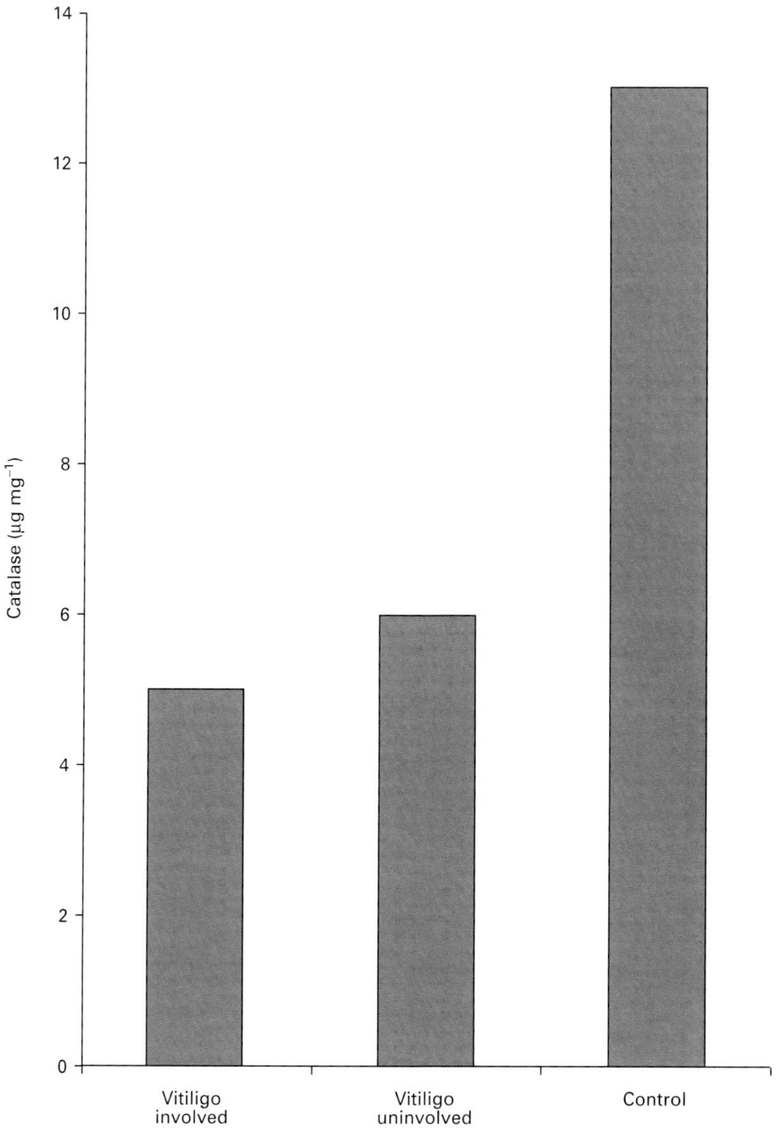

Fig 23.1 Catalase levels in vitiligo patients. The presence of low catalase levels in epidermal cell extracts of patients with vitiligo (involved n = 12, uninvolved n = 10) compared to healthy controls (n = 7)

high concentrations of H_2O_2 (10^{-3} M) lead to deactivation (Aronoff 1965). Taking these results into consideration they would favour direct deactivation of catalase and as a consequence explain low levels of this enzyme in vitiligo.

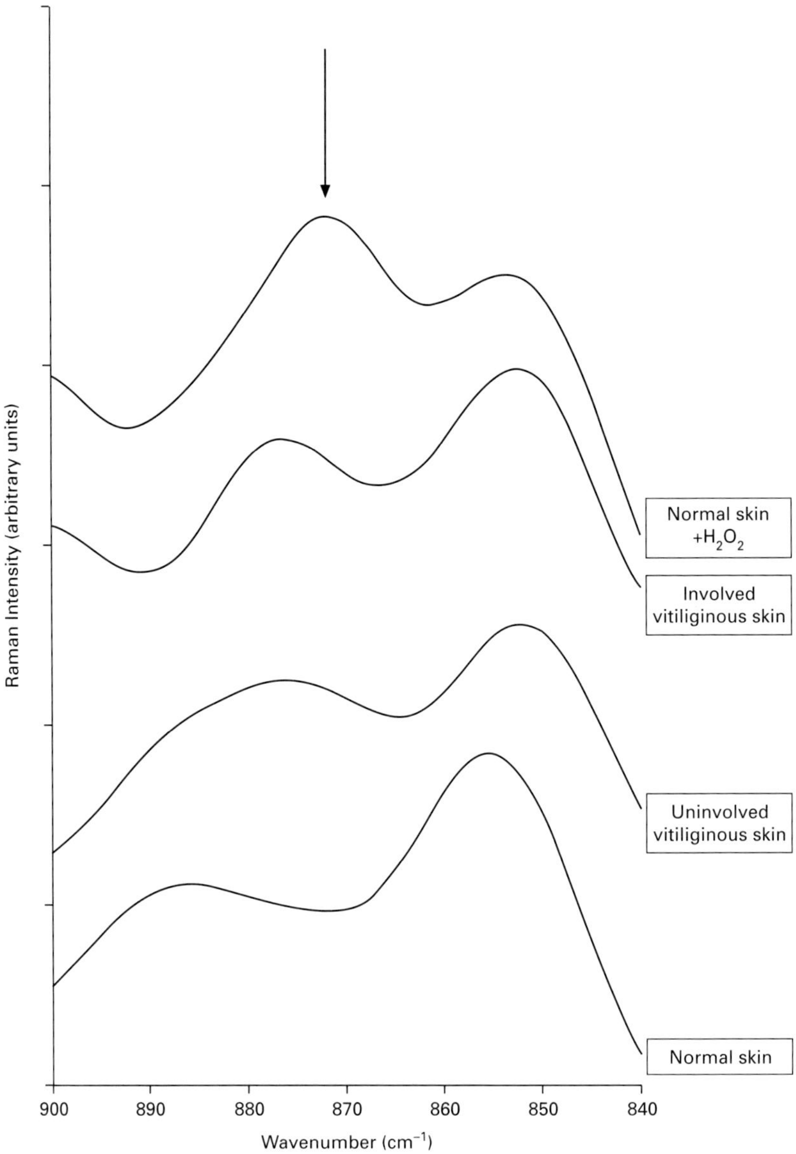

Fig. 23.2 FT-Raman spectra of the skin. *In vivo* FT-Raman spectra from the skin show the presence of H_2O_2 in the epidermis at 875 cm^{-1} in one patient with vitiligo compared to a healthy control with the same photo skin type before and after exposure to a H_2O_2 (33×10^{-3} M).

Identified sources of epidermal H_2O_2 in patients with vitiligo

To date there are at least five recognized pathways involved in the overproduction of H_2O_2 in vitiligo.

Increased *de novo* synthesis and defective recycling of the essential cofactor (6R)-L-erythro-5,6,7,8-tetrahydrobiopterin ($6BH_4$)

One consequence of increased *de novo* synthesis of $6BH_4$ and a decreased 4a-carbinolamine dehydratase in the recycling process in vitiligo is the accumulation of micromolar levels of the 7 isomer ($7BH_4$) (Schallreuter *et al.* 1994b, c). This event leads to the inhibition of phenylalanine hydroxylase with concomitant increased production of H_2O_2 from the intermediate 4a-peroxy-$6BH_4$ yielding quinonoid dihydropterin via a short circuit (Davis *et al.* 1992). H_2O_2 rapidly oxidizes $6BH_4$ to 6-biopterin, which has been shown to be cytotoxic to normal melanocytes (Schallreuter *et al.* 1994a). Hence the control of the redox status is crucial to melanocyte survival. It has been shown that the redox status can be under regulation of the important antioxidant system thioredoxin/thioredoxin reductase (Schallreuter-Wood & Wood 1995; Wood *et al.* 1995).

Increased catecholamine biosynthesis in association with increased levels of monoamine oxidase A (MAO A)

In patients with vitiligo, significantly increased norepinephrine plasma levels as well as urinary levels of catecholamine metabolites have been well documented by various investigators (Morrone *et al.* 1992; Schallreuter *et al.* 1994c; Orecchia *et al.* 1996). Moreover, these findings correlate with increased epidermal MAO A and catechol-O-methyltransferase activities (Schallreuter *et al.* 1996). One consequence of increased MAO A activities is the accumulation of H_2O_2.

Inhibition of thioredoxin/thioredoxin reductase by calcium

Thioredoxin and thioredoxin reductase are highly expressed in both melanocytes and keratinocytes, in the cytosol as well as in the cell membranes (Schallreuter *et al.* 1986). This effective antioxidant system reduces H_2O_2 to water and its activity is allosterically regulated by calcium via a single specific EF-hands binding domain (Schallreuter & Wood 1991). It has been realized that oxidative stress induces the expression of the system. These results are in agreement with the observation of increased membrane associated thioredoxin reductase activities in vitiligo. The lower activities in the involved skin compared to the uninvolved skin in the same patient could be reconciled on the basis of increased extracellular calcium due to a defective uptake of this ion in both melanocytes and keratinocytes

(Schallreuter & Pittelkow 1988; Schallreuter *et al.* 1994b; Schallreuter-Wood *et al.* 1996).

Increased NADPH oxidase activities by the cellular infiltrate

The presence of a nonspecific perilesional cellular infiltrate in the skin of patients with vitiligo has been well documented. Therefore the 'oxygen burst' of these cells could add to the oxidative stress in vitiligo.

Increased nitric oxide synthase (NOS) activities

NOS catalyses the conversion of L-arginine to L-citrulline yielding nitric oxide or superoxide anion. Inducible as well as constitutive NOS require $6BH_4$ as an essential cofactor and allosteric regulator for their activities (Mayer & Werner 1995). Since $6BH_4$ is overproduced in vitiligo, it was anticipated that NOS activities may be induced in this disorder. Consequently this overproduction could lead to increased H_2O_2 production due to the disproportionation of superoxide anions. Recently we have found a significant expression of both isoenzymes in melanocytes and keratinocytes established from involved and uninvolved epidermis of these patients (K.U. Schallreuter, unpublished data). These findings would support NOS induced H_2O_2 production.

Oxidative stress and calcium homeostasis in vitiligo

It has been well established that oxidative stress can significantly influence calcium homeostasis at the cellular level (Marks *et al.* 1996). An imbalance of this important second messenger has been identified in melanocytes and keratinocytes from involved epidermis of patients with vitiligo compared to healthy controls using the isotope ^{45}calcium (Schallreuter & Pittelkow 1988; Schallreuter-Wood *et al.* 1996). However, it is noteworthy that this imbalance can be corrected upon the addition of 10^{-2} M calcium under *in vitro* conditions.

Pseudocatalase for substitution of impaired catalase in vitiligo

Over twenty years ago Ya Sychev *et al.* (1977) discovered that simple manganese bicarbonate complexes are able to disproportionate H_2O_2 to oxygen and water. The importance of the bicarbonate group to catalase activity by manganese complexes was confirmed by Stadtmans' group (Stadtman *et al.* 1990). Binuclear manganese-containing enzymes with excellent catalase activities were identified in bacteria by Kono and Fridovich (1983). Similar mixed valent binuclear manganese complexes were developed for the oxidative removal of stains from clothes by the detergent industry (Hage *et al.* 1994). Based on these observations we used a bis (Mn)(EDTA) bicarbonate complex (Pseudocatalase, Patent No. EPO58417 1 A) for the removal of H_2O_2 in the epidermis of patients with vitiligo (Schallreuter *et al.* 1995). This pseudocatalase functions as a pro-drug requiring UV light for the full activation of the complex. The efficacy of the successful degradation of epidermal H_2O_2 has been followed *in vivo* using FT Raman spectroscopy. This effective catalytic process is presented in Fig. 23.3.

Successful repigmentation after treatment with a topical pseudocatalase and calcium in combination with low dose UVB

In a pilot study, 33 patients with vitiligo (12 males, 21 females; mean age 41 ranging from 4 to 68 years) have been treated with a topical application of pseudocatalase, calcium and a short-term narrow-band (311 nm) UVB exposure (Schallreuter *et al.* 1995). The majority of the group had photo skin type III (Fitzpatrick classification). Twenty patients had the most common form of generalized vitiligo vulgaris. The mean duration of the disease in the patient group was 14 years (range 1–38). All patients had active disease at the beginning of the treatment. The activity of the disease correlated with the expression of the yellow/green fluorescence upon Wood's light examination, indicative of high epidermal levels of 7-biopterin (Schallreuter *et al.* 1995) (see Fig. 19.1, p 152).

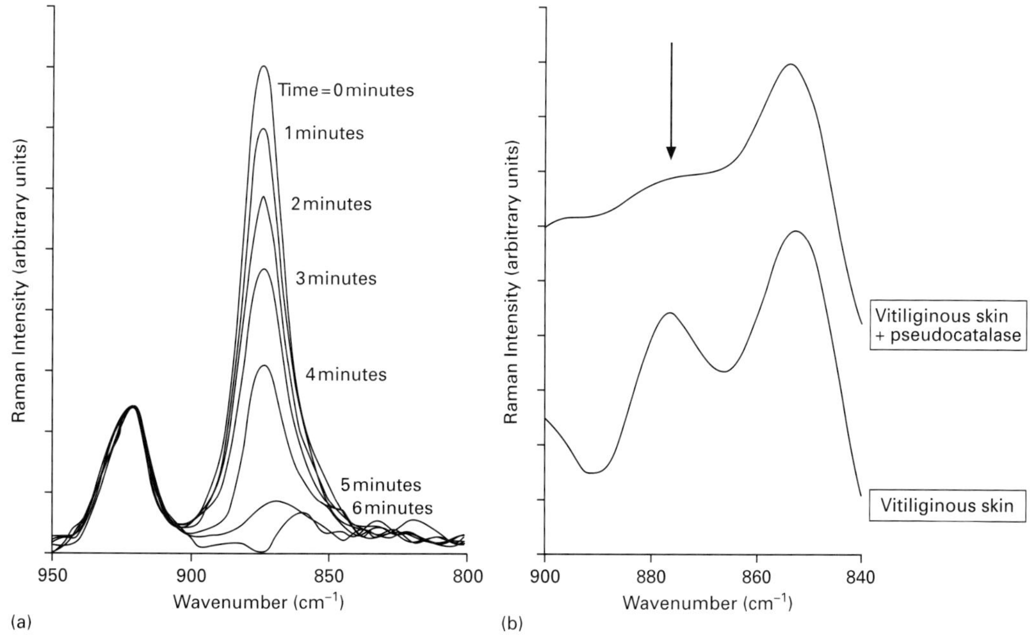

Fig. 23.3 FT-raman spectra of H_2O_2 *in vitro* and *in vivo*. (a) FT-Raman spectra demonstrate the rapid time-dependent removal of H_2O_2 from the solution upon the effect of pseudocatalase following the decrease of the O-O stretch at 875 cm^{-1}. (b) FT-Raman spectroscopy shows the effective H_2O_2 degradation *in vivo* in involved vitiliginous epidermis after the topical application of pseudocatalase containing an active bis (Mn)(EDTA) bicarbonate catalyst.

The treatment protocol included the topical application of the pseudocatalase/calcium formulation twice a day on the total body surface. In addition patients received narrow band (311 nm) UVB radiation with the fixed dose of 0.3 Joule cm^{-2} twice to three times a week. The study was conducted over a period of 36 months.

There were two fundamental observations:

1 The active depigmentation process was stopped in all patients of this group.

2 First repigmentation was observed in the majority after 2–4 months. Focal vitiligo showed 90–100% repigmentation in all cases, in the segmental type the repigmentation was considerably slower and the vulgaris type was usually fastest in the face. There was no repigmentation of the finger tips and the feet. Figures 23.4 and 23.5 present examples before and after treatment with pseudocatalase.

This treatment modality has been used in a sizeable group of patients since the pilot study with less exciting results. There are several explanations for the less successful results of this large trial carried out in London, UK. There is accumulating evidence that the substitution with a pseudocatalase in association with low dose UVB or natural sunlight can successfully correct the epidermal oxidative stress in vitiligo. The close follow up of the repigmentation process in suction blister material as well as in full skin biopsies has clearly proven a reduction of the oxidative damage in the epidermis of these patients. However, the latest results also show that this treatment has, apparently, to be continued until the full repigmentation has taken place because only then does the depigmentation process seem to be fully arrested. In addition, there is now increasing evidence that patients with a significantly inhibited phenylalanine hydroxylase activity in association with an accumulation of epidermal L-phenylalanine do not show any significant repigmentation without correction of this metabolic block (Schallreuter *et al.* 1998). In our experience this patient group represents approximately 40% of the vitiligo population studied so far. It is also noteworthy that these patients do not show any progress of the depigmentation underlining the importance of H_2O_2 in the pathogenesis of this disease (Schallreuter *et al.* 1998). At the present time it is still unclear whether the accumulation of H_2O_2 is the cause or the consequence of a metabolic cascade in this depigmentation disorder.

Recently it was reported that narrow band UVB radiation (311 nm) 3 times per week alone is an efficient treatment for patients with vitiligo (Westerhof & Nieuweboer-Krobotova 1997). The authors compared this treatment to topically applied PUVA and found no significant differences in the efficacy. The average single dose (J cm^{-2}) for this approach was approximately twenty times the dose used in the pseudocatalase trial. During our studies a group of 20 patients treated with 0.3 J cm^{-2} twice a week did not demonstrate any significant improvement after 6 and 12 months (K.U.Schallreuter, unpublished data). However, taking into consideration that UVB generates H_2O_2 and O_2^- it could be possible that the

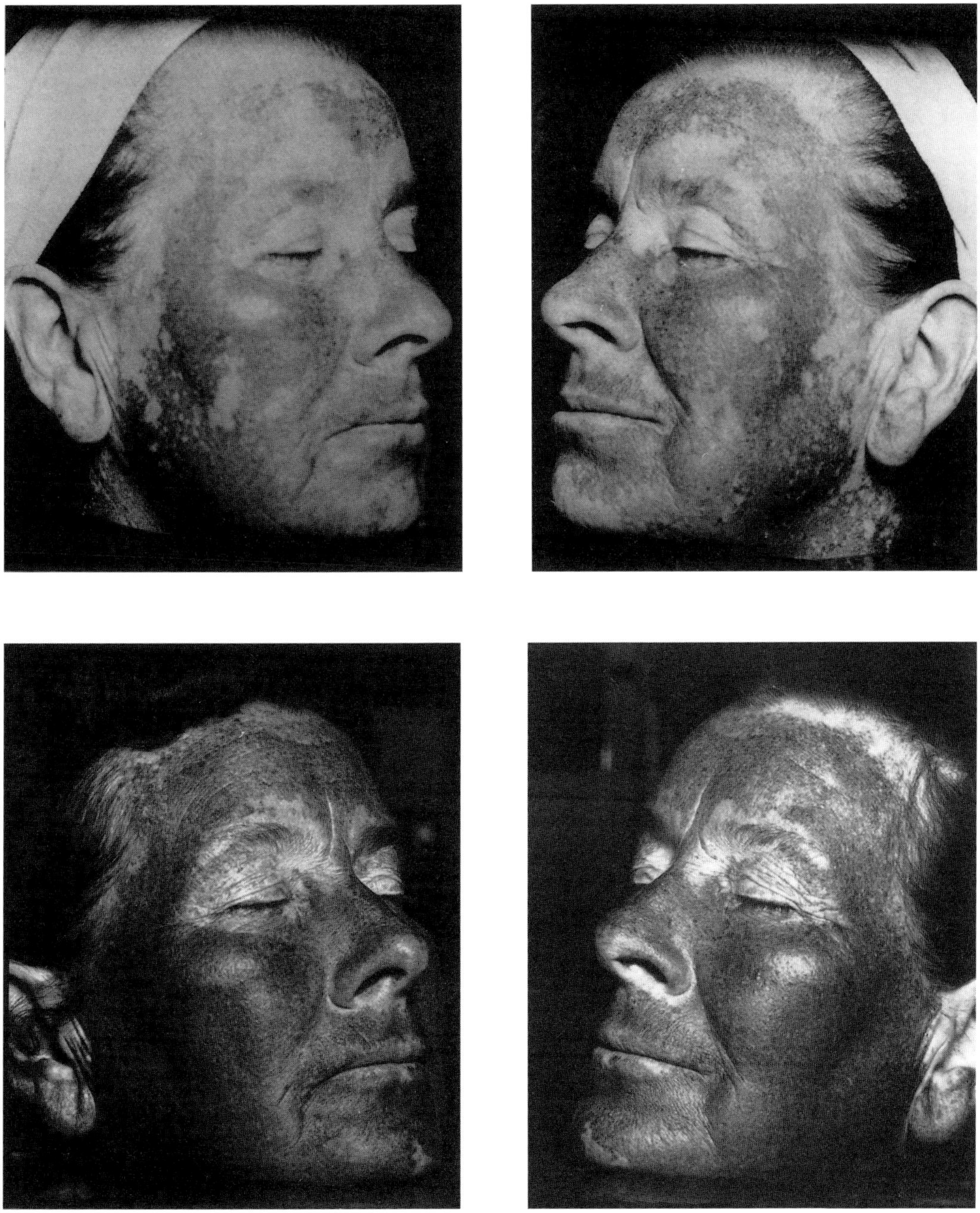

Fig. 23.4 Photographic documentation of pseudocatalase treatment. Facial vitiligo (photo skin type III) after 8 months treatment with pseudocatalase/calcium and UVB (0.3 Joule cm^{-2}) twice per week. The photos are taken with UVA exposure at 351 nm to enhance the contrast between involved and uninvolved skin.

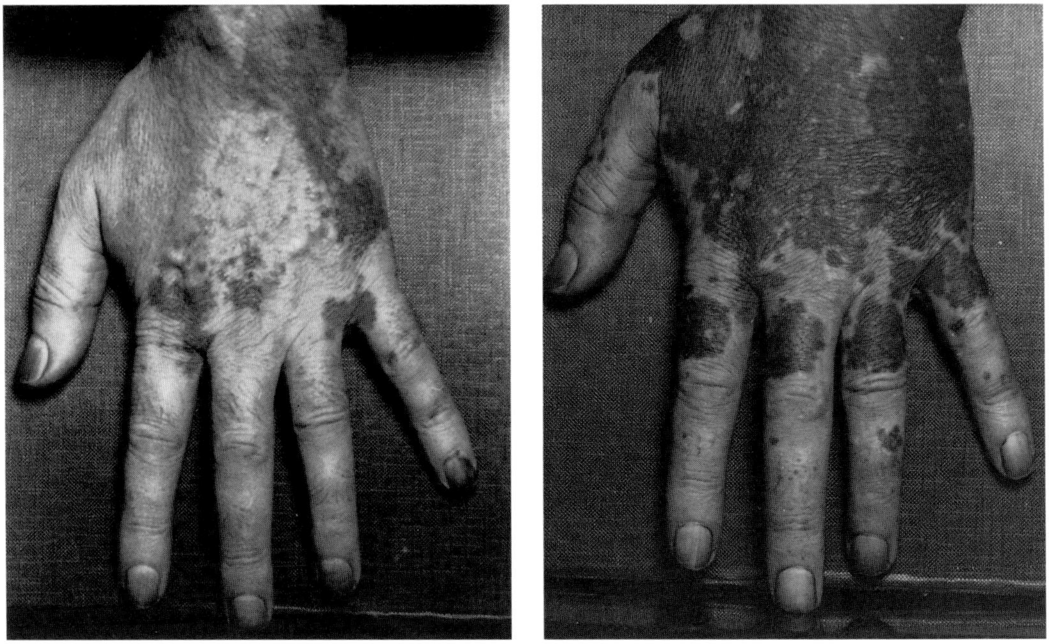

Fig. 23.5 Photographic documentation of pseudocatalase treatment. Extensive vitiligo of the hands (photoskin type III) before and after 12 months treatment with pseudocatalase/calcium and UVB (0.3 Joule cm^{-2}) twice a week (documentation is as described in Fig. 23.4).

amount produced would be insufficient to fully oxidize $6BH_4$–6-biopterin. Under these conditions 7,8-dihydroxanthopterin could be preferentially generated. This metabolite has been claimed to be photoprotective (Armarego *et al.* 1983).

This work needs further investigation.

References

Armarego, W.L.F., Randles, D. & Taguchi, H. (1983) Peroxidase catalyzed aerobic degradation of 5,6,7,8-tetrahydrobiopterin at physiological pH. *European Journal of Biochemistry* **135**, 393–403.

Aronoff, S. (1965) Catalase: kinetics of photo-oxidation. *Science* **150**, 72–73.

Bhawan, J. & Bhutani, L.K. (1983) Keratinocyte damage in vitiligo. *Journal of Cutaneous Pathology* **10**, 207–212.

Boissy, R., Liu, Y.Y., Medrano, E.E. & Nordlund, J.J. (1991) Structural aberration of the rough endoplasmic reticulum and melanosome compartmentalisation in long term cultures of melanocytes from vitiligo patients. *Journal of Investigative Dermatology* **97**, 395–404.

Davis, M.D., Ribeiro, P., Tipper, J. & Kaufman, S. (1992) '7-Tetrahydrobiopterin', a naturally occurring analogue of tetrahydrobiopterin is a cofactor for, and a potential inhibitor of the aromatic amino acid hydroxylases. *Proceedings of the National Academy of Sciences, USA* **89**, 10108–10113.

Hage, R., Iburg, J.E., Kerschner, J. *et al.* (1994) Efficient manganese catalysts for low temperature bleaching. *Nature* **369**, 637–639.
Kono, Y. & Fridovich, I. (1983) Isolation and characterization of the pseudocatalase of Lactobacillus plantarum. *Journal of Biological Chemistry* **258**, 6015–6019.
Maresca, V., Roccella, M., Camera, E. *et al.* (1997) Increased sensitivity to peroxidative agents as a possible pathogenic factor of melanocyte damage in vitiligo. *Journal of Investigative Dermatology* **109**, 310–313.
Marks, D.B., Marks, A.D. & Smith, C.M. (1996) Oxygen metabolism and oxygen toxicity. In: *Basic Medical Biochemistry: a Clinical Approach*, pp. 327–340. Williams & Wilkins, Baltimore, Maryland.
Mayer, B. & Werner, E.R. (1995) Why tetrahydrobiopterin? *Advances in Pharmacology* **34**, 251–261.
Medrano, E.E. & Nordlund, J.J. (1990) Successful culture of adult human melanocytes obtained from normal and vitiligo donors. *Journal of Investigative Dermatology* **95**, 441–445.
Moellman, G., Klein-Angerer, S., Scollay, D.A., Nordlund, J.J. & Lerner, A. (1982) Extracellular granular material and degeneration of keratinocytes in normally pigmented epidermis of patients with vitiligo. *Journal of Investigative Dermatology* **79**, 321–330.
Morrone, A., De Picardo, M., Luca, C. *et al.* (1992) Catecholamines and vitiligo. *Pigment Cell Research* **5**, 58–62.
Nordlund, J.J. & Abdel-Malek, Z. (1988) Progress in clinical and biological research. In: *Mechanisms for Post-Inflammatory Hyperpigmentation and Hypopigmentation* (ed. J. Bagnara), pp. 219–236. Alan R. Liss, New York.
Nordlund, J.J. & Ortonne, J.P. (1992) Vitiligo and depigmentation. *Current Problems in Dermatology* **4**, 3–30.
Orecchia, G., Frattini, P., Cucchi, M.L. & Santagostino, G. (1996) Normal-range plasma catecholamines in patients with generalised and acrofacial vitiligo: preliminary report. *Dermatology* **192**, 191–192.
Ortonne, J.P. & Bose, S.K. (1993) Vitiligo: Where do we stand? *Pigment Cell Research* **8**, 61–72.
Schallreuter, K.U. & Pittelkow, M.R. (1988) Defective calcium uptake in keratinocyte cell cultures from vitiliginous skin. *Archives of Dermatological Research* **280**, 137–139.
Schallreuter, K.U. & Wood, J.M. (1991) EF-hands calcium-binding regulates the thioredoxin reductase/thioredoxin electron transfer in human keratinocytes and melanocytes. In: *Novel Calcium-Binding Proteins* (ed. C. Heizmann), pp. 339–360. Springer Verlag, Berlin.
Schallreuter, K.U., Pittelkow, M.R. & Wood, J.M. (1986) Free radical reduction by thioredoxin reductase at the surface of normal and vitiliginous human keratinocytes. *Journal of Investigative Dermatology* **87**, 728–732.
Schallreuter, K.U., Wood, J.M. & Berger, J. (1991) Low catalase levels in the epidermis of patients with vitiligo. *Journal of Investigative Dermatology* **97**, 1081–1085.
Schallreuter, K.U., Büttner, G., Pittelkow, M.R., Wood, J.M., Swanson, N.N. & Körner, C. (1994a) The cytotoxicity of 6-biopterin to human melanocytes. *Biochemical and Biophysical Research Communications* **204**, 43–48.
Schallreuter, K.U., Wood, J.M., Pittelkow, M.R. *et al.* (1994b) Regulation of melanin biosynthesis in the human epidermis by tetrahydrobiopterin. *Science* **263**, 1444–1446.
Schallreuter, K.U., Wood, J.M., Ziegler, I. *et al.* (1994c) Defective tetrahydrobiopterin and catecholamine biosynthesis in the depigmentation disorder vitiligo. *Biochimica et Biophysica Acta* **1226**, 181–192.
Schallreuter, K.U., Wood, J.M., Lemke, K.R. & Levenig, C. (1995) Treatment of vitiligo with a topical application of pseudocatalase and calcium in combination with short term UVB exposure: a case on 33 patients. *Dermatology* **190**, 223–229.
Schallreuter, K.U., Wood, J.M., Pittelkow, M.R. *et al.* (1996) Increased monoamine oxidase A activity in the epidermis of patients with vitiligo. *Archives of Dermatological Research* **288**, 14–18.

Schallreuter, K.U., Zschiesche, M., Moore, J. *et al.* (1998) *In vivo* evidence for compromised phenylalanine metabolism in vitiligo. *Biochemical and Biophysical Research Communications* **243**, 395–399.

Schallreuter-Wood, K.U. & Wood, J.M. (1995) Control of melanogenesis in the human epidermis by the redox-status of tetrahydrobiopterins. *Pteridines* **6**, 104–107.

Schallreuter-Wood, K.U., Pittelkow, M.R. & Swanson, N.N. (1996) Defective calcium transport in vitiliginous melanocytes. *Archives of Dermatological Research* **288**, 11–13.

Schallreuter, K.U., Moore, J., Wood, J.M., Beazley, W.D., Gaze, D.C. *et al.* (1999) *In vivo* and *in vitro* evidence for hydrogen peroxide (H_2O_2) accumulation in the epidermis of patients with vitiligo and its successful removal by a UVB activated pseudocatalase. *Journal of Investigative Dermatology, Symposium Proceedings* **4**, 91–96.

Stadtman, E.R., Bertlett, B.S. & Chock, P.B. (1990) Manganese dependent disproportionation of hydrogen peroxide in bicarbonate buffer. *Proceedings of the National Academy of Sciences USA* **87**, 384–388.

Westerhof, W. & Nieuweboer-Krobotova, L. (1997) Treatment of vitiligo with UVB radiation vs topical psoralen plus UV-A. *Archives of Dermatology* **133**, 1525–1528.

Wood, J.M., Schallreuter-Wood, K.U., Lindsey, N.J. *et al.* (1995) A specific tetrahydrobiopterin binding domain on tyrosinase controls melanogenesis. *Biochemical and Biophysical Research Communications* **206**, 480–485.

Ya Sychev, A., Isak, V.G. & Van Lap, D. (1977) Catalytic properties of carbonate complexes of manganese (II) and cobalt (II) in the decomposition of hydrogen peroxide. *Zhornal Fizicheskoi Khimii* **51**, 363–366.

Yohn, J.J., Norris, D.A., Yrastorza, G. *et al.* (1991) Disparate antioxidant enzyme activities in cultured human cutaneous fibroblasts, keratinocytes and melanocytes. *Journal of Investigative Dermatology* **97**, 405–409.

24: Surgical Therapies for Vitiligo

RAFAEL FALABELLA

Introduction

In spite of all available medical therapies for vitiligo, a significant number of patients fail to respond with appropriate repigmentation, and yet they want additional treatment. Failure is probably due to:

1 a too strong and active depigmentation process for which medical treatment is relatively weak to induce repigmentation;

2 the melanocyte reservoir located in the hair follicle (Ortonne *et al.* 1980; Cui *et al.* 1991, Chapter 20) is completely depleted, and/or spared melanocytes from epidermis, or those located at the border of lesions, cannot be fully stimulated because of badly understood factors.

Grafting and transplantation of melanocytes may be an answer to this situation, by artificially creating a new source of pigment cells on depigmented skin, from which melanocytes proliferate and spread originating repigmentation of affected areas. However, an important condition to be considered before trying surgical repair is to determine the depigmentation activity in the affected patient with vitiligo, since a stable disease must be established in order to achieve repigmentation by these methods. Although a precise characterization is lacking, stable vitiligo may be defined according to several parameters:

1 no further depigmentation or enlargement of old maculae for about 2 years;

2 no Koebner's phenomenon developing during the same period of time;

3 spontaneous repigmentation around or within achromic lesions;

4 a positive minigrafting test, where a repigmentation halo occurs around small 1–2 mm minigrafts implanted 3–4 mm apart within the recipient site (Falabella *et al.* 1995a).

Indications and contraindications for surgical repair

Not every patient with vitiligo is a good candidate for surgical repigmentation and the key for success is an appropriate selection of patients, since there are specific criteria that must be fulfilled for such therapies.

Indications

1 The best indication is unilateral vitiligo, either segmental or focal, when this condition has come to a halt and stable disease, as defined previously, is observed. A success rate of about 95% in these patients may be anticipated (Falabella *et al.* 1995a).
2 Bilateral vitiligo, when stable, may also respond in about 48% of selected patients (Falabella *et al.* 1995a).
3 Other skin conditions with depigmentation that may respond to surgical methods are: piebaldism (Falabella *et al.* 1995b), achromia due to monobenzyl ether of hydroquinone toxicity, leukoderma post burn or trauma, and healed discoid lupus erythematosus (LE) (Falabella 1986).

Contraindications

1 An absolute contraindication for surgery of vitiligo is progression of the depigmenting process, mainly observed in bilateral vitiligo. In this clinical presentation it is compulsory to define the complete stability before any surgical attempt is made.
2 A keloidal diathesis, mainly if the upper dermis is manipulated with surgical procedures.
3 A hyperpigmentation tendency to minor trauma, since relatively dark skin following surgical repigmentation procedures may be aesthetically unacceptable.

Selection of patients

Patients qualifying for surgical procedures should be carefully evaluated. Once the condition has been established as refractory to medical therapy and there are clear indications for surgical repair, several things should be considered before treatment is initiated (Falabella 1989):

Age of patient. Surgical procedures should be preferably performed after adolescence; nevertheless some younger patients may accept correction of achromic defects.

Emotional stability. Surgical repigmentation is an invasive procedure, which may originate pigmentary imperfections. These changes may not be well accepted by emotionally unstable patients, who are excessively concerned about their aesthetic alterations.

Patient's expectations. Every effort should be made by explaining to the patient about anticipated results of surgical repigmentation. Although remarkable improvement is frequently achieved, minor changes such as incomplete repigmentation, slight hyperpigmentation or minor scars at donor or recipient sites should be discussed with the patient to avoid confusion or misunderstanding.

Size and location of lesions. The preferred lesions to be treated are those located on exposed and more visible areas; extensive depigmentation is difficult to restore and treatment is usually prolonged; in such patients the cost benefit is questionable.

Minigrafting test. It is recommended that only patients with a positive test, in whom an appropriate response to therapy may be anticipated, should be treated. This test offers reassurance to both patient and physician about future results of surgical therapy.

Side-effects. Although unpredictable, the possibility of developing hyperpigmentation or hypopigmentation, secondary infection, lack of graft survival and minor scars should be mentioned to patients, so that they fully understand and collaborate to solve or accept these minor problems when they occur.

Technique and donor area. In spite of being technical items, advantages or disadvantages should be discussed with the patient before therapy. Sometimes minor but permanent changes may occur in the donor area, mainly when the dermis is manipulated.

Serial procedures. Repigmentation, as a rule, is not achieved in a single procedure, and several sessions should be planned to obtain acceptable cosmetic results. Minor additional sessions may be required.

Methods

Several methods are suitable for surgical repigmentation.

Epidermal suspensions

A donor skin sample is obtained from the scalp by superficial shaving (Gauthier & Surleve-Bazeille 1992) and treated with trypsin 0.25% until an epidermal suspension containing keratinocytes and melanocytes is obtained. After washing these cells with saline solution, the suspension is inoculated into blisters raised with liquid nitrogen or spread onto achromic skin previously denuded by superficial dermabrasion. Repigmentation occurs by coalescence of cell grafted areas within the following months.

Suction epidermal grafting

Initially described for stable leukoderma other than vitiligo (Falabella 1971,

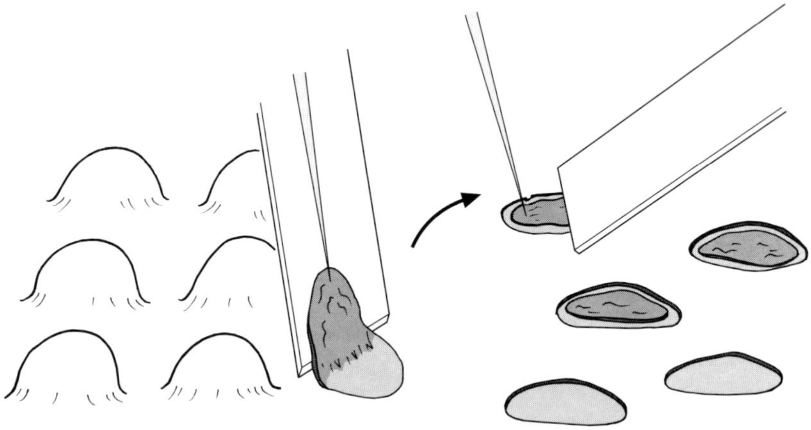

Fig. 24.1 Suction epidermal grafting. (a) After 2 or 3 three hours of suction, or 1 hour if heat is simultaneously applied (42°C), donor blisters suitable for grafting are obtained; (b) these epidermal grafts are transferred to recipient sites, previously treated with liquid nitrogen 2 days earlier, and denuded on the day of grafting.

1984), this method has been used in recent years by others for stable vitiligo with noticeable success (Suvanprakorn *et al.* 1985; Koga 1988; Matsumura *et al.* 1993; Mutalik 1993; Hann *et al.* 1995). This method is performed in two stages. First, denuding the recipient site by either blistering with liquid nitrogen which is done two days prior to grafting, and secondly, harvesting the grafts by raising the donor epidermis with suction at a negative pressure of 200–300 mmHg during 2–3 hours. If heat up to 42°C is applied to the donor site during suction, blistered grafts may be obtained in 45–60 minutes (Skouge *et al.* 1992). Grafts are freed from donor site with iris scissors and transferred to the recipient bed with a microscope glass slide used as a carrier spatula. The epidermis is preferably implanted as small 0.5–1.0 cm grafts separated from each other by similar distance, and covered with nonadherent dressings (Fig. 24.1); repigmentation occurs after several months by proliferation of melanocytes and pigment spread from grafts originating coalescence of treated areas. Sunlight exposure or PUVA therapy enhance the repigmentation process (Hann *et al.* 1995; Skouge & Morison 1995). The advantages of this method are the absence of scarring, and the possibility of reusing the donor site for future treatments. Care should be taken in avoiding this procedure in active vitiligo because besides failure, koebnerization of the donor site may occur (Hatchome *et al.* 1990).

Thin dermo-epidermal grafts

Initially described in India for treating long-standing, quiescent vitiligo (Behl 1964). The purpose of this method is to remove the achromic epidermis and superficial papillary dermis of a depigmented area of vitiligo by

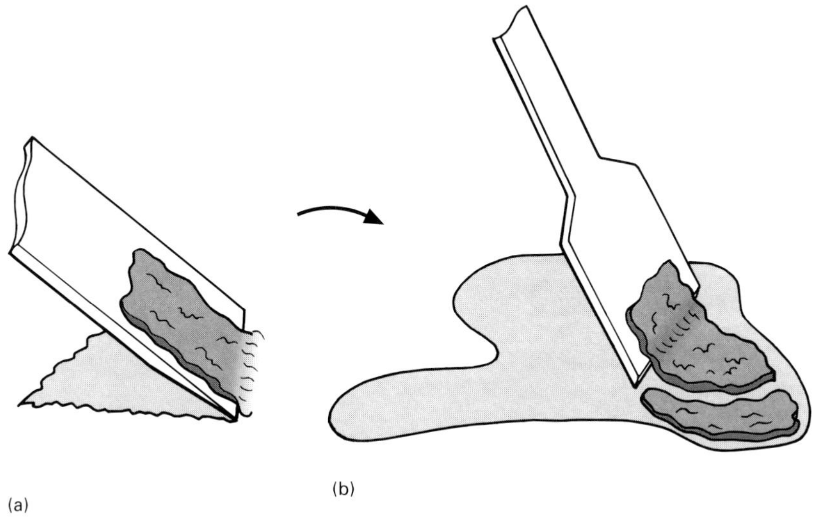

Fig. 24.2 Thin dermo-epidermal grafts. (a) Harvesting thin split 0.03 mm thickness grafts is performed with dermatome; (b) grafts are then transferred with a grafting spatula onto a depigmented area where the epidermis was previously removed by superficial dermabrasion.

dermabrasion, and replace it with very thin dermo-epidermal grafts of about 0.03 mm thickness harvested from normally pigmented donor skin (Fig. 24.2); the treated lesion usually repigments within several weeks (Kahn & Cohen 1995). Although the method is simple, care should be taken to avoid harvesting grafts of excessive thickness to prevent unaesthetic results and/or hypopigmentation or slight scarring at donor site.

Minigrafting

This is the simplest method that can be carried out by any dermatologist without special training; besides, minimal equipment is required. It consists of implanting very small punch grafts of 1.0–1.2 mm within achromic areas, separated 3–4 mm from each other (Falabella 1988) (Fig. 24.3); repigmentation occurs by melanocyte and pigment spread up to 2 mm from the edge of each minigraft, covering an area of about 4–5 mm in diameter, corresponding to approximately 20–25 times its original size (Falabella 1986). Grafts may be harvested from hidden areas such as gluteal regions, although other areas are also suitable for this method. Once grafted, the recipient site is covered with Micropore® adhesive tape and left in place for 2 weeks; 2 mm punch grafts have also been tried with success (Boersma *et al.* 1995). Repigmentation occurs by coalescence of pigmentation arising from the small grafted dermoepidermal islands within several months, but sunlight exposure for 10–15 min daily is important to stimulate melanocyte migration. Serial procedures are frequently required for restoring pigmentation in the average patient (Fig. 24.4). One of the disadvantages of this method is the development of minute and punctiform scars at the donor site, which can be

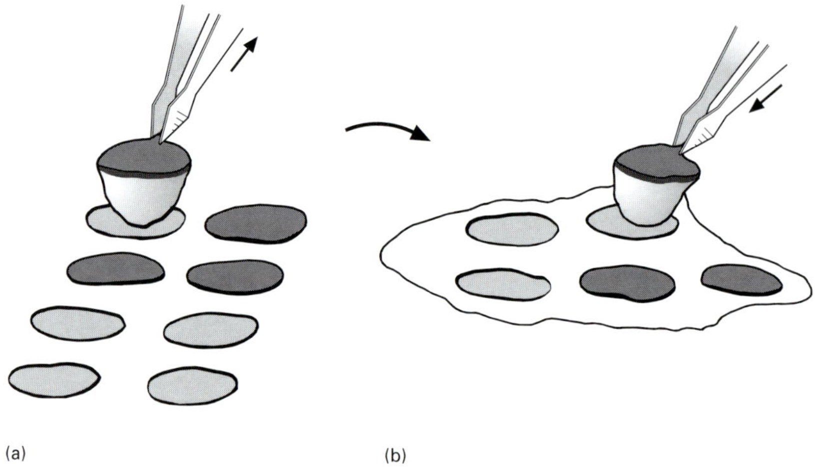

Fig. 24.3 Minigrafting. (a) Small, 1.0–1.2 mm punch grafts are harvested very close to each other from the gluteal region, and collected on a nonadhering dressing moistened with physiologic saline solution; (b) minigrafts are then transferred to the recipient site, where small perforations separated 3–4 mm apart were performed prior to harvesting the minigrafts. The treated area is covered with Micropore adhesive tape for 2 weeks.

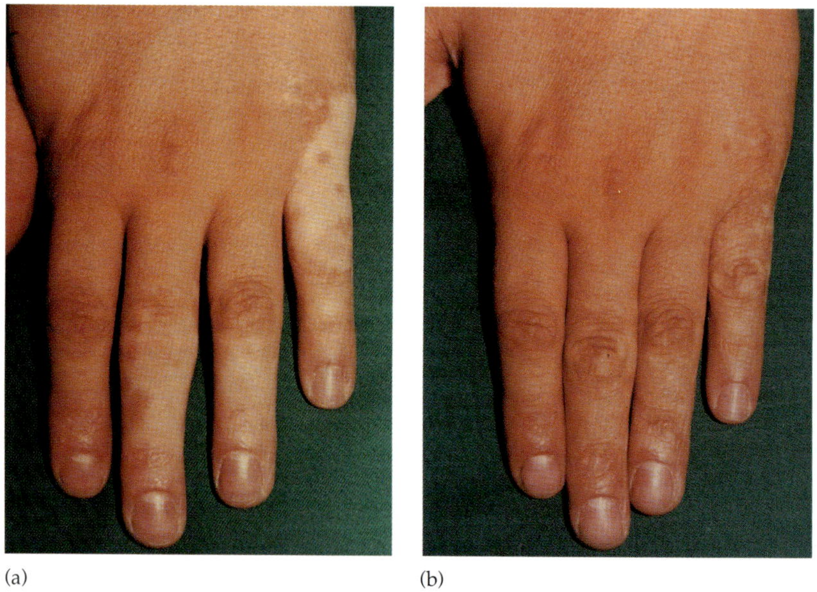

Fig. 24.4 (a) Minigrafting. A 35-year-old patient developed unilateral vitiligo on the dorsum of his last three right fingers. Achromic skin became refractory to medical therapy and remained stable for the last 3 years. (b) After several minigrafting sessions and a few additional minigrafts where required, nearly complete repigmentation was achieved in this difficult anatomical location.

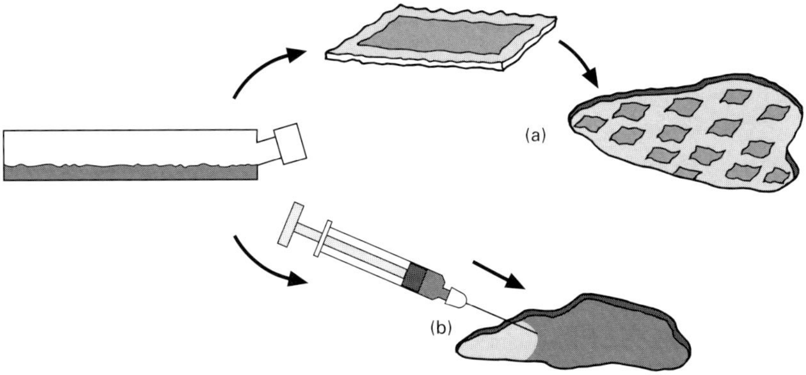

Fig. 24.5 *In vitro* cultured epidermis and melanocyte suspensions. (a) Cultured cells are obtained by trypsinization of a small donor skin sample, and processed with different methods to form either epidermal membranes or melanocyte cell suspensions; (b) membranes are transferred to donor leukodermic sites previously denuded with liquid nitrogen as for epidermal grafting, or cell suspensions are inoculated and spread onto similar areas previously prepared by superficial dermabrasion.

more noticeable with minigrafts larger than 1.2 mm. Nevertheless, the benefit achieved by repigmenting the achromic defect is far more rewarding than this minor side-effect. Minigrafts of 1.0 mm are recommended in facial lesions of young patients to prevent the possibility of 'cobblestoning', a side-effect observed in minigrafting due to slight protrusion of minigrafts on the surface of the treated achromic defect (Falabella 1986, 1988).

In-vitro cultured epidermis and melanocyte suspensions

Although at present these methods are at a stage of development, newer technologies by culturing cells *in vitro* have been successfully used for repigmenting vitiligo and piebaldism. Two basic methods have been reported:

1 Cultured epidermal sheets with melanocytes, which are transplanted onto achromic skin with similar procedures as described for epidermal grafting (Brysk *et al.* 1989; Falabella *et al.* 1989, 1992), and

2 Cultured melanocyte suspensions, which are transplanted onto depigmented areas previously denuded with dermabrasion or liquid nitrogen blistering, by spreading cells onto the surface of these areas (Fig. 24.5).

Repigmentation usually occurs after several months by re-colonization of pigment cells within the basal cell layer of the new epidermis (Lontz *et al.* 1994; Olsson & Juhlin 1995). The enormous future potential of this technology for treating vitiligo has been demonstrated by transplantation of cryopreserved cultured autologous melanocytes in several patients, followed by repigmentation of achromic defects (Olsson *et al.* 1994). However, more knowledge on the biology and safety of *in vitro* cultured cells is necessary before cultured cells are used in daily practice (Falabella 1994).

Combination method

Repigmentation methods are selected individually for each patient depending on the available technology and physician's experience; however, combination of surgical procedures may be useful, particularly in small areas that did not become repigmented with any of the previously described methods; partially repigmented defects can be additionally treated by implanting a few extra minigrafts in such areas devoid of pigmentation until complete restoration of affected areas is achieved (Falabella *et al.* 1995a).

Repigmentation of leukotrichia

During surgical repigmentation of vitiligo with *in vitro* cultured grafts, it was observed that depigmented hairs on treated areas recovered their normal pigmentation. An explanation for this phenomenon was the possible migration of pigment cells from the grafted epidermis towards the hair follicle walls and from this site towards the hair bulb, where melanocytes incorporated normal pigment into the hair shaft (Falabella *et al.* 1992). Later on, successful repigmentation of hairs was also achieved on areas of leukotrichia by implanting epidermal grafts followed by PUVA (Hann *et al.* 1992, 1995) and thin dermo-epidermal grafts (Agrawal & Agrawal 1995).

Finally, surgical methods for repigmenting vitiligo are important therapeutic options for depigmented skin, but medical failure and stable disease are *conditio sine qua non* for considering these procedures as the main therapy; besides, careful selection of patients is a definitive clue for success.

References

Agrawal, K. & Agrawal, A. (1995) Vitiligo: Repigmentation with dermabrasion and split thickness skin graft. *Dermatologic Surgery* **21**, 295–300.

Behl, P.N. (1964) Treatment of vitiligo with homologous thin Thiersch skin grafts. *Current Medical Practice* **8**, 218–221.

Boersma, B.R., Westerhof, W. & Bos, J.D. (1995) Repigmentation in vitiligo vulgaris by autologous minigrafting: Results in nineteen patients. *Journal of the American Academy of Dermatology* **33**, 990–995.

Brysk, M.M., Newton, R.M., Rajaraman, S. *et al.* (1989) Repigmentation of vitiliginous skin by cultured cells. *Pigment Cell Research* **2**, 202–207.

Cui, J., Shen, L. & Wang, G. (1991) Role of hair follicles in the repigmentation of vitiligo. *Journal of Investigative Dermatology* **97**, 410–416.

Falabella, R. (1971) Epidermal grafting. An original technique and its application in achromic and granulating areas. *Archives of Dermatology* **104**, 592–600.

Falabella, R. (1984) Repigmentation of leukoderma by autologous epidermal grafting. *Journal of Dermatologic Surgery and Oncology* **10**, 136–144.

Falabella, R. (1986) Repigmentation of stable leukoderma by autologous minigrafting. *Journal of Dermatologic Surgery and Oncology* **12**, 172–179.

Falabella, R. (1988) Treatment of localized vitiligo by autologous minigrafting. *Archives of Dermatology* **124**, 1649–1655.

Falabella, R. (1989) Grafting and transplantation of melanocytes for repigmenting vitiligo and other types of leukoderma. *International Journal of Dermatology* **28**, 363–369.

Falabella, R. (1994) Vitiligo (Letter). *Acta Dermato-Venereologica (Stockholm)* **74**, 147–156.

Falabella, R., Escobar, C. & Borrero, I. (1989) Transplantation of *in-vitro* cultured epidermis bearing melanocytes for repigmenting vitiligo. *Journal of the American Academy of Dermatology* **21**, 257–264.

Falabella, R., Borrero, I. & Escobar, C. (1992) Treatment of refractory and stable vitiligo by *in-vitro* cultured epidermal autografts bearing melanocytes. *Journal of the American Academy of Dermatology* **26**, 230–236.

Falabella, R., Arrunátegui, A., Barona, M.I. & Alzate, A. (1995a) The minigrafting test for vitiligo: Detection of stable lesions for melanocyte transplantation. *Journal of the American Academy of Dermatology* **32**, 228–232.

Falabella, R., Barona, M.I., Escobar, C., Borrero, I. & Arrunátegui, A. (1995b) Surgical combination therapy for vitiligo and piebaldism. *Dermatologic Surgery* **21**, 852–857.

Gauthier, Y. & Surleve-Bazeille, J.E. (1992) Autologous grafting of non cultured melanocytes: a simplified method for treatment of depigmented lesions. *Journal of the American Academy of Dermatology* **26**, 191–194.

Hann, S.K., Im, S., Park, Y.K. & Hur, W. (1992) Repigmentation of leukotrichia by epidermal grafting and systemic psoralen plus UVA (Letter). *Archives of Dermatology* **128**, 998–999.

Hann, S.K., Im, S., Bong, H.W. & Park, Y.K. (1995) Treatment of stable vitiligo with autologous epidermal grafting and PUVA. *Journal of the American Academy of Dermatology* **32**, 943–948.

Hatchome, N., Kato, T. & Tagami, H. (1990) Therapeutic success of epidermal grafting in generalized vitiligo is limited by the Koebner phenomenon. *Journal of the American Academy of Dermatology* **22**, 87–91.

Kahn, A. & Cohen, M.J. (1995) Vitiligo: Treatment by dermabrasion and epithelial sheeth grafting. *Journal of the American Academy of Dermatology* **33**, 646–648.

Koga, M. (1988) Epidermal grafting using the tops of suction blisters in the treatment of vitiligo. *Archives of Dermatology* **124**, 1656–1658.

Lontz, W., Olsson, M.J., Moellman, G. & Lerner, A. (1994) Pigment cell transplantation for treatment of vitiligo: a progress report. *Journal of the American Academy of Dermatology* **30**, 591–597.

Matsumura, Y., Furukawa, F. & Imamura, S. (1993) Epidermal grafting for treatment of vitiligo. Associations among success rate, clinical type and autoantibodies. *Journal of Dermatologic Treatment* **4**, 109–112.

Mutalik, S. (1993) Transplantation of melanocytes by epidermal grafting. An Indian experience. *Journal of Dermatologic Surgery and Oncology* **19**, 231–234.

Olsson, M.J. & Juhlin, L. (1995) Transplantation of melanocytes in vitiligo. *British Journal of Dermatology* **132**, 587–591.

Olsson, M.J., Moellman, G., Lerner, A. & Juhlin, L. (1994) Vitiligo repigmentation with cultured melanocytes after cryostorage. *Acta Dermato-Venereologica (Stockholm)* **74**, 226–228.

Ortonne, J.P., Schmitt, D. & Thivolet, J. (1980) PUVA-induced repigmentation of vitiligo: scanning electron microscopy of hair follicles. *Journal of Investigative Dermatology* **74**, 40–42.

Skouge, J.W., Morison, W.L., Diwan, R.V. & Rotter, S. (1992) Autografting and PUVA. *Journal of Dermatologic Surgery and Oncology* **118**, 357–360.

Skouge, J.W. & Morison, W.L. (1995). Vitiligo treatment with a combination of PUVA therapy and epidermal autografts. *Archives of Dermatology* **131**, 1257–1258.

Suvanprakorn, P., Dee-Ananlap, S., Pongsomboon, C. & Klaus, S.N. (1985) Melanocyte autologous grafting for treatment of leukoderma. *Journal of the American Academy of Dermatology* **13**, 968–974.

25: Micropigmentation

REBAT M. HALDER

Many patients with vitiligo respond favourably to treatment modalities such as topical corticosteroids and PUVA therapy. Even in these patients, certain areas such as the lips, distal digits, elbows and knees continue to respond poorly. Various preparations such as makeup and dyes are available to cover these areas. However, these are not permanent or waterproof. Moreover, other areas such as the axilla and genitals are not amenable to PUVA therapy because of their sensitivity to the treatment.

The technique of permanent dermal micropigmentation using a non-allergenic iron oxide pigment can be used to cover recalcitrant areas of vitiligo (Halder *et al.* 1989; Bolognia 1993; Bose 1995; Halder & Nordlund 1998). This is an adaptation of the technique of permanent eyeliner tattooing (Patipa 1987). The pigment is tattooed into the skin by means of a cluster of needles attached to a high speed reciprocating apparatus. The apparatus used consists of a hand piece equipped with a needle holder tip which is connected to a power unit. A foot pedal is used to activate the hand piece. The hand piece is capable of variable speeds up to 9200 strokes per minute and the depth of needle penetration is adjustable from 1 to 1.75 mm.

The iron oxide pigments are available in a variety of colours and shades from various manufacturers. It is advisable to avoid colours that contain black or grey pigments as these will result in a Tyndall effect causing a blue or purple hue to appear in areas of micropigmentation. As will be discussed later, there is fading of the dye by about 20% within the first few weeks (Mazza & Rager 1993). However, because the dye is being applied to a completely achromic area, the colour will appear darker than the surrounding normal skin upon initial application (Halder *et al.* 1989). Thus, when the micropigmentation technique is used for vitiligo, it is best to choose a colour that actually closely matches the surrounding normal skin.

A 9-cluster needle consisting of a rosette of 9 needle tips and measuring approximately 1 mm in diameter is used (Fig. 25.1).

In preparation for the procedure, the patient is positioned for comfort while allowing for good exposure and stabilization of the skin area of interest. This area is carefully prepared with an antiseptic solution such as 70% isopropyl alcohol or 10% povidone-iodine solution. Sterile towels are draped around it. The skin is anaesthetized by infiltrating with a 1%-2% lidocaine solution with or without epinephrine (1 : 100 000 v/v) subcutaneously. Epinephrine should not be used in local anaesthesia of the ear, tip of the nose, or fingers because of the risk of ischaemia. For extensive vitiligo involvement of the fingers or lips, nerve block anaesthesia is used.

The micropigmentation process is carried out at cycles of 9200 strokes per minute. The hand piece is set at 1.75 mm. At this setting the pigments have been shown histologically to penetrate to the level of the dermis (Tse *et al.* 1985; Papita *et al.* 1986; Patipa 1987). Best results are obtained by repeated gentle jabbing motions with the needle perpendicular to the skin surface until a confluent layer of abutting pigment dots is deposited (Fig. 25.2). The force applied with each jabbing motion to achieve proper needle penetration depends on the firmness and thickness of the skin being tattooed. Fingertips and areas over bony prominences require virtually no force, whereas firm pressure with the hand piece is necessary on the lips. An antibiotic ointment is used as needed to wipe away the excess pigment during the procedure. Freshly micropigmented areas are either dressed

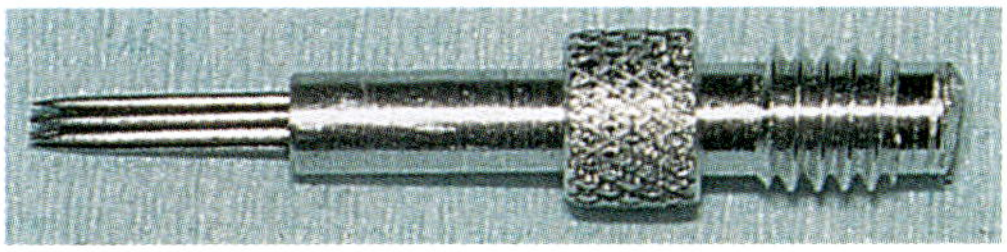

Fig. 25.1 Cluster needle used for micropigmentation.

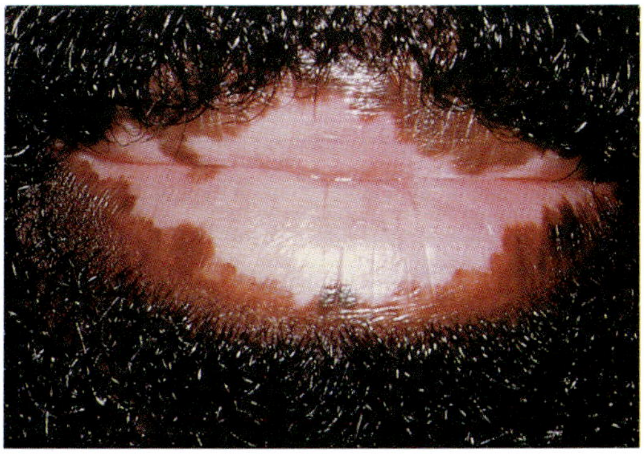

(a)

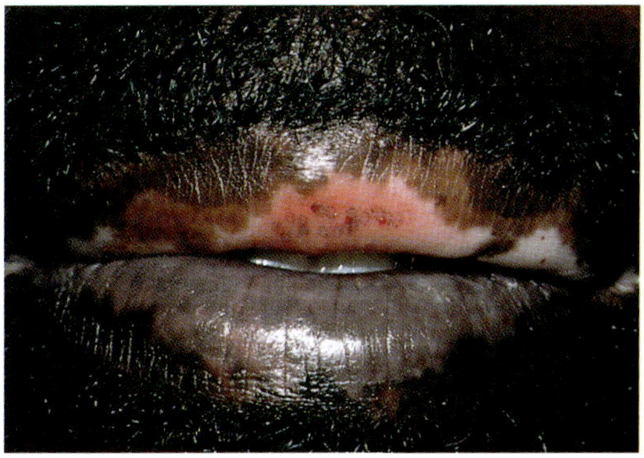

(b)

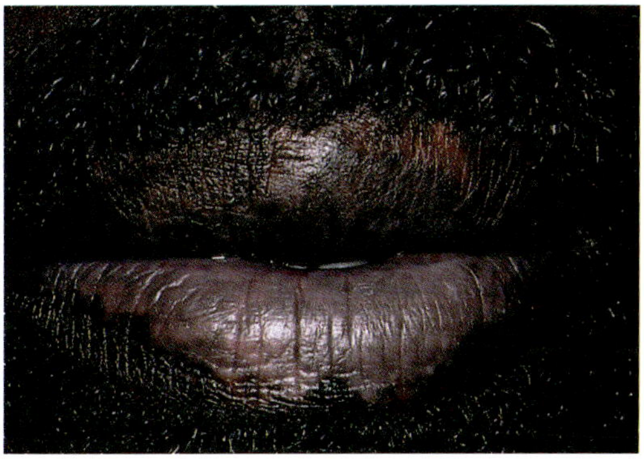

(c)

Fig. 25.2 (a) Vitiligo of the lips unresponsive to PUVA therapy. (b) Micropigmentation of lower lip completed. Note rosette formation of pigment being placed in upper lip. (c) Micropigmentation completed of upper and lower lip. Tyndall effect is seen on lower lip.

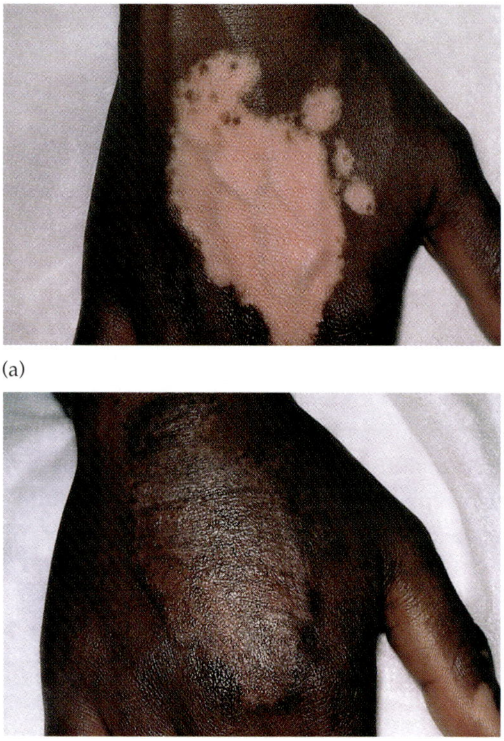

(a)

(b)

Fig. 25.3 (a) Vitiligo of dorsum of hand. (b) Hand after micropigmentation. Note the fading of colour in treated area.

with the antibiotic ointment and sterile nonadherent dressings or, for the lips, application of antibiotic ointment alone is sufficient. Written instructions are given to keep the dressing clean and dry and to remove it after 24 hours. Thereafter, the micropigmented areas are left exposed while keeping them as dry as possible for the next 5 days, except for the application of antibiotic ointment twice a day. Specific instructions are made against exposing these areas to alcohol, acetone, detergents, and other cleaning agents except for mild soap for at least 1 week if necessary. All patients are routinely instructed to return for weekly follow-up for the first 2 weeks and then monthly if no complications occur.

The immediate result of micropigmentation is a dramatic aesthetic improvement (Figs 25.2 & 25.3). Fading does occur, however. For the majority of cases only a moderate degree of fading occurs. In some cases, especially those involving the fingertips there is a significant loss of pigment. Generally, the most precipitous loss of pigment occurs within 1 week of the procedure with maximal fading occurring within 6 weeks. The pigment that remains usually persists with minimal to no further fading, although a slight bluish hue is noted in most cases, evidence of the Tyndall effect (Fig. 25.3).

Short-term complications are few, mild, localized and generally occur immediately following the procedure with complete resolution within 1 week. These include serous oozing from scattered points of puncture usually lasting several hours. Moderate swelling of the lips invariably occurs, however, with resolution within 24 hours. Herpes simplex infection of the lips has been reported to be reactivated following the procedure (Halder *et al.* 1989). It is essential to inquire about previous herpes simplex infection. Patients with such a history should not have micropigmentation of the lips or should be treated with prophylactic antiviral drugs. Bacterial infection rarely occurs in a treated area (Halder *et al.* 1989).

Long-term complications of micropigmentation include Koebnerization at the site of micropigmentation with enlargement of the borders of the treated area (Halder *et al.* 1989). There have been rare reports of allergy to the pigments used (Larson 1996). X-ray analysis has shown titanium and talc particles in addition to iron oxide in some dyes (Simons *et al.* 1988). These contaminants or iron oxide itself may be the cause of allergic reactions. A scratch test and patch test to detect pigment allergy should be done 10–14 days prior to the procedure. Sarcoid-like granulomas at tattooed sites have been reported as another long-term complication of micropigmentation (Larson 1996). It has been noted that some people who have had micropigmentation with iron oxide pigments have swelling in a treated area following magnetic resonance imaging (MRI) (Jackson & Aker 1987; Carr 1995; Larson 1996). This may be due to the fact that magnetically active substances injected into the skin act as conductors (Sacco 1987). It is advised that patients who have micropigmentation done be warned about and be reminded to mention this if they later have MRI to a treated area.

Micropigmentation for vitiligo is overall a safe procedure and is especially useful for sites that have a poor rate of repigmentation with other modalities. The permanent and waterproof nature of the pigment has obvious advantages over the inconveniences inherent with the use of make up to cover vitiligo areas. By allowing the patient to perform their daily activities with added confidence and convenience, it positively affects the psychosocial well-being of the individual. Disadvantages include the invariable fading of the pigment which requires additional treatments with the procedure. It can be difficult to match the patient's skin colour perfectly. As well, the colour does not adjust to seasonal changes of uninvolved sites (LePoole & Boissy 1997). There have been no studies that have shown the protective effect of iron oxide pigments against ultraviolet light so that patients should be cautioned about sun exposure to treated areas. Removal of unwanted or unsatisfactory micropigmentation tattoos has been reported with the use of super-pulsed CO_2, alexandrite, flashlamp pigment and Q-switched Nd:YAG lasers (Watts *et al.* 1992; Fitzpatrick *et al.* 1994). However, flesh-coloured tattoo pigment (iron oxide) will reduce to black upon laser impact.

References

Bolognia, J. (1993) Therapeutics in pigmentary disorders medical, surgical and physical approaches. In: *Pigmentation and Pigmentary Disorders* (ed. N.Levine), pp. 492–524. CRC Press, Boca Raton.

Bose, S. (1995) Is micropigmentation surgery an answer to stable bindi-induced depigmentation? *Journal of Dermatology* **22**, 533–534.

Carr, J. (1995) Danger in performing MR imaging on women who have tattooed eyeliner or similar types of permanent cosmetic injections. *American Journal of Roentgenology.* **165**, 1546–1547.

Fitzpatrick, R., Goldman, M. & Dierick, C. (1994) Laser ablation of facial cosmetic tattoos. *Aesthetic Plastic Surgery* **18**, 91–96.

Halder, R. & Nordlund, J. (1998) Surgical treatment of pigmentary disorders. In: *The Pigmentary System: Physiology and Pathophysiology* (eds J.Nordlund, R.Boissy, V.Hearing, R.King & J.-P.Ortonne), pp. 997–998. Oxford University Press, Oxford.

Halder, R., Pham, H., Breadon, J. & Johnson, B. (1989) Micropigmentation for the treatment of vitiligo. *Journal of Dermatological Surgery and Oncology* **15**, 1092–1098.

Jackson, J.G. & Acker, J. (1987) Permanent eyeliner and MR imaging. *American Journal of Roentgenology* **149**, 1080.

Larson, D. (1996). Micropigmentation. *Annals of Plastic Surgery* **36**, 193.

LePoole, C. & Boissy, R. (1997) Vitiligo. *Seminars in Cutaneous Medicine and Surgery* **16**, 3–14.

Mazza, J.F. & Rager, C. (1993) Advances in cosmetic micropigmentation. *Plastic and Reconstructive Surgery* **92**, 750–751.

Patipa, M. (1987) Eyelid tattooing. *Dermatologic Clinics* **5**, 335–348.

Patipa, M., Jakobiec, F. & Krebs, W. (1986) Light and electron microscopic findings with permanent eyeliner. *Ophthalmology* **93**, 1361–1365.

Sacco, D. (1987) Permanent eyeliner and MR imaging [reply]. *American Journal of Roentgenology* **149**, 1080.

Simons, K., Payne, C. & Heyde, R. (1988) Blepharopigmentation: histopathologic observation and X-ray microanalysis. *Ophthalmologic Plastic Reconstructive Surgery* **4**, 57–62.

Tse, D., Folberg, R. & Moore, K. (1985) Clinicopathologic correlate of a fresh eyelid pigment implantation. *Archives of Ophthalmology* **103**, 1515–1517.

Watts, M., Downes, R., Collins, J. & Walker, N. (1992) The use of Q-switched Nd: YAG laser for removal of permanent eyeliner tattoo. *Ophthalmologic Plastic Reconstructive Surgery* **8**, 292–294.

26: Depigmentation for the Treatment of Extensive Vitiligo

JAMES J. NORDLUND

Depigmentation

Indications for depigmentation

The basic defect causing depigmentation of vitiligo is absence of melanocytes. Without melanocytes, melanin cannot be synthesized and the skin becomes white (see Chapter 2). Such skin is cosmetically unattractive, a problem for most patients with vitiligo (see Chapter 13), and the skin is physiologically abnormal (see Chapter 31).

There are two different approaches to the treatment of patients with vitiligo. The best treatment is to replace the missing melanocytes. If successful, repigmentation restores both the morphological and physiological aberrations found in the depigmented skin (see Chapter 5 and Chapter 31). However, repigmentation is not always possible. It requires a reservoir of melanocytes within the hair follicle. By definition glabrous skin lacks a reservoir. Hair-bearing skin that has white hair also lacks a reservoir (see Chapter 20). Both types of skin, glabrous skin or that with white hairs, cannot be repigmented with medical therapies like PUVA or topical steroids. Surgical approaches for treating such skin are appropriate but at times are contraindicated because some of these patients have progressive vitiligo (see Chapter 24). At times vitiligo is too extensive for surgical therapies or there are other contraindications. For some or all of these patients the second approach is often a good solution.

The second type of treatment is depigmentation by means of which the remaining melanocytes in the normal-appearing skin are destroyed by applications of the chemical monobenzone (monobenzyl ether of hydroquinone). Depigmentation solves the cosmetic problem caused by vitiligo, namely, spotted skin colour. From a patient's perspective, the best situation is to have one's own colour; the second best is to have a single colour. The worst condition is to have spotted, multicoloured skin like those who have vitiligo. For those for whom repigmentation is not possible, depigmentation is an excellent treatment because its end point is a single colour, i.e. white skin. Biologically it aggravates or extends the basic problem, i.e. loss of melanocytes. But like amputation of a gangrenous limb, removal of the residual melanocytes at times is the best option. Depigmentation is easy to initiate but difficult to achieve. Application of the monobenzone for a few weeks will not effect depigmentation. In fact depigmentation almost always requires the application of the medication for extended periods, from months to a year or two. Thus the patients must be chosen correctly and carefully.

Patient selection

Patients should be chosen carefully. Depigmentation is reserved usually for adults or at least those who are old and mature enough to recognize that depigmentation will alter their appearance very significantly. And the patient will require some time to adjust to the new image he/she will have of himself or herself. Children and teenagers usually cannot understand the implications of a depigmented appearance. However on rare occasion a child or teenager is subject to cruelty and taunting that makes his/her life unbearable. With proper advice from a psychiatrist and careful input from parents, teachers and colleagues involved, depigmentation can be implemented successfully even in young people or children.

The patient needs to have a relatively good self image, reasonable coping skills (see Chapter 13) and he/she must have realistic expectations for depigmentation. Depigmentation will not solve the social and psychological problems of a patient with vitiligo. It can assist in their feeling better about their image and in making the daily use of cosmetics less burdensome or unnecessary. Depigmentation is an assistance to having a pleasant life, not the way to solve a person's personal and social problems. A psychiatrist or psychologist at times might be very helpful in evaluating the expectations of the patient with vitiligo.

The patient must be well informed about the outcome and must understand that depigmentation also requires lifelong care of the skin. When depigmentation is complete the patient is susceptible to sunburn and will need to be cautious for the remainder of their life about using sunscreens, wearing appropriate protective clothing and avoiding excessively sunny environments. Photographs of depigmented patients and talking to those who have successfully completed a programme of depigmentation are very useful techniques to help the patient understand the process and outcome.

Often patients are told that depigmentation from monobenzone is permanent. Indeed the major loss of melanocytes usually is permanent but not always. Following a sunburn or even intense sun exposure, many patients note repigmentation on the face or arms. It can be minimal and easily removed by re-treatment with monobenzone. However, on occasion repigmentation can be very marked and widespread. Such patients are very disappointed that their efforts to depigment have been reversed partially making their appearance again unattractive. Thus the patient must be committed to long-term protection of the skin from sunlight.

Most physicians seem inappropriately concerned about the risk of skin cancers in patients with vitiligo. The most dangerous skin cancer is melanoma that has a propensity to metastasize and kill the patient. But melanomas cannot occur in a patch of vitiligo. Melanomas are neoplasms arising from melanocytes which are not located in the depigmented skin. Keratinocyte-derived cancers, i.e. squamous and basal cell epitheliomas, can occur in depigmented skin of vitiligo (Ortonne 1978; Ortonne *et al.* 1978; Calanchini-Postizzi & Frenk 1987) but rarely seem to do so (Nordlund & Ortonne 1998). Even if they were to occur in a patch of vitiligo, these particular two cancers are readily detectable at an early stage and are almost invariably curable. Thus they present essentially no risk or danger to the patient who understands their biology and who will seek medical attention when appropriate. Patients must be carefully instructed about cancers, sunlight and other aspects of vitiligo. For those who desire depigmentation and understand its implications, it is an excellent choice of treatment.

Patients of any skin type or ethnic background can be depigmented with good results. Those with darker skins must be prepared for the greater change in appearance although most individuals with dark skin who are seeking depigmentation already are so disfigured that the loss of pigment is very desirable. Individuals without vitiligo who are seeking depigmentation for social reasons or because they wish to mimic another race are usually very poor candidates for treatment with monobenzone. With rare exception, monobenzone is not indicated for any other condition except for vitiligo.

Methods

Selection and preparation of patient

The people and colleagues who are close to and important to the patient must be informed of the procedures outlined here and ideally should be shown photographs of a person of the same gender and skin colour who has depigmented. It is desirable to loan the patient some colour photos to take home for a week or two to show to his/her family. If a spouse or parents accompany the patient, it is very useful to ensure that everyone is satisfied. It is very helpful to have the patient talk by telephone or in person with a successfully depigmented patient. Only the patient can make the decision to depigment or not to depigment. But the decision is facilitated greatly with support of the family and the doctor.

Patient instructions

The patient is instructed in need for the lifelong use of sunscreens, protective clothing and the risks of skin cancers.

Purchase of monobenzone

The patient buys monobenzone available as Benoquin™ from Elder

Pharmaceuticals, Cosa Mesa, CA. Some pharmacists are able to prepare 20% ointment of monobenzone.

Patch test

A patch test is applied for 48–72 hours to detect contact sensitivity to monobenzone.

Therapy

If there is no contact sensitivity, the patient is instructed to apply the Benoquin sparingly twice daily to normal skin on the hands, arms, neck, face and ears only. Some women will desire to treat the lower parts of the legs during the first sessions, a request that is reasonable. The physician should warn the patient that application of monobenzone is time consuming and the medication is expensive. Because of this, most patients do not choose to depigment their trunk, just the exposed skin. Applications continue until depigmentation is complete, occasionally just a period of 3–4 months, more commonly a period of 6–12 months. Treating too large an area is simply too laborious.

Follow up

The patient is examined about every 2–3 months for progress. The pigment fades away slowly. Usually the pigmented macules do not enlarge. Physicians must support and encourage the patient when the colour fades slowly.

Precautions

The patient is instructed in avoiding exposure of others to monobenzone directly or inadvertently. The patient washes hands with soap and water immediately after application and the patient avoids direct contact of treated skin with another person for 30–60 minutes after application. Spouses apply the medication 1 hour before bedtime. Mothers apply monobenzone after children have left for school. The tube is carefully stored so that children cannot handle it. Inadvertent exposures are treated by washing the area with soap and water.

Exigencies

The patient calls the physician for problems (see Complications below).

Patients who continue the therapy sufficiently long will gradually lose all pigment in the treated areas and achieve a very attractive cosmetic appearance (Figs 26.1 and 26.2).

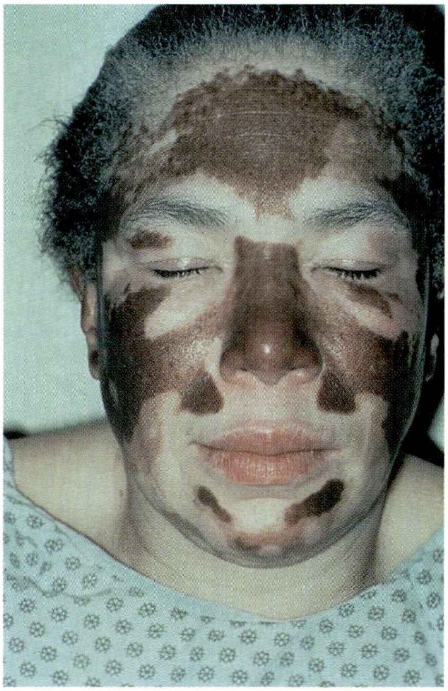

Fig. 26.1 Extensive depigmentation disfiguring the face of an African-American woman. (From Halder & Nordlund (1998). With permission from R. Halder and Oxford University Press.)

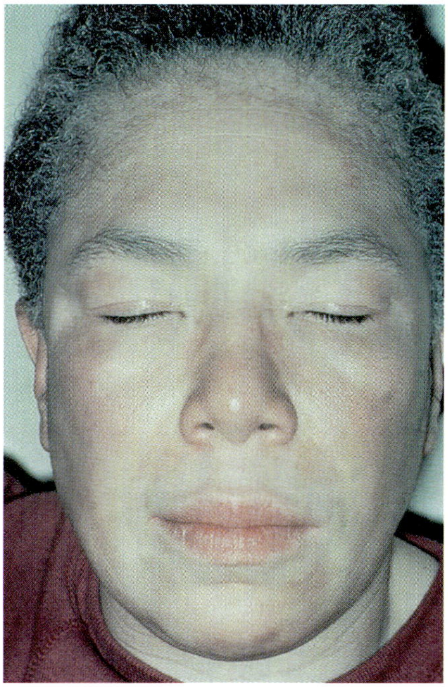

Fig. 26.2 Successful depigmentation from application of monobenzone. (From Halder & Nordlund (1998). With permission from R. Halder and Oxford University Press.)

Complications

There are few complications. The most common is dermatitis (Nordlund *et al.* 1985). It is restricted exclusively to the pigmented skin. On the neck it sometimes is an irritant dermatitis and is easily treated with applications of a steroid like triamcinolone acetonide 0.1% or a comparable preparation. At times dilution of the 20% monobenzone to 10% or 5% solves the problem of irritant dermatitis.

Sometimes monobenzone seems to cause a true allergic contact dermatitis (Nordlund *et al.* 1985). This author has not found a way to continue depigmenting a patient who is allergic to monobenzone. Most affected individuals are very sensitive to the medication and develop a vesicular dermatitis that is very pruritic. It is treated like any other allergic contact dermatitis. This complication means that the person must discontinue therapy without recourse to any other depigmenting or repigmenting treatments. Applications of topical steroids to suppress the allergy in conjunction with applications of monobenzone have not been successful for those with true allergic dermatitis.

Sunburn requires appropriate use of sunscreens with an SPF of 20–25 and judicious use of protective clothing such as Solumbra™.

Spontaneous repigmentation of treated skin manifested as perifollicular freckles can be treated with applications of monobenzone or one of the other techniques noted below.

Other methods of depigmenting skin

A few patients will have small areas on the face, hands or arms that resist depigmenting in response to monobenzone. Melanocytes are susceptible to injury by freezing. Gentle freezing of the pigmented skin with a cryospray several times over the period of some weeks or months can cause the residual pigment to disappear without complications or problems. This cryotherapy is limited to small areas of pigmented skin. It is uncomfortable and the patient must be tolerant of the discomfort.

There have been reports of laser being effective in destroying residual pigmentation although not all dermatologists have had good success (Renfro & Geronemus 1992; Thissen & Westerhof 1997).

Conclusions

Depigmentation or removal of residual pigmentation is a very good way to treat a few patients with extensive vitiligo or with pigment loss unresponsive to repigmentation. But the patients must be carefully chosen, prepared prudently and monitored. The end result is excellent in abrogating cosmetic disfigurement.

References

Calanchini-Postizzi, E. & Frenk, E. (1987) Long-term actinic damage in sun-exposed vitiligo and normally pigmented skin. *Dermatologica* **174** (6), 266–271.

Halder, R. & Nordlund, J. H. (1998) Topical treatment of pigmentary disorders. In: *The Pigmentary System. Physiology and Pathophysiology* (eds J.J. Nordlund, R.E. Boissy, V.J. Hearing, R.A. King & J.P. Ortonne) Oxford University Press, New York pp. 969–975.

Nordlund, J.J. & Ortonne, J.P. (1998) Vitiligo vulgaris. In: *The Pigmentary System: Physiology and Pathophysiology* (eds J.J. Nordlund, R. Boissy, V. Hearing, R.A. King & J.P. Ortonne), pp. 513–553. Oxford University Press, New York.

Nordlund, J.J., Forget, B., *et al.* (1985). Dermatitis produced by applications of monobenzone in patients with active vitiligo. *Archives of Dermatology* **121** (9), 1141–1144.

Ortonne, J.P. (1978) Vitiligo et epitheliomas cutanes. *Annales de Dermatologie et de Venereologie* **105**, 1063–1064.

Ortonne, J.P., Pelletier, N., *et al.* (1978) [Vitiligo and cutaneous epitheliomas]. *Annales de Dermatologie et de Venereologie* **105** (12), 1063–1064.

Renfro, L. & Geronemus, R.G. (1992) Lack of efficacy of the Q-switched ruby laser in the treatment of vitiligo [letter]. *Archives of Dermatology* **128** (2), 277–278.

Thissen, M. & Westerhof, W. (1997) Laser treatment for further depigmentation in vitiligo. *International Journal of Dermatology* **36** (5), 386–388.

27: Ancillary Therapies: Helping the Patient with Vitiligo to Adjust

JUDITH PORTER

The physical disfigurement of vitiligo, caused by uneven pigmentation, stigmatizes the victim and often makes him or her the object of discrimination by others. The staring, rude remarks, and other types of negative interaction may have an impact on the patient's personality and may lead to discomfort, depression, or reinforce low self-esteem. Thus, therapy for vitiligo must emphasize not only the medical but also take account of the psychological stress reported by two-thirds of a large sample of patients in a recent study (Porter & Beuf 1991). There are two basic strategies for handling the psychological distress of vitiligo: concealing the condition and supportive therapy.

For those patients who manifest psychological ill effects due to vitiligo, it often helps to conceal the condition so that it is not so visible. There are several concealment strategies. Vitiligo is most noticeable when normal skin is tanned, since the contrast between the tanned skin and the vitiligo makes the depigmentation more visible. Patients can be advised to stay out of the sun at peak periods except during treatment time or use a strong sun screen. Sun protection products are numbered according to the sun protection factor (SPF), with the higher numbers giving more protection. Patients with vitiligo should use a sunscreen with an SPF of 15 or higher. During treatment, an SPF of 8–10 protects against sunburn but does not block the UVA needed for treatment. Sunscreens should be reapplied after swimming or perspiring.

Another helpful strategy is to conceal the vitiligo with clothing, if it is possible to do so. In one study, more than half the patients reported that they wore special clothing, often using a combination of hats, gloves, long stockings, and long sleeves in order to conceal effectively the depigmented skin and avoid negative reactions from others (Porter *et al.* 1986, 1987).

Concealment of the depigmented areas by cosmetics is another common strategy utilized by patients. Although appearance is a central part of the feminine role definition, studies of patients with vitiligo show no significant gender differences with regard to degree of disturbance by vitiligo. This is due in part to the fact that women are more likely than men to use makeup which covers the vitiligo. Greater problems for women than men in psychological adjustment, however, have been found in psoriasis patients, where the disorder cannot be disguised cosmetically (Roengik & Roengik 1978; Porter *et al.* 1986, 1990). Patients should be reassured that cosmetics are not only for women nor are they only for the face. Anyone, including men and children, can wear them anywhere on the body (Porter & Beuf 1988). It is especially important for parents to recognize the helpful effects of cosmetology for children who are bothered by their appearance. Cosmetics exist in a wide range of skin tones, many are waterproof, and many do not rub off. There are also special dermatological cosmetics that patients even with severe vitiligo can find useful. In extreme cases where cosmetics are ineffective, dyes and stains may be utilized, but patients should be advised to consult a dermatologist for the names of suitable commercial products (Porter & Beuf, undated).

Although concealment may be a helpful adjustment strategy for some individuals, helping to return the appearance to normal, psychological counselling and support are extremely important for many patients. Although most patients in one study claimed that their families were emotionally supportive, upon closer investigation, 20% of the families were more concerned about the effects of vitiligo on themselves (contagion, inheritability) rather than its effect on the patient (Porter *et al.* 1987; Porter 1989). Psychological support from the physician treating vitiligo was deemed extremely important by these patients; however, seeing a dermatologist was not a guarantee of successful resolution of problems. Patients continued to harbour unanswered questions about the prognosis, treatment, and social limitations of vitiligo. Yet many patients thought that doctors were reluctant to answer their questions. From 25–30% of this sample felt that physicians had not adequately explained the cause, course and treatment of the disease or had not answered questions adequately, in part because doctors were too busy (Porter & Beuf, undated).

Lowered self-esteem, however, is a frequent result of vitiligo, and simply answering the patient's questions does not ensure that the psychological needs will be met. An understanding physician can deal with milder psychological reactions by being a good listener and giving some advice on treatment and the use of cosmetics to camouflage the disorder. Vitiligo support groups can also be helpful. Data from a recent study suggest that informal support groups, formed in a vitiligo clinic when patients were scheduled at the same general time period, helped patients adjust to the disease. Because of the racial implications of 'turning white', African-American physicians or a hospital environment where there are other African-American vitiligo patients may provide support for African-Americans with vitiligo (Porter & Beuf 1991, 1994).

Patients with more profound psychological reactions should be referred for counselling. Research reveals that we can predict which patients are particularly in need of emotional support or psychiatric referral. The patients most at risk of suffering adverse psychological effects are those with underlying low self-esteem or depression, conditions that are often present prior to the onset of vitiligo. For such people, vitiligo is often 'the straw that breaks the camel's back'. Individuals with feelings of personal inadequacy cope poorly with vitiligo, feel that the prognosis is hopeless, and think that neither family nor physician care about them. They are also less likely to trust the judgement of their doctor. These perceptions create a vicious cycle, driving the patient deeper into depression. Patients who have poor self-esteem or underlying feelings of worthlessness should be referred for psychiatric help. The underlying depression must be treated if the patient is to cope adequately with the disease or even to continue in dermatological treatment for vitiligo (Porter & Beuf 1991).

Young adults, those with severe vitiligo, and those for whom appearance is very important are also high-risk categories for psychological disturbance by vitiligo (Porter & Beuf 1991). The physician should carefully evaluate the emotional reaction of individuals in these categories, giving them emotional support, reassurance, and, if necessary, referrals to psychological counselling or support groups. There is a stereotype that males are less concerned about impaired appearance than are females. Research with vitiligo patients indicates this is a myth. Men are as concerned about their impaired appearance as women but are less likely to tell their physicians about it or express their emotions about their stigma. Thus, physicians should take the initiative with male patients, exploring their emotional reactions and giving advice about concealment strategies (Porter & Beuf, undated).

American society places a high value on appearance. The patient who fears the social consequences of vitiligo is responding to a very real situation of discrimination and resulting low self-esteem. The use of concealment strategies, physician support, support groups and, if necessary, psychological counselling are important supplementary therapies in treating the vitiligo patient.

References

Lerner, A. & Moellmann, G. (undated) *Vitiligo*. National Vitiligo Foundation, Tyler, Texas.

Porter, J. (1989) Psychosocial effects of skin disease, pp. 388–390. In: *Medical and Health Annual: 1989*. Encyclopedia Britannica Inc., Chicago, Illinois.

Porter, J. & Beuf, A. (undated) *Vitiligo: a Handbook for Patients*. National Vitiligo Foundation, Tyler, Texas.

Porter, J. & Beuf, A. (1994) *Vitiligo: a Manual for Physicians*. National Vitiligo Foundation, Tyler, Texas.

Porter, J. & Beuf, A. (undated) The effect of a racially consonant medical context on adjustment of African-American patients to physical disability. *Medical Anthropology* **16**, 1–16.

Porter, J. & Beuf, A. (1991) Racial variation in reaction to physical stigma: a study of degree of disturbance by vitiligo among black and white patients. *Journal of Health and Social Behavior* **32**, 192–204.

Porter, J. & Beuf, A. (1988) Response of older people to impaired appearance: The effect of age on disturbance by vitiligo. *Journal of Aging Studies* **2**, 167–181.

Porter, J., Beuf, A., Lerner, A. & Nordlund, J. (1990) The effect of vitiligo on sexual relationships. *Journal of the American Academy of Dermatology* **22**, 221–222.

Porter, J., Beuf, A., Lerner, A. & Nordlund, J. (1987) Response to cosmetic disfigurement: Patients with vitiligo. *Cutis* **39**, 493–494.

Porter, J., Beuf, A., Lerner, A. & Nordlund, J. (1986) The psychosocial effect of vitiligo: a comparison of vitiligo patients with 'normal' controls, with psoriasis patients, and with patients with other pigmentary disorders. *Journal of the American Academy of Dermatology (Part 1)* **15**, 220–225.

Roengik, R. & Roengik, H. (1978) Sex differences in the psychological effects of psoriasis. *Cutis* **21**, 529–533.

28: Sunscreens and Sun Protection

JAMES J. NORDLUND

Vitiligo vulgaris is characterized by the disappearance of melanocytes from the epidermis (Chapters 1 and 2). The affected skin typically is depigmented, i.e. completely white. The pigmentary system in the skin is one of the major mechanisms by which the skin is protected from the damaging effects of sunlight, i.e. the production of cancers most commonly squamous or basal cell carcinomas (for review see Nordlund *et al.* 1998). (Completely depigmented skin containing no melanocytes cannot be the source of a melanoma.) Thus such skin is subject to injury by sunlight. Interestingly, the number of cancers in vitiligo skin seems to be few (Nordlund & Ortonne 1998) although the explanation for this paucity of cancers is not known. Regardless, vitiligo skin can and does burn and occasionally does transform into keratinocyte-derived malignancies (Nordlund & Ortonne 1998). In addition, tanning of the normally pigmented skin accentuates the contrast between the white and dark skin. The patients find this marked contrast cosmetically unattractive. Thus depigmented skin, like all light coloured skin, needs to be protected with sunscreens or sun blocks and appropriate clothing.

It is well known that UVB spectrum (290 nm–320 nm) can cause erythema and burn in skin. It has become clear more recently that longer UVA spectrum (320 nm–400 nm) also can produce erythema but the dose of UVA required is about 1000 times greater than that needed for UVB erythema.

Patients with vitiligo might be exposed to ultraviolet light in many settings. Their exposed skin on the face, neck, hands and forearms is subject to sunlight routinely during the daylight hours. Less easily exposed skin such as that on the trunk and proximal parts of the extremities is likely to be exposed during outdoor recreational activities such as sunbathing or swimming. In addition the entire integument will be exposed during treatments of vitiligo with PUVA or sunlight.

Skin protection

Sunscreens are chemicals with the capacity to absorb ultraviolet light. Usually the chemical has a rather specific absorption spectrum. Thus there are UVB screens (Diffey & Farr 1991) and UVA screens (Gange *et al.* 1986; Lowe *et al.* 1987; Kaidbey & Barnes 1991; Roelandts 1991; Leenutaphong 1992; Cole 1994). There is no single chemical currently obtainable with the capacity to absorb both spectra in their entirety, although some commercially available preparations contain a variety of chemicals that absorb parts or most of both spectra. There are other chemicals such as titanium dioxide that do not absorb ultraviolet light, but rather block its penetration into the epidermis, i.e. sun blocks (Diffey & Farr 1991). These products are also useful to protect the skin.

UVB sunscreens and blocks are marketed with a sun protective factor. The factor is a measure of the absorptive or blocking capacity of the product and the abrogation of the sun's burning potential. For a person with a type I or II skin (reviewed in Nordlund *et al.* 1998), during summer months at noon the sun can burn the skin in about 10 minutes. A preparation with an SPF 2 will retard burning by absorption of 50% of the incident ultraviolet light and require 20 minutes exposure before a burn occurs. An SPF of 25 absorbs or blocks 96% of the sun and requires 250 minutes exposure to burn. An SPF of 50 absorbs 98% and requires 500 minutes exposure to direct sun, a difference from the SPF 25 that is not of much practicality. Thus screens with an SPF of 20–25 are considered sufficient for most practical conditions. This measure of the blocking capacity of a preparation designated as SPF is not used for UVA screens.

For routine daily activities during which the person is outdoors only transiently, the exposed skin depigmented by any cause including vitiligo should be protected by applications each morning of a sunscreen or block with an SPF of 20–25. UVA screens are advisable when available. For those living in southern climates where the sun is intense all year long, the sunscreen should be used daily and a UVA screen might be added. For those in temperate climates where the winter sun is not intense the preparations need be used during the summer months only. Summer means from the spring equinox (April 21) through to the autumn equinox (September 21).

For outdoor activities during summer when sun exposure will be prolonged and intense (including outdoor types of work), the person should apply both a UVB and UVA screen (Gange *et al.* 1986; Lowe *et al.* 1987; Leenutaphong 1992; Anonymous 1993, 1994; Cole 1994). Most patients with depigmentation from vitiligo will observe that even applications of sunscreens are not sufficiently protective and they will observe erythema following prolonged sun exposure. Hats with a wide brim, attractive beach clothes or special clothing such as Solumbra™ are necessary to minimize sunburn. Caution must be taken even on cloudy days or in the shade where there is sufficient UVA to cause erythema.

Recently it has become apparent that UVB as a single modality might be useful for the treatment of vitiligo. Westerhof found monochromatic UVB 311 nm to be as effective as topical PUVA for treating vitiligo (Westerhof & Nieuweboer-Krobotova 1997). In Italy, the Ratokderm™ facility has used full spectrum UVB successfully for the same purpose. This author has observed extensive repigmentation following exposure to natural sunlight with a concomitant mild erythema. Thus natural sunlight might be a useful therapeutic modality for those with vitiligo if used cautiously to prevent burning. Patients are instructed to go outdoors into the full sun around noon for 20 minutes after applying a sunscreen with an SPF of 2–4. The surrounding normal skin should be treated also. The duration of exposure can be increased daily until very mild erythema is noted. This is a way to provide phototherapy even to children without the restraints of artificial light and the limitations imposed by oral psoralens.

PUVA and skin protection

Patients with vitiligo often are treated with PUVA, a combination of psoralens and exposure to ultraviolet light (for review see Halder & Nordlund 1998; Nordlund & Ortonne 1998). Generally physicians prefer to use artificial sources of UVA to treat patients with vitiligo because it is easier to control the amount of UVA delivered. Following ingestion of psoralens, the skin is highly susceptible to the burning effects of UVA including that in sunlight. UVA does penetrate through window glasses in homes and cars. Thus it is necessary to consider a patient's potential exposure to UVA and sometimes it is advisable to treat the skin with UVA protective blocks on the days psoralens are taken by mouth or applied topically (Anonymous 1989; Roelandts 1991; Antoniou & Katsambas 1992; Leenutaphong 1992; Anonymous 1993, 1994; Cole 1994; Tokura *et al.* 1994; Nordlund *et al.* 1996). The administration of PUVA requires appropriate training and should be done only by those with sufficient knowledge of its safe and effective use.

It is also possible to use psoralens with natural sunlight. Natural sunlight has both UVB and UVA. To use psoralens with natural sunlight, it is advisable to apply a UVB sunscreen with an SPF of 4–6 to prevent UVB erythema. The dose of sunlight is carefully controlled by limiting the time the patient is out in the sun and by titration of the dose of psoralen taken by mouth. Topical psoralens probably should not be used with natural sunlight except in special circumstances to avoid a severe burn.

PUVA and eye protection

Psoralens do penetrate into the eyes as well as the skin. There is concern that PUVA might be an aggravating or contributing factor for cataracts in the lens (El-Mofty & El-Mofty 1979; Antoniou & Katsambas 1992; Stern 1994). Thus all patients receiving PUVA should wear eyeglasses that absorb UVA on the days when taking psoralens by mouth. These should be worn from the time of ingestion of the pills until evening time of the same day (Nordlund *et al.* 1996). Such eyeglasses are available in sports shops, from optometrists and from dermatologists engaged in providing PUVA.

References

Anonymous (1989) Photoplex—a broad spectrum sunscreen. *Medical Letter on Drugs and Therapeutics* **31** (794), 59–60.

Anonymous (1993) Shade UVAGuard—a second broad-spectrum sunscreen. *Medical Letter on Drugs and Therapeutics* **35** (898), 53–54.

Anonymous (1994) British Photodermatology Group guidelines for PUVA. *British Journal of Dermatology* **130** (2), 246–255.

Antoniou, C. & Katsambas, A. (1992) Guidelines for the treatment of vitiligo. *Drugs* **43** (4), 490–498.

Cole, C. (1994) Multicenter evaluation of sunscreen UVA protectiveness with the protection factor test method. *Journal of the American Academy of Dermatology* **30** (5 Part 1), 729–736.

Diffey, B.L. & Farr, P.M. (1991) Sunscreen protection against UVB, UVA and blue light: an *in vivo* and *in vitro* comparison [published erratum appears in Br J Dermatol 1991 December; 125 (6): 609]. *British Journal of Dermatology* **124** (3), 258–263.

El-Mofty, A.M. & El-Mofty, A. (1979) Retrospective ocular study of patients receiving oral 8-methoxypsoralen and solar irradiation for the treatment of vitiligo. *Annals of Ophthalmology* **11**, 946–948.

Gange, R.W., Soparkar, A., Matsinger, E., Dromgoole, S.H., Sefton, J. & DeGryse, R. (1986) Efficacy of a sunscreen containing butyl methoxydibenzoyl-methane against ultraviolet A radiation in photosensitized subjects. *Journal of the American Academy of Dermatology* **15** (3), 494–499.

Halder, R. & Nordlund, J.J. (1998) Phototherapy for Pigmentary Disorders. In: *The Pigmentary System: Physiology and Pathophysiology* (eds J.J.Nordlund, R.E.Boissy, V.J.Hearing, R.A.King & J.P.Ortonne), pp. 977–983. Oxford University Press, New York.

Kaidbey, K.H. & Barnes, A. (1991) Determination of UVA protection factors by means of immediate pigment darkening in normal skin. *Journal of the American Academy of Dermatology* **25** (2 Part 1), 262–266.

Leenutaphong, V. (1992) Evaluating the UVA protection of commercially available sunscreens. *Journal of the Medical Association of Thailand* **75** (11), 619–624.

Lowe, N.J., Dromgoole, S.H., Sefton, J., Bourget, T. & Weingarten, D. (1987) Indoor and outdoor efficacy testing of a broad-spectrum sunscreen against ultraviolet A radiation in psoralen-sensitized subjects. *Journal of the American Academy of Dermatology* **17** (2 Part 1), 224–230.

Nordlund, J.J. & Ortonne, J.-P. (1998) Vitiligo vulgaris. In: *The Pigmentary System: Physiology and Pathophysiology* (eds J.J.Nordlund, R.E.Boissy, V.J.Hearing, R.A.King & J.P.Ortonne), pp. 513–549. Oxford University Press, New York.

Nordlund, J.J., Grimes, P.E., Halder, R. & Minus, H.R. (1996) Guidelines of care for vitiligo vulgaris. *Journal of the American Academy of Dermatology* **35**, 620–626.

Nordlund, J.J., Boissy, R.E., Hearing, V.J., King, R.A. & Ortonne, J.-P., eds. (1998) *The Pigmentary System: Physiology and Pathophysiology*. Oxford University Press, New York.

Roelandts, R. (1991) Which components in broad-spectrum sunscreens are most necessary for adequate UVA protection? *Journal of the American Academy of Dermatology* **25** (6 Part 1), 999–1004.

Stern, R.S. (1994) Ocular lens findings in patients treated with PUVA. Photochemotherapy Follow-Up-Study. *Journal of Investigative Dermatology* **103** (4), 534–538.

Tokura, Y., Yagi, H. *et al.* (1994) Evaluation of ultraviolet-A protection by sunscreen agents using a mouse model of contact photoallergy. *Journal of Dermatological Science* **7** (1), 39–44.

Westerhof, W. & Nieuweboer-Krobotova, L. (1997) Treatment of vitiligo with UV-B radiation vs. psoralen plus UV-A. *Archives of Dermatology* **133**, 1525–1528.

29: Alternative Therapies for Vitiligo

GIOVANNI E. ORECCHIA

Dedication: to my son Pietro

The wide range of possible treatments confirms that the therapy of this disorder is still a difficult problem for both the doctor and the patient. Conventional therapies, such as psoralens plus UVA (PUVA) or surgical treatments (see Chapters 21–26) with skin grafts are not always able to bring about a complete repigmentation. Often only one-third of patients achieve satisfactory results. Moreover these treatments are time consuming and costly.

Therefore it is suitable to consider other nontraditional treatments (Lemke 1993) either as first line therapies or as alternative approaches for patients who either have failed or are unsuitable for the above therapies. It is important that every patient try several modalities of therapy before the disease is considered resistant or untreatable.

Heliotherapy

Heliotherapy (from the Greek word 'Hélios', the sun) is the most simple and ancient way of treating vitiligo, even though some modern day dermatologists advise their patients to avoid sun because tanning accentuates the contrast with the normal surrounding skin. It is an economical treatment easily accepted during leisure time and is particularly suitable for children. It is relatively safe because of the absence of a significant increase of chronic actinic damage (Calanchini-Postizzi & Frenk 1987) and because of the rareness of skin cancer reported to develop in patients with vitiligo (Ortonne *et al.* 1978).

The normal skin should be protected by broad-spectrum sunscreens with a high sun protection factor (SPF) to reduce contrast with vitiliginous skin. Burns to the normal-appearing skin might induce the isomorphic (Koebner's) phenomenon and is at risk for photoaging. The vitiligo areas should be exposed to sunlight just enough to achieve an asymptomatic erythema. A mild inflammatory reaction is necessary for the replication and migration of melanocytes from the follicles and the edges of the lesion into the depigmented skin. Between treatments the vitiliginous areas should be protected to avoid sunburns.

Usually heliotherapy is combined with other treatments, such as applications of topical steroids or ingestion of various vitamins. Exposure to the sun can follow the topical applications or oral consumption of other agents such as psoralens, Melagenina, khellin (KUVA) or the amino acid phenylalanine.

The mode of action of heliotherapy is unknown but sunlight has been shown to stimulate proliferation of melanocytes in normal skin and this effect presumably is what is observed in those with vitiligo. Heliotherapy has been reported to influence some enzymes in the blood serum of patients (Dimov *et al.* 1976) and in particular copper metabolism (Zlatkov *et al.* 1972). It re-establishes the normal tyrosinase activity possibly by reducing serum copper level and plasma ceruloplasmin (Zlatkov *et al.* 1971).

UVB

UVB radiation is known to be an important factor in stimulating the synthesis of melanin pigmentation in the skin by increasing tyrosinase activity and stimulation of proliferation of melanocytes (Abdel-Malek *et al.* 1993). UVB produced by a variety of commercially available lamps and phototherapy boxes can induce repigmentation in patches of vitiligo. UVB alone has been used successfully in 14 of 24 (57%) patients who showed more than 75% of repigmentation after 12 months treatment. Like other treatments, UVB produced the best results in facial lesions of individuals with skin types V and VI (Koster & Wiskerman 1990). The indications, possible mechanisms, results, acute and chronic side-effects have been discussed in detail (Honigsmann 1990).

In order to reduce the carcinogenic and photoaging effects of the broad-spectrum UVB, other investigators proposed using monochromatic 311 nm band for treating psoriasis (Van Weelden *et al.* 1988, 1990) and vitiligo. The results have been promising (Westerhof & Nieuweboer-Krobotova 1997). In fact the 311 nm lamps induce less erythema than broad-spectrum UVB bulbs, while treatment response is still high. It seems to be better than topical psoralen plus UVA.

Advantages of monochromatic light include no photocontact allergenicity, less phototoxicity, itching, and xerosis, no hyperkeratosis, shorter sessions (usually no longer than 5 minutes) and suitability during pregnancy (Westerhof & Nieuweboer-Krobotova 1997).

UVB has been used in combination with topical vitamin C (Nakamura *et al.* 1997) purportedly to reduce the deleterious effects on cutaneous immunity. Others have suggested that UVB in combination with vitamin B_{12} (Juhlin & Olsson 1997) is more effective than UV alone but there are insufficient data to confirm these assumptions. However, the maximum safe cumulative doses have not yet been established and it is difficult to decide when phototherapy should be discontinued (Park *et al.* 1996).

In the past few years in Italy, a new way of using UVB has been instituted by Ratokderm with success. Beams of UVB with a diameter of few mm to 30 mm are focused on the depigmented patches until erythema develops. The depigmented skin gains colour after a number of sessions in both treated and nontreated areas. Melanogenesis and proliferation of melanocytes at sites distal to the area of radiation with UVB have been reported both in animals and humans (Stierner *et al.* 1989; Nordlund & Ortonne 1998).

That sunlight, UVB or monochromatic UVB can induce repigmentation is an important observation. There are numerous unsubstantiated claims for the efficacy of various drugs as outlined in this chapter and other monographs. It is possible that either sunlight or UVB is responsible for many of the claims for therapeutic success of vitamins, herbs or even the results obtained with Food and Drug Agency (of the USA) approved medications.

Human placental extracts

Melagenina was first used in Cuba in the 1970s for the treatment of vitiligo, psoriasis and alopecia. It is a hydroalcoholic extract of the human placenta and the active ingredient is said to be an α-lipoprotein produced by and extracted from the cotyledons of placenta with 95% ethanol (Cao *et al.* 1989). Melagenina should be applied three times a day before exposure to ultraviolet light, sunlight or infrared light. The timing of the application is said to be critical and must be administered at 8 hour intervals. The treatment takes from months to as long as 10 years.

Preliminary results from one study on 732 patients with vitiligo claimed that 84% of patients achieved total repigmentation. These excellent results could not be repeated. In a second study, only 31% of 200 patients were said to be totally repigmented. It is stated that cured patients had no residual depigmentation, had no recurrences and that hands and feet also responded to this therapy. However 40% of those treated in one study (on 732 patients) showed new spots of vitiligo while data on treatment and long-term follow-ups were not presented.

An analysis of the claims for Melagenina has been published (Nordlund & Halder 1990) and the authors could not obtain sufficient data to verify that Melagenina was either an effective treatment or that it contained trophic factors for melanocytes. The best success seemed to occur mainly in the Caribbean basin or in other areas of high sun intensity, because the patients who noted repigmentation in Cuba lost any beneficial effect on returning home. Experiments repeated in other laboratories in the United States and other countries have not been able to confirm the animal and laboratory data claimed by the Cuban workers (Nordlund & Halder 1990; Nordlund 1992).

Results of other clinical studies in Venezuela, Mexico, India and Trinidad (Suite & Quamina 1991) confirm the lack of efficacy of Melagenina. In San Marino, Melagenina was distributed by a private clinic which stopped a couple of years ago because the treatment was said to be expensive and the results disappointing. Nevertheless, this medication has had its partisans (Azambuja 1992). Other researchers have attributed its efficacy to 21-amino acid peptide, endothelin. Endothelins are potent cytokines that are able to stimulate melanocyte motility and growth (Pal *et al.* 1995).

Khellin (KUVA)

Khellin is extracted from the seeds of the plant *Ammi visnaga*. Since 1982 Khellin has been proposed as another oral photochemotherapy treatment for vitiligo (Abdel-Fattah *et al.* 1982). Results of recent studies on the use of oral or topical khellin suggest that it has real potential as a therapy for vitiligo (Ortel *et al.* 1988). It is a furanochromone with a chemical structure closely resembling the psoralen family and having similar photobiological, photochemical and phototherapeutic properties (Morliere *et al.* 1988; Pathak & Dalle Carbonare 1989). It seems to have fewer phototoxic effects (Dell'Acqua *et al.* 1981; Abeysekera *et al.* 1983). Furthermore, Khellin has no photochemical effects on DNA (Trabalzini *et al.* 1990) and does not induce detectable DNA mutations (Riccio *et al.* 1992).

It is recommended that khellin be given orally at the doses of 50–100 mg, 2.5 hours prior to exposure to sun or UVA up to 15 J cm^{-2}. On this protocol, during the first two months of treatment, 25% of patients showed a mild elevation of liver transaminases which returned to normal within 5–12 weeks without any sign of progressive liver disease (Ortel *et al.* 1988). Other side-effects reported were nausea (in 21% of cases), orthostatic hypotension (in 7%) (Ortel *et al.* 1988) and porphyria cutanea tarda (Jansen *et al.* 1995).

Because of the toxicity, the interest of most research has been concentrated on the use of topical preparations (Orecchia & Perfetti 1992). Mixtures of solvents, like water/2-propanol/propylene glycol, have provided a very effective system able to solubilize khellin (Giordano *et al.* 1994; Orecchia *et al.* 1994). Preliminary clinical data, with 1% of this gel formulation applied 30 minutes prior to UVA exposure, seem to offer promising results (Orecchia & Giordano 1996; Orecchia *et al.* 1998). Iontophoresis can further improve the penetration of the drug (Marconi *et al.* 1997) and, hopefully, its efficacy.

The mechanism of action of Khellin is probably similar to that of the psoralens (Kao & Yu 1992). Khellin could also involve some growth factors on the melanocyte membrane (Laskin & Laskin 1988) or elicit an intracellular response via the G_i alpha protein (Distefano *et al.* 1996). Additionally Khellin has the capacity to interfere with the noradrenaline-sensitive mechanisms responsible for loading and releasing calcium stores (Schallreuter & Pittelkow 1988; Ubeda & Villar 1989) and/or calcium transport in vitiliginous melanocytes (Schallreuter-Wood *et al.* 1996). Since Khellin produces a concentration dependent inhibition of noradrenaline (Ubeda *et al.* 1991), it may also counteract the effects of the catecholamine excess reported in vitiligo (Schallreuter *et al.* 1994a, b). Furthermore, Khellin inhibition of noradrenaline results in vasodilation (Ubeda & Villar 1989).

Topical and systemic phenylalanine

Phenylalanine is a natural, essential amino acid and a precursor of tyrosine which is required for the synthesis of melanin. It is a major component of daily dietary protein and there is little danger of experiencing serious side-effects due to its administration. (Patients with phenylketonuria, liver disease and other disorders must not undertake this therapy. See contraindications to use of phenylalanine noted below.) It was proposed for photochemotherapy by Cormane *et al.* (1985) who reported a dense follicular repigmentation in 26.3% of the patients and a sparse one in 68.4%, after 8 months of oral treatment with phenylalanine. They prescribed 50 mg/kg body weight 45 minutes prior to UVA exposure, given twice a week. In a previous, preliminary work the Cormane group used 200 mg/kg on a three times a week schedule with comparable results (Cormane *et al.* 1983).

These data were confirmed by other investigators who prescribed 50–100 mg/kg body weight (Frisch & Milbradt 1988; Antoniou *et al.* 1989). Improved results have been reported when this therapy was combined with topical phenylalanine (Antoniou *et al.* 1989; Thiele 1991; Siddiqui *et al.* 1994; Camacho 1995), with UVB (Biella & Haustein 1990), or with 5-MOP (Beretti *et al.* 1989). Promising results were also reported in children (Schulpis *et al.* 1989). However, recurrences were reported after suspension of treatment ranging in magnitude from 12% (Schulpis *et al.* 1989) to 64% (Greiner *et al.* 1994). The evaluation of its efficacy is not uniform. Other investigators are sceptical (Orecchia *et al.* 1992) or disappointed (Pruvot-Sentous *et al.* 1992; Rosenbach *et al.* 1993) with the results.

Contraindications

One author has warned about the risks of this therapy in normal subjects (Thomas & Largillière 1988). Absolute therapeutic contraindications are phenylketonuria, skin cancer, impaired liver and renal function, pregnancy, lactation, prior radiation therapy and arsenic exposure.

The mechanism of action of phenylalanine is still unknown. Besides the hypothesis that phenylalanine stimulates repigmentation directly (Cormane *et al.* 1983; Frisch & Milbradt 1988; Schulpis *et al.* 1989), it also could act by inhibiting antibody synthesis (Ryan & Carver 1963) or by reducing the number of Langerhans cells (Westerhof *et al.* 1986).

Topical and systemic tyrosine or L-DOPA

L-Tyrosine has been unsuccessfully tried to treat patients with vitiligo (given orally in combination with UVA) (Cormane *et al.* 1983). Topical tanning products and tan accelerators containing tyrosine failed to demonstrate any efficacy in repigmenting vitiligo lesions (Jakorsky *et al.* 1987). Levodopa has shown efficacy in the control of parkinsonism, a disorder in which neuromelanin is lost from the substantia nigra. Because neurones and melanocytes share the same neural crest origin, levodopa has been tried also for the treatment of vitiligo. It was applied twice daily in 10% and 20% alcoholic solutions with some evidence of repigmentation in 25% of patients (Woolfson & Finn 1972). Levodopa was also given orally at the doses of

125–1500 mg daily in association with ultraviolet light. The results of these trials have been poor (Goolamali 1973).

Cysteine

Cysteine is an amino acid prescribed for treating vitiligo by many Italian dermatologists for use before sun exposure. However its efficacy has not been demonstrated to be superior to heliotherapy alone (Orecchia & Perfetti 1989).

Other readily available photosensitizers

Since psoralens are not available in Nigeria, George (1989) tried other photosensitizers such as 'Fa' soap which contains psoralens and exposure to sunlight. He reported some success.

Vitamins and trace elements

This treatment approach is based on the rationale that vitiligo is caused by a deficiency of some nutritional element(s) and that it can be cured by replacing the lacking nutrients. Deficiency of vitamin B_{12}, associated with vitiligo, was reported many years ago (Bleifeld & Gehrmann 1969; Banerjee *et al.* 1970), probably due to defective absorption (Bleifeld & Gehrmann 1967). Moreover, it is common opinion that vitiligo is associated with autoimmune disorders and, in particular, with pernicious anaemia, although these associations might be more apparent than real (Nordlund & Majumder 1997).

Montes and coworkers investigated 15 patients suffering from vitiligo who had diminished serum levels of folic acid (11 patients), vitamin B_{12} (5 patients) and ascorbic acid (in the plasma of 4 patients). He treated them orally with 2 mg of folic acid and 500 mg of vitamin C twice a day along with 100 mg of vitamin B_{12} every two weeks, administered intramuscularly. He reported steady and significant repigmentation in eight of these 15 patients after several years of therapy (Montes *et al.* 1992).

Very recently folic acid and vitamin B_{12} have been used in association with sun exposure in summer and artificial UVB irradiation in winter with results better than for either the vitamins or radiation alone (Juhlin & Olsson 1997). It was suggested that the pteridine part of folic acid could interfere with the recycling of the reduced pterins in vitiligo (Schallreuter *et al.* 1994a, b), and that vitamin B_{12} down-regulates the formation of homocysteine, which seems to cause the depigmentation in vitiligo. However, since the patients had normal serum level of both vitamins, it appears that their deficiency is not a significant factor in inducing vitiligo (Juhlin & Olsson 1997).

Vitamins C and E are used in vitiligo for their antioxidant properties. Because copper is a critical cofactor in the pathway for melanin synthesis, copper sulphate has been tried to treat 45 patients (Kalampalikis *et al.* 1992). It should be noted that copper in excessive quantities is toxic.

Antioxidants

It has been proposed that vitiligo and the loss of melanocytes is caused by formation of free radicals related to a deficiency of antioxidants (Picardo *et al.* 1994; Maresca *et al.* 1997). Canthaxantine, a food-colouring agent, was used as a pigment to darken and photoprotect vitiliginous skin (Gupta *et al.* 1985). It was also used in combination with β-carotene (Pietzcker & Kuner-Beck 1979) to obtain a more natural brown reddish colouring in order to decrease the disturbing contrast between the lesions and the surrounding skin (Raab *et al.* 1985). However canthaxantine intake can produce yellow crystalline deposits in the retina which have been seen to persist for 13 years after stopping the drug (H.F.Haberman, unpublished).

α-Tochopherol was given in combination with PUVA in order to shorten the duration of the treatment (Koshevenko 1989). α-Tochopherol cream combined with weak to moderate topical corticosteroids or PUVA was proposed and used with success by Mandel *et al.* (1997). Topical vitamin C appears to reduce the erythema of UV radiation and to abrogate the deleterious effects of UVB on cutaneous immunity (Nakamura *et al.* 1997). The author has suggested that this vitamin could be a useful complementary tool for the various forms of ultraviolet treatments.

Some patients with active or stable disease were treated with an antioxidant pool (tocopherol acetate, ubiquinone, selenio-methionine, methionine) in order to increase both enzymatic and nonenzymatic antioxidant pattern. After three months of therapy, the progression of the vitiligo was stopped and, in some cases, repigmentation of the most recent lesions was observed (Picardo *et al.* 1997).

Pentoxifylline was tried in three patients for three months at the dose of 1.2 g a day without success (Goldstein *et al.* 1992). Flavonoids were tried in vitiligo patients by the author without evidence of significant improvement.

Immunomodulators

One of the theories for the causation of vitiligo is an autoimmune attack against melanocytes. Thus the use of immunosuppressive or immunomodulating agents seems reasonable.

Cyclophosphamide

Cyclophosphamide was given orally 50 mg, twice a day to 33 patients (Gokhale 1979). An improvement was reported in 82% of the patients who had never been treated before. There seemed to be 'definite improvement' in 95% of those previously treated in different ways. Repigmentation was noticed also on sites not easily amenable to treatment, such as dorsa of fingers, toes and lips. Hair loss, leukopenia and nausea were the transient side-effects of this treatment. This treatment is not recommended for general use and, if indicated, should be undertaken only by those expert in the use of this medication (Gokhale & Parakh 1983).

Mechlorethamine

Mechlorethamine can cause hyperpigmentation of the skin after topical application by increasing the number of melanocytes. Van Scott and Yu (1975) noticed some repigmentation in a black man with hypopigmentation treated with topical nitrogen mustard for mycosis fungoides. He observed in a black woman with vitiligo unresponsive to PUVA punctate repigmentation after 1 month and 'substantial repigmentation' after 3 months of topical mechlorethamine. This compound is reported to be carcinogenic when topically applied.

Cyclosporin

Cyclosporin-A (6 mg/kg per day) was given for 5–30 weeks to treat 12 different dermatoses including vitiligo. Vitiligo showed no response (Gupta *et al.* 1990). A case of polyglandular autoimmune syndrome (type II) with vitiligo healed completely and did not recur after cyclosporin-A treatment was discontinued (Csaszar & Patakfalvi 1992).

Inosiplex

Repigmentation was observed in six of 12 patients after 6 months of treatment with Isoprinosine, a result thought to be due to its immunomodulatory effects (Grimes 1993). The author confirms these data. Isoprinosine is thought to potentiate photochemotherapy in some patients given 50 mg/kg per day for 14 days consecutively and then for 3 days per week for 4 months (Galbraith *et al.* 1984).

In another trial, four patients unresponsive to other treatments did not respond to 4 g a day of Isoprinosine administered for 4 months (Mandel *et al.* 1997).

Anapsos

Anapsos is a saponine composed of a ketosteroid and a desoxyhexose, with immunomodulatory properties. It is extracted from the rhizomes of the fern *Polypodium leucotomos* found in Central America, especially in Honduras. Known as Calaguala, this fern has been used for centuries in the popular medicine.

A few years ago it was reported to be efficacious, at the oral dose of 360 mg per day for 5 months, in healing vitiligo patients (Mohammed 1989). Later other studies were conducted with topical and oral administrations

(Corrales *et al.* 1994; Jaen *et al.* 1994). It may act also through several mechanisms, such as antioxidant effect and depletion of Langerhans cells in the skin, i.e. with an immunosuppression mechanism (Westerhof *et al.* 1986; Gonzalez *et al.* 1997). The author had some patients who underwent this treatment for 6 months without success.

Levamisole

Because of its immunomodulator activity, this anthelmintic drug has been used in 64 patients in an oral dose of 150 mg on two consecutive days every week for up to 48 months. It was effective when given alone, and even more so when combined with topical steroids (fluocinolone acetonide acetate or clobetasol propionate), in controlling and reducing limited and slow spreading vitiligo (Pasricha & Khera 1994). Side-effects were minimal, except severe vomiting in two cases.

Fluorouracil

Topical fluorouracil used for treating tumours of the skin can cause an increase of pigmentation. It has been tried for vitiligo in combination with dermabrasion.

On day one, epidermal abrasion was performed in 28 cases using an electrical dermabrader. Then 5% fluorouracil cream was applied daily for 7–10 days with an occlusive dressing. Antiseptic creams were used to prevent secondary infection. After 1 week there was epithelization and after 1 or 2 more weeks repigmentation started. 64% of patients had complete or almost complete repigmentation, 18% had partial response and 18% did not respond. Only minimal pain was reported (Tsuji & Hamada 1983). In a later trial, 2.5% fluorouracil dissolved in 8% dimethylsulphoxide to enhance the absorption was tried in eight patients. The preparation was applied twice daily for 2–3 months without response (Monk 1985). Partial results were obtained by other investigators. Only bilateral, symmetrical vitiligo responded, whereas segmental vitiligo failed to respond (Szekeres & Morvay 1985). Stripping the epidermis with cellophane tape before fluorouracil was tried but without success (Mandel *et al.* 1997). Dermabrasion or sanding seem important in inducing repigmentation in combination with fluorouracil.

Melanocyte stimulating hormone

α-Melanocyte stimulating hormone (α-MSH) has a moderate darkening effect on normal skin, but had no effect on vitiliginous skin, when injected intramuscularly into a 29-year-old subject with vitiligo who had undergone a cervical sympathectomy. Local injection in patches of vitiligo did not change pigmentation of normal or vitiliginous skin (Lerner *et al.* 1966). The use of α-MSH or its derivatives cannot be recommended for vitiligo, because all the effects of these hormones are not yet known (Nordlund 1991).

Anti-leprosy drugs

Clofazimine

Clofazimine is an aposafranin, also known as B.663 and marketed as Lamprene (Geigy) for the treatment of leprosy. Patients receiving this phenazine dye develop some degree of darkening of the skin which becomes blackish-brown or purplish-black. The longer the treatment, the deeper the coloration which is due to the increase of both the thickness of the pigmented epidermal layers and the deposition of the drug in both the epidermis and in dermis. Bor (1973) used clofazimine (100 mg daily) and sunlight in eight white females. He noted that after 6–8 weeks there was some perifollicular repigmentation that lasted for many years. However, repigmentation does not seem due to the presence of melanocytes nor to the crystals of the drug in the tissues, but due to melanin migrating from functioning melanocytes of surrounding areas. These results were not confirmed by two other investigators. One investigator noted repigmentation in only two out of 20 patients and concluded that sun exposure had as good an effect as the combination (Shukla 1981). The second author reported that the cosmetic result did not satisfy his 20 patients and, in one case, a Dubreuilh-like lesion was stimulated by Lamprene (Shuppli 1981).

The drug seems to be rather safe except for the peculiar pigmentation that it causes (Kumar *et al.* 1987), however, exacerbation of vitiligo has been recently reported (Brown-Harrel *et al.* 1996).

Thiambutosine BP

Thiambutosine BP (CIBA 1906) is another drug used in the treatment of leprosy which can cause hyperpigmentation both of hypopigmented areas and normal skin. However a trial on five patients (2 g 30 minutes before UV exposure) failed to produce any improvement (Verbov 1972).

Anti-malarial drugs

Chloroquine

Chloroquine diphosphate was administered in daily doses of 500 mg to improve light sensitivity in a 49-year-old man suffering from vitiligo (Christiansen 1955). The patient noticed, after 1 week, an increased light tolerance. After 4 weeks of treatment, repigmentation appeared in perifollicular patches and, 5 months later, some macules showed 50–90% repigmentation, the better result noted on the face. The total dose of chloroquine was 30 g (Christiansen 1955). Chloroquine has been reported to be responsible for vitiligo appearance (Christiansen 1995).

Penicillamine

One case of vitiligo responded to oral therapy with penicillamine during the treatment for rheumatoid arthritis. Repigmentation failed to remain when the drug was suspended (Alarcon Segovia 1982).

Tar

Coal tar has both anti-inflammatory-immunosuppressive and melanogenic properties. Crude coal tar, 300 mg/mL in a mixture of polysorbate (Zetar bath oil emulsion) was applied at weekly intervals to vitiligo macules and allowed to stay on for at least two hours. About 50% of patients noted repigmentation after 10–20 treatments (Urbanek 1983). However, other investigators disagree with these results (Goldstein *et al.* 1992). Apart from its use in vitiligo, tar has also been used as an alternative treatment for other dermatoses (Leong 1990).

Lasers

Low energy laser irradiation influences catecholamine synthesis in some dermatological conditions such as vitiligo (Mandel 1982). Clinical trials with lasers showed beneficial effects in 18 vitiligo patients (Mandel 1984). The low energy laser exposure was administered 5 times per week in a dose of 20 mW cm^{-2}, for 10 minutes. Marked repigmentation was observed in 63.9% of patients (Mandel *et al.* 1997). Very recently ultrapulse carbon dioxide laser has been recommended in association with PUVA therapy for vitiligo treatment (Knoell *et al.* 1997). The short pulsed carbon dioxide laser has been successfully tried for removal of the epidermis before grafting with a split-thickness skin graft (Kahn *et al.* 1996).

The Ruby laser has been proposed as an effective, fast and safe method for removing cosmetically disturbing remnants of normal pigment in vitiligo patients with a positive Koebner's phenomenon, to reach a permanent state of depigmentation (Thissen & Westerhof 1997).

Folk medicine

Anacarcin forte oil

This oil has been used in India for treating 10 patients with vitiligo (Punshi 1980). Seven cases were reported to show excellent results in 6–12 weeks, while two showed only erythema and oozing and one had urticarial rash. anacarcin forte oil contains active principles of *Semicarpus anacardium* nuts, a deciduous tree of sub-Himalayan area. The juice of the pericarp of the nut is used in indigenous medicine externally and internally for rheumatism and various skin diseases. In the treatment of vitiligo the oil was applied during the night and then the areas were exposed to the sun at

8 a.m. next morning. Toxicity studies on a proprietary preparation of *Semecarpus anacardium* have been reported (Vaishnav *et al.* 1983).

Chinese herbal medications

Extracts of herbs have been reported to be useful in treating vitiligo when administered by both oral and topical routes (Cheng & Shi 1987; Shao & Ye 1995). The real nature of these compounds is unknown and toxicological studies are not available. The safety and efficacy are based on the Chinese traditional principles such as Liqi, Ziyin, Huoxue and Qufeng. Plants which are used include *Astragalus membranaceous, Codonopsis pilosula, Eclipta prostrata, Polygonum multiforum* and *Tribuluo terrestris*. They are cooked and drunk as decoctions, taken in tablet form or given by injection (Shao & Ye 1995).

Angelica sinensis root is another herb commonly used in traditional Chinese medicine. However, one study failed to demonstrate its efficacy on mouse melanocyte proliferation in culture (Raman *et al.* 1996). Its mechanism of action is still unclear, although an immune modulator effect has been demonstrated in atopic eczema (Sheehan & Atherton 1992; Xu *et al.* 1997), which is prevalent in vitiligo (Perfetti *et al.* 1991).

The belief that herbs, as natural products available without a prescription, are harmless, is commonplace and may lead to abuse of these compounds. Herbs containing potent pharmacologically active substances are dispensed in unknown quantities and combinations to faithful and vulnerable patients, without being subjected to drug licensing, toxicity monitoring and surveillance procedures (Ferguson *et al.* 1997). Six cases of serious hepatotoxicity from herbs have been reported in the United Kingdom in the past 4 years (Davis *et al.* 1990; Graham-Brown 1992). Moreover, Chinese herbs were responsible for inducing severe cardiomyopathy that persisted despite discontinuation of treatment (Ferguson *et al.* 1997).

Other herbs

Roots and stalks are reported to be used with success in some regions of Africa (e.g. Burkina Faso). They are soaked in water for a few days then the patient bathes the vitiligo macules. There are good reasons for suspecting that the effectiveness of such treatments is due to the presence of psoralens such as in *Picrorhiza kurroa* (Bedi *et al.* 1989). Patients must be warned about the injudicious use of such herbs because of the risk of severe phototoxic dermatitis (Ossenkopele *et al.* 1991).

Minoxidil

Vitiligo repigmentation occurs first in the perifollicular areas, therefore stimulation of hair growth seemed a valid approach (Sriniva *et al.* 1990). One group tried topical minoxidil in combination with PUVA to retain hair in anagen phase and consequently to obtain an acceleration of repigmentation. In fact, hair darkening was reported after oral (15 mg twice daily) (Burton & Marshall 1979) and topical minoxidil (Fiedler-Weiss 1987; Headington 1987).

This rationale had already been tried 10 years before by a group of French investigators (Gianadda *et al.* 1980), who combined PUVA with dinlitrochlorobenzine (DNCB) to stimulate hair follicles but without any benefit. Our personal experience failed to demonstrate any influence of minoxidil in potentiating repigmentation (Orecchia *et al.* 1994), perhaps because its action is mainly directed to the hair bulb, whose melanocytes do not relate to the vitiligo repigmentation (Ortonne *et al.* 1980; Cui *et al.* 1991).

References

Abdel-Fattah, A., Aboul-Enein, M.N., Wassel, G.M. & El-Menshawi, B.S. (1982) An approach to the treatment of Vitiligo by Khellin. *Dermatologica* **165**, 136–140.

Abdel-Malek, A., Swope, V. & Dixon, K. (1993) A possible unique mechanism for UVB induced hyperpigmentation. (Abstract) *XV International Pigment Cell Conference;* London. 26–30 September, Pg 5.

Abeysekera, B.F., Abramowsky, Z. & Towers, G.H.M. (1983) Genotoxicity of the natural furochromones, Khellin and Visnagin and the identification of a Khellin-thymine photoadduct. *Photochemistry and Photobiology* **38**, 311–315.

Alarcon Segovia, D. (1982) Repigmentation of vitiligo under penicillamin therapy for rheumatoid arthritis. *Archives of Dermatology* **118**, 962.

Antoniou, C., Schulpis, H., Michas, T. *et al.* (1989) Vitiligo therapy with oral and topical phenylalanine with UVA exposure. *International Journal of Dermatology* **28**, 545–547.

Azambuja, R.D. (1992) Melagenina and vitiligo (letter). *Dermatology* **184** (2), 153–155.

Banerjee, A.K., Banerjee, D.K. & Chaudhury, D.S. (1970) Serum vitamin B_{12} level in vitiligo. A preliminary study. *Bulletin of the Calcutta School of Tropical Medicine* **18**, 73–75.

Bedi, K.L., Zutshi, U., Chopra, C.L. & Amla, V. (1989) Picrorhiza kurroa, an ayurvedic herb, may potentiate photochemotherapy in vitiligo. *Journal of Ethnopharmacology* **27**, 347–352.

Beretti, B., Grupper, C.H., Bermejo, D. *et al.* (1989) PUVA 5-MOP and PUVA 5-MOP + Phenylalanine in the treatment of vitiligo. In: *Psoralens: Past, Present, and Future of Photochemoprotection and Other Biological Activities* (eds T.B.Fitzpatrick, P.Forlot, M.A.Pathak & F.Urbach), pp. 103–108. Libbey, Eurotex, Paris.

Biella, U. & Haustein, U.F. (1990) Die Behandlung der Vitiligo mit UV und Phenylalanin. *Deutsche Dermatologie* **38**, 1063–1064.

Bleifeld, W. & Gehrmann, G. (1967) Vitamin B_{12} Resorptionsstudien bei Vitiligo. *Deutsche Medizinische Wochenschrift* **92**, 1072–1074.

Bleifeld, W. & Gehrmann, G. (1969) Vitamin B_{12} Mangel und Vitiligo. *Blut* **19**, 223–225.

Bor, S. (1973) Clofazimine (Lamprene) in the treatment of vitiligo. *South African Medical Journal* **47**, 1451–1454.

Brown-Harrell, V., Nitta, A.T. & Goble, M. (1996) Apparent exacerbation of vitiligo syndrome in a patient with pulmonary Mycobacterium avium complex disease who received clofazimine therapy. *Clinical Infectious Diseases* **22**, 581–582.

Burton, J.L. & Marshall, A. (1979) Hypertrichosis due to minoxidil. *British Journal of Dermatology* **101**, 593–595.

Calanchini-Postizzi, E. & Frenk, E. (1987) Long-term actinic damage in sun-exposed vitiligo and normally pigmented skin. *Dermatologica* **174**, 266–271.

Camacho, F. (1995) L-fenilalanina en el tratamiento del vitiligo. *Monographs in Dermatology* **8**, 190–204.

Cao, C.M., Taboas, M., Garcia, G. & Gonzales, E. (1989) Estudio experimental y clinico del efecto pigmentante epidermico del extracto placentario humano. In: *Melagenina Seleccion de Trabajos de Investigation Publicados Y Presentados En Eventos Cientificos, 1976–89,Palacio de Las Convenciones de Cuba, Havana, Cuba*, pp. 21–30.

Cheng, Y.Q. & Shi, D.R. (1987) Clinical analysis of the effects of a combined therapy with Vernonia anthelmintica and others on 329 cases of vitiligo. *Chung Hsi Chieh Ho Tsa Chih* **7**, 350–351.

Christiansen, J.V. (1955) Chloroquine-induced vitiligo. a case report and review of the literature (letter). *Acta Dermato-Venereologica (Stockholm)* **76**, 166–167.

Cormane, R.H., Anwar, H., Siddiqui, A.H. & Nengerman, I.M. (1983) Photochemotherapy of vitiligo with oral phenylalanine. *Journal of Investigative Dermatology* **80**, 367. (Abstract).

Cormane, R.H., Siddiqui, A.H., Westerhof, W. & Schutgens, R.B.H. (1985) Phenylalanine and UVA light for the treatment of vitiligo. *Archives of Dermatological Research* **277**, 126–130.

Corrales, H., Pathak, M.A., Fitzpatrick, T.B. & Gonzales, S. (1994) The use of oral and topical Polypodium leucotomos (Difur[R]) in the treatment of vitiligo. American Academy of Dermatology: Scientific Poster Exhibit 38.

Csaszar, T. & Patakfalvi, A. (1992) Treatment of polyglandular autoimmune syndrome with cyclosporin-a. *Acta Medica Hungarica* **49**, 187–193.

Cui, J., Shen, L.Y. & Wang, G.C. (1991) Role of hair follicles in the repigmentation of vitiligo. *Journal of Investigative Dermatology* **97**, 410–416.

Davis, E.G., Pollock, I. & Steep, H.M. (1990) Chinese herbs for eczema (Letter). *Lancet* **336**, 177.

Dell'Acqua, F., Vedaldi, D., Boccichetti, F. & Bordin, F. (1981) Photochemotherapy of skin disease: comparative study of the photochemical and photobiological properties of various mono and bifunctional agents. *Il Farmaco* **36**, 519–535.

Dimov, D., Petkov, I., Zlatkov, N.B., Durmisev, A. & Jordanova, J. (1976) Determination of some enzymes in the blood serum of patients with vitiligo before and after heliotherapy. *Ceskoslovenska Dermatologie* **51** (3), 148–152.

Distefano, A., Lagaetana, R., Bovalini, L., Lusini, P. & Martelli, P. (1996) Pertussis toxin reverses the inhibition of the adenylyl cyclase system by Khellin in HeLa cells. *Biochimica et Biophysica Acta* **1314** (1–2), 105–108.

Ferguson, J.E., Chalmers, R.J.G. & Rowlands, D.J. (1997) Reversible dilated cardiomyopathy following treatment of atopic eczema with Chinese herbal medicine. *British Journal of Dermatology* **136**, 592–593.

Fiedler-Weiss, V.C. (1987) Potential mechanisms of minoxidil-induced hair growth in alopecia areata. *Journal of the American Academy of Dermatology* **16**, 653–656.

Frisch, W. & Milbradt, R. (1988) Photochemotherapie der Vitiligo mit L- Phenylalanin. *Aktuelle Dermatologie* **14**, 361–364.

Galbraith, G.M.P., Thiers, B.H. & Fudenberg, H.H. (1984) An open-label trial of immunomodulation therapy with inosiplex (Isoprinosine) in patients with alopecia totalis and cell mediated immunodeficiency. *Journal of the American Academy of Dermatology* **11**, 224–230.

George, A.O. (1989) The use of readily available photosensitizers for vitiligo in Nigeria. *International Journal of Dermatology* **28**, 475–477.

Gianadda, B., Ortonne, J.P. & Thivolet, J. (1980) Essai de traitement du vitiligo par l'association DNCB ´PUVA. *Annales de Dermatologie et de Venereologie* **107**, 197–198.

Giordano, D., Rillosi, M., Benelli, P. *et al.* (1994) Preformulation studies and formulation strategies on khellin, an old/new antivitiligo agent: interaction with cyclodestrins, solubility in mixed solvent systems and permeation through artificial membranes. *European Journal of Pharmaceutics and Biopharmaceutics* **40** (4), 232–236.

Gokhale, B.B. (1979) Cyclophosphamide and vitiligo. *International Journal of Dermatology* **18**, 92.

Gokhale, B.B. & Parakh, A.P. (1983) Cyclophosphamide in vitiligo. *Indian Journal of Dermatology* **28**, 7–10.

Goldstein, E., Haberman, H.F., Menon, I.A. & Pawloski, D. (1992) Non-psoralen treatment of vitiligo. Part II. Less commonly used and experimental therapies. *International Journal of Dermatology* **5**, 314–319.

Gonzalez, S., Pathak, M.A., Cuevas, J., Villarubia, V.G. & Fitzpatrick, T.B. (1997) Topical or oral administration with an extract of Polypodium leucotomos prevents acute sunburn and psoralen-induced phototoxic reactions as well as depletion of Langerhans cells in human skin. *Photodermatology Photoimmunology and Photomedicine* **13**, 50–60.

Goolamali, S.K. (1973) Levodopa in vitiligo. *Lancet* **i**, 675–676.

Graham-Brown, R. (1992) Toxicity of Chinese herbal remedies (Letter). *Lancet* **340**, 673.

Greiner, D., Ochsendorf, F.R. & Milbradt, R. (1994) Vitiligo-Therapie mit Phenylalanin/UVA. Katamnestische Untersuchungen nach funf Jahren. *Hautarzt* **45**, 460–463.

Grimes, P.E. (1993) Vitiligo. An overview of therapeutic approach. *Dermatologic Clinics* **11**, 325–338.

Gupta, A.K., Haberman, H.F., Pawloski, D., Shulman, G. & Menon, I.A. (1985) Canthaxantin. *International of Journal of Dermatology* **24**, 528–532.

Gupta, A.K., Ellis, C.N., Nickoloff, B.J. *et al.* (1990) Oral cyclosporine in the treatment of inflammatory and noninflammatory dermatosis. A clinical and immunopathological analysis. *Archives of Dermatology* **126**, 339–350.

Headington, J.T. (1987) Hair follicle biology and topical minoxidil: possible mechanism of action. *Dermatology* **175** (Suppl. 2), 19–22.

Honigsmann, H. (1990) Phototherapy and photochemotherapy. *Seminars in Dermatology* **9**, 84–90.

Jaen, P., Alonso, M.L., Martin, M., Fitzpatrick, T.B. & Pathak, M.A. (1994) The potential use of the fern Polypodium leucotomos in the treatment of vitiligo. American Academy of Dermatology: Scientific Poster Exhibit 39.

Jakorsky, C., Ratz, J.L. & Dijkstra, J.W.E. (1987) Efficacy of tan accelerators. *Journal of the American Academy of Dermatology* **16**, 769–771.

Jansen, T., Megahed, M., Holzle, E. & Plewig, C. (1995) Provocation of porphyria cutanea tarda by KUVA-therapy of vitiligo. *Acta Dermato-Venereologica (Stockholm)* **75**, 232–233.

Juhlin, L. & Olsson, M.J. (1997) Improvement of vitiligo after oral treatment with vitamin B_{12} and folic acid and the importance of sun exposure. *Acta Dermato-Venereologica (Stockholm)* **77**, 460–462.

Kahn, A.M., Ostad, A., Moy, R.L. & Wheeland, R. (1996) Grafting following short pulse carbon dioxide laser de-epithelization. *Dermatologic Surgery* **22**, 965–968.

Kalampalikis, D., Ioannides, D., Teknetzis, A. & Minas, A. (1992) Treatment of vitiligo with sulphuric copper. A study of 45 cases. *Proceedings of the European Academy of Dermatology and Venereology An* vol, pp.

Kao, C.H. & Yu, H.S. (1992) Comparison of the effect of 8- methoxypsoralen (8-MOP) plus UVA (PUVA) on human melanocytes in Vitiligo vulgaris and *in vitro*. *Journal of Investigative Dermatology* **98**, 734–740.

Knoell, K.A., Schreiber, A.J. & Milgraum, S. (1997) Treatment of vitiligo with the ultrapulse carbon dioxide laser in patients concomitantly receiving oral psoralen plus UVA therapy. *Archives of Dermatology* **133**, 1605–1606.

Koshevenko, I.N. (1989) Alpha-tocopherol in the combined treatment of vitiligo. *Vestnik Dermatologii I Venerologii (Moskva)* **10**, 70–72.

Koster, W. & Wiskerman, A. (1990) Phototherapie mit UVB bei Vitiligo. *Zeitschrift für Hautkrankheiten* **65**, 1022–1024.

Kumar, B., Kaur, S., Kaur, I. & Gangowar, D.N. (1987) More about clofazimine: 3 years experience and review of literature. *Indian Journal of Leprosy* **59**, 63–74.

Laskin, J.D. & Laskin, D.L. (1988) Role of psoralens receptors in cell growth regulation. In: *Psoralen and DNA Photobiology. Vol 2.* (ed. F.P. Gasparro), p. 135. CRC Press, Boca Raton, Florida.

Lemke, R. (1993) Alternative therapien der Vitiligo. *Aktuelle Dermatologie* **19**, 129–132.

Leong, L.Y. (1990) How I use coal tar in dermatology. *Singapore Medical Journal* **31**, 614–615.
Lerner, A.B., Snell, R.S., Chanco-Turner, M.L. & McGuire, G.S. (1966) Vitiligo and sympathectomy. *Archives of Dermatology* **94**, 269–278.
Mandel, A.S.H. (1982) the influence of laser therapy on the content of serotonin and dopamine in patients with local scleroderma. *Vestnik Dermatologii I Venerologii (Moskva)* **8**, 13–17.
Mandel, A.S.H. (1984) Skin repigmentation after laser therapy. *Vestnik Dermatologii I Venerologii (Moskva)* **9**, 26–29.
Mandel, A.S.H., Haberman, H.F., Pawlowsky, D. & Goldstein, E. (1997) Non PUVA non surgical therapies for vitiligo. *Clinics in Dermatology* **15**, 907–919.
Marconi, B., Mancini, F., Colombo, P., Orecchia, G. & Santi, P. (1997) Distribuzione della kellina nella pelle umana sottoposta a ionoforesi transdermica. Simposio 1997 AFI-ISPE. Montecatini Terme, 21–23 maggio.
Maresca, V., Roccella, M., Roccella, F. *et al.* (1997) Increased sensitivity to peroxidative agents as a possible pathogenic factor of melanocyte damage in vitiligo. *Journal of Investigative Dermatology* **109**, 310–313.
Mohammed, A. (1989) Vitiligo repigmentation with anapsos (Polypodium leucotomos) (letter). *International Journal of Dermatology* **28**, 479.
Monk, B. (1985) Topical fluorouracil in vitiligo. *Archives of Dermatology* **121**, 25–26.
Montes, L.F., Diaz, M.L., Lajous, J. & Garcia, N.J. (1992) Folic acid and vitamin B_{12} in vitiligo: a nutritional approach. *Cutis* **50**, 39–42.
Morliere, P., Honigsmann, H., Averbeck, D. *et al.* (1988) Phototherapeutic, photobiologic and photosensitizing properties of khellin. *Journal of Investigative Dermatology* **90**, 720–724.
Nakamura, T., Pinnell, S.R., Darr, D. *et al.* (1997) Vitamin C abrogates the deleterious effects of UVB radiation on cutaneous immunity by a mechanism that does not depend on TNF-alfa. *Journal of Investigative Dermatology* **109**, 20–24.
Nordlund, J.J. (1991) Alfa-melanocyte stimulating hormone: a ubiquitous cytokine with pigmenting effects. *JAMA* **266**, 2753–2754.
Nordlund, J.J. (1992) Melagenina and vitiligo (Reply). *Dermatology* **184** (2), 154–155.
Nordlund, J.J. & Halder, R. (1990) Melagenina. An analysis of published and other available data, *Dermatologica* **181**, 1–4.
Nordlund, J.J. & Majumder, P.P. (1997) Recent investigations on vitiligo vulgaris. *Dermatologic Clinics* **15**, 69–78.
Nordlund, J.J. & Ortonne, J.P. (1998) Milan treatment procedure (Report). Vitiligo. *The Newsletter of the National Vitiligo Foundation Inc.* **6**, 9.
Orecchia, G. & Giordano, F. (1996) A new preparation of khellin in the topical treatment of vitiligo (Abstract). *Journal of Investigative Dermatology* **106**, 944.
Orecchia, G. & Perfetti, L. (1989) Cystine in the treatment of vitiligo. *G Ital Dermatol Venereol* **124**, 529–531.
Orecchia, G. & Perfetti, L. (1992) Photochemotherapy with topical khellin and sunlight in vitiligo. *Dermatology* **184**, 120–123.
Orecchia, G., Perfetti, L., Borghini, F. & Malagoli, P.G. (1992) Phenylalanine in the treatment of vitiligo. *Annali Italiani Dermatologia Clinicae Sperimentale* **46**, 143–146.
Orecchia, G., Malagoli, P.G. & Santagostino, L. (1994) Topical minoxidil does not potentiate the effect of sunlight in vitiligo repigmentation. *Ann Ital Dermatol Clin Sper* **48**, 81–83.
Orecchia, G., Sangalli, M.E., Gazzaniga, A. & Giordano, F. (1998) Topical photochemotherapy of vitiligo with a new khellin formulation: preliminary clinical results. *Journal of Dermatologic Treatment* **9**, 65–69.
Ortel, B., Tanew, A. & Honigsman, H. (1988) Treatment of Vitiligo with Khellin and ultraviolet a. *Journal of the American Academy of Dermatology* **18**, 693–701.
Ortonne, J.P., Pelletier, N., Chabanon, M. & Thivolet, J. (1978) Vitiligo et épitéliomas cutanés. *Annales de Dermatologie et de Venereologie (Paris)* **105**, 1063–1064.

Ortonne, J.P., Schmitt, D. & Thivolet, J. (1980) PUVA-induced repigmentation of vitiligo: scanning electron microscopy of hair follicles. *Journal of Investigative Dermatology* **74**, 40–42.

Ossenkopele, P.M., van der Sluis, W.G. & van Vloten, W.A. (1991) Phototoxic dermatitis following the use of Ammi majus fruit for vitiligo. *Nederlands Tijdschrift Voor Geneeskunde* **135** (11), 478–480.

Pal, P., Roy, R., Dutta, A.K., Biswas, B. & Bhadra, R. (1995) Hydroalcoholic human placental extract: skin pigmenting activity and gross chemical composition. *International Journal of Dermatology* **34** (1), 61–66.

Park, S.H., Hann, S.K. & Park, K. (1996) Ten-year experience of phototherapy in Yonsei Medical Center. *Yonsei Medical Journal* **37** (6), 392–396.

Pasricha, J.S. & Khera, V. (1994) Effect of prolonged treatment with levamisole on vitiligo with limited and low-spreading disease. *International Journal of Dermatology* **33** (8), 584–587.

Pathak, M.A. & Dalle Carbonare, M. (1989) Melanogenetic potential of various furocoumarins in normal and vitiliginous skin. In: *Psoralens: Past, Present and Future of Photochemoprotection and Other Biological Activities* (eds T.B.Fitzpatrick, P.Forlot, M.A.Pathak & F.Urbach), p. 87. Libbey, Paris.

Perfetti, L., Cespa, M., Nume, A. & Orecchia, G. (1991) Prevalence of atopy in vitiligo. Preliminary report. *Dermatologica* **182**, 218–220.

Picardo, M., Passi, S., Morrone, A., Grandinetti, M., Di Carlo, A. & Ippolito, F. (1994) Antioxidant status in the blood of patients with active vitiligo. *Pigment Cell Research* **7**, 110–115.

Picardo, M., Camera, E., Maresca, V., Pittarello, A., Feonetti, F. & Passi, S. (1997) Antioxidant treatment in vitiligo? (Abstract). *Pigment Cell Research* **10**, 360.

Pietzcker, F. & Kuner-Beck, V. (1979) 'Pigmentausgleich' durch beta-Karotin oral. Ein neues therapeutisches Prinzip in der kosmetischen Dermatologie. *Hautarzt* **30**, 308–311.

Pruvot-Sentous, D., Loesche, C., Léonard, F., Thomas, P. & The Group of Phototherapy Research of, S.F.P.D. (1992) PUVA–therapy and association of phenylalanine and UVA therapy in vitiligo. A multicentre study of 81 observations. *European Journal of Dermatology* **2**, 469–474.

Punshi, S.K. (1980) Topical use of Anacarcin Forte (R) oil in vitiligo. *Indian Journal of Dermatology Venereology and Leprology* **46**, 102–103.

Raab, W.P., Tronnier, H. & Wiskemann, A. (1985) Photoprotection of skin coloring by oral carotenoids. *Dermatologica* **171**, 371–373.

Raman, A., Lin, Z.X., Sviderskaya, E. & Kowalska, D. (1996) Investigation of the effect of Angelica sinensis root extract on the proliferation of melanocytes in culture. *Journal of Ethnopharmacology* **54**, 165–170.

Riccio, M.L., Coratza, G., Bovalini, L. & Martelli, P. (1992) Investigation of mutagenic activity in Salmonella typhimurium of the furochromone Khellin, proposed as therapeutic agents for skin diseases. *Mutation Research* **279** (2), 103–108.

Rosenbach, T., Wellenreuther, U., Nurnberger, F. & Czarnetzki, B. (1993) Vitiligobehandlung mit Phenylalanin und UV-a. *Hautarzt* **44**, 208–209.

Ryan, W. & Carver, M. (1963) Inhibition of antibody synthesis by L- phenylalanine. *Science* **43**, 479–480.

Schallreuter, K.U. & Pittelkow, M.R. (1988) Defective calcium uptake in keratinocyte cell cultures from vitiliginous skin. *Archives of Dermatologic Research* **280**, 137–139.

Schallreuter, K.U., Buttner, G., Pittelkow, M.R., Wood, J.M., Swanson, N.N. & Koerner, C. (1994a) The cytotoxicity of 6-biopterin to human melanocytes. *Biochemical and Biophysical Research Communications* **204**, 432–438.

Schallreuter, K.U., Wood, J.M., Ziegler, I., Lemke, K.R., Pittelkow, M.R. & Gutlich, M. (1994b) Defective tetrahydrobiopterin and catecholamine biosynthesis in the depigmentation disorder vitiligo. *Biochimica et Biophysica Acta* **1226**, 181–192.

Schallreuter-Wood, K.U., Pittelkow, M.R. & Swanson, N.N. (1996) Defective calcium transport in vitiliginous melanocytes. *Archives of Dermatologic Research* **288**, 11–13.

Schulpis, C.H., Antoniou, C., Michas, T. & Stratigos, J. (1989) Phenylalanine plus ultraviolet light: preliminary report of a promising treatment for childhood vitiligo. *Pediatric Dermatology* **6**, 332–335.
Shao, C. & Ye, G. (1995) Current treatment of vitiligo in China. *Chinese Medical Journal (Engl)* **108**, 647–649.
Sheehan, M.P. & Atherton, D.J.A. (1992) Controlled trial of Chinese medicinal plants in widespread non-exudative atopic eczema. *British Journal of Dermatology* **126**, 179–184.
Shukla, S.R. (1981) Evaluation of clofazimine in vitiligo. *Dermatologica* **163**, 169–171.
Shuppli, R. (1981) Lampren bei vitiligo. *Dermatologica* **163**, 487–489.
Siddiqui, A.H., Stolk, L.M.L., Bhaggoe, R., Hu, R., Schutgens, R.B.H. & Westerhof, W. (1994) L- Phenylalanine and UVA irradiation in the treatment of vitiligo. *Dermatology* **188**, 215–218.
Srinivas, C.R., Shenoi, S.D. & Balachandran, C. (1990) Acceleration of repigmentation in vitiligo by topical minoxidil in patients on photochemotherapy. *International Journal of Dermatology* **29**, 154–155.
Stierner, U., Rosdahl, I., Augistsson, A. & Kagedal, B. (1989) UVB irradiation induces melanocyte increase in both exposed and shielded human skin. *Journal of Investigative Dermatology* **92**, 561–564.
Suite, M. & Quamina, D.B. (1991) Treatment of vitiligo with topical melagenina—a human placental extract. *Journal of the American Academy of Dermatology* **24** (6 Part 1), 1018–1019.
Szekeres, E. & Morvay, M. (1985) Repigmentation of vitiligo macules treated topically with Efudix cream. *Dermatologica* **171**, 55–59.
Thiele, B. (1991) Photochemotherapie mit L-phenylalanin und UV-a-licht (PAUVA) als alternatives Therapiekonzept bei Vitiligo. *Aktuelle Dermatologie* **17**, 53–57.
Thissen, M. & Westerhof, W. (1997) Laser treatment for further depigmentation in vitiligo. *International Journal of Dermatology* **36**, 386–388.
Thomas, P. & Largillière, C. (1988) La phénylalanine est-elle vraiment inoffensive dans le traitement du vitiligo? (letter). *Annales de Dermatologie et de Venereologie* **115**, 195.
Trabalzini, L., Martelli, P., Bovalini, L., Dall'Acqua, F. & Sage, E. (1990) Photosensitization of DNA of defined sequence by furochromones, Khellin and visnagin. *Photochemistry and Photobiology* **7**, 317–336.
Tsuji, T. & Hamada, T. (1983) Topically administered fluorouracil in vitiligo. *Archives of Dermatology* **119**, 722–727.
Ubeda, A. & Villar, A. (1989) Relaxant actions of khellin on vascular smooth muscle. *Journal of Pharmacy and Pharmacology* **41** (4), 236–241.
Ubeda, A., Tejerin, T., Tamargo, J. & Villar, A. (1991) Effects of Khellin on contractile responses and 45Ca2+ movements in rat isolated aorta. *Journal of Pharmacy and Pharmacology* **43** (1), 46–48.
Urbanek, R.W. (1983) Tar vitiligo therapy (letter). *Journal of the American Academy of Dermatology* **8**, 755.
Vaishnav, R., Sankaranarayanan, A., Chaudhury, R.R., Mathur, V.S. & Chakravarti, R.N. (1983) Toxicity studies on a proprietary preparation of Semecarpus anacardium. *Indian Journal of Medical Research* **77**, 902–908.
Van Scott, E.J. & Yu, R.J. (1975) Melanogenesis from topical mechlorethamine and analogues in skin hairless mice and in vitiligo. *Journal of Investigative Dermatology* **65**, 476–478.
Van Weelden, H., de La Faille, H.B., Young, E. & Van der Leun, J.C. (1988) A new development in UVB phototherapy of psoriasis. *British Journal of Dermatology* **119**, 11–19.
Van Weelden, H., de La Faille, H.B., Young, E. & Van der Leun, J.C. (1990) Comparison of narrow- band UV-B phototherapy and PUVA photochemotherapy in treatment of psoriasis. *Acta Dermato-Venereologica (Stockholm)* **70**, 212–215.
Verbov, J. (1972) Use of CIBA 1906 (Thiambutosine BP) n in vitiligo. *British Journal of Dermatology* **87**, 81–82.
Westerhof, W. & Nieuweboer-Krobotova, L. (1997) Treatment of vitiligo with UV-B radiation vs topical psoralen plus UV-a. *Archives of Dermatology* **133**, 1525–1528.

Westerhof, W., Groot, I., Krieg, S.R., Bos, J.D. & Cormane, R.H. (1986) Langerhans' cell population studies with OKT6 and HLA-DR monoclonal antibodies in vitiligo patients treated with oral phenylalanine loading and UVA irradiation. *Acta Dermato-Venereologica (Stockholm)* **259**, 74.

Woolfson, H. & Finn, O.A. (1972) Topical levodopa in vitiligo. *Lancet* **i**, 598.

Xu, X.J., Banerjee, P., Rustin, M.H.A. & Poulter, L.W. (1997) Modulation by Chinese herbal therapy of immune mechanisms in the skin of patients with atopic eczema. *British Journal of Dermatology* **136**, 54–59.

Zlatkov, N.B., Petkov, I., Genov, D. & Bozhkov, D. (1971) Copper metabolism in vitiligo patients after heliotherapy. *Dermatologica* **143** (2), 115–120.

Zlatkov, N.B., Petkov, I., Genov, D. & Bozhkov, D. (1972) Effects of heliotherapy on copper exchange in vitiligo. *Zeitschrift für Physiotherapie* **24** (6), 461.

PART 5
TOPICS RELATED TO VITILIGO

30: Depigmentation Other Than Vitiligo

JEAN-CLAUDE BYSTRYN

Introduction

Localized, spontaneous and complete depigmentation of the skin that resembles the depigmentation of vitiligo can occur in association with pigmented naevi and with melanoma (Kopf *et al.* 1965; Bystryn & Xie 1998). The depigmentation may occur within the lesion, around it, or at a distal site (see Table 30.1). Loss of pigmentation within a lesion is normally associated with regression of the depigmented part of the lesion. Depigmentation around a lesion is referred to as a leukoderma acquisitum centrifugum, and can occur around various benign pigmented naevi or primary or metastatic melanoma (Kopf *et al.* 1965). Halo naevus is the specific type of leukoderma acquisitum centrifugum which occurs around a pigmented naevus (Kopf *et al.* 1965). Depigmentation distal to a pigmented lesion, that resembles vitiligo but is not otherwise explained, is referred to as vitiligo-like depigmentation. It is, at times, associated with melanoma.

Depigmentation in these different leukodermas probably results from different mechanisms as it involves the destruction of different types of pigment cells (normal or malignant melanocytes, normal or atypical naevus cells); occurs in different locations (at the site of, adjacent to, or distal to the cells that initiated the process); and is associated with different histological abnormalities (the presence or absence of a dense cellular infiltrate). The possible causes are discussed subsequently.

Halo naevi and leukoderma acquisitum centrifugum

A halo naevus is a pigmented naevus surrounded by a ring of depigmentation that may progress to spontaneous disappearance of the naevus (Wayte *et al.* 1968). It is the most common form of leukoderma acquisitum centrifugum. Leukoderma acquisitum centrifugum is a generic term that applies to other forms of acquired depigmentation around pigmented lesions and should not be used to refer specifically to halo naevus.

Clinical features

Halo naevi occur in approximately 1% of the population (Ortonne *et al.*

Table 30.1 Leukodermas associated with neoplasia.

Within the neoplasm (associated with regression)
halo naevi
congenital naevi
melanoma, primary and metastatic
Around the neoplasm (leukoderma acquisitum centrifugum)
halo naevi
congenital naevi
spitz naevi
blue naevi
neurofibromas
melanoma
Distal from the neoplasm (vitiligo-like depigmentation)
melanoma

1983). It involves all races, may occur at any age, but is most common in children and young adults (Wayte *et al.* 1968). Eighty-five to 90% of cases occur during the first three decades of life (Wayte *et al.* 1968). The typical halo naevus consists of a pigmented naevus surrounded by a macule of complete depigmentation (Fig. 30.1). The central naevus is usually an acquired naevus cell naevus, sometimes a dysplastic naevus, and rarely a congenital naevus. There are usually three phases in the evolution of a halo naevi—appearance of the halo, regression of the central naevus, and disappearance of the halo. Halo naevi typically begin with a circular or oval ring of depigmentation around a pre-existing naevus. The pigment loss occurs in days to weeks and is asymptomatic. The underlying skin is normal in appearance. The margin between depigmented and normally pigmented skin is well defined. There is no relation between the size of the naevus and that of the depigmentation. In 3% to 50% of patients, the central naevus eventually disappears after several months to years. Halo naevi occur predominantly on the trunk, particularly the upper torso. Their distribution is

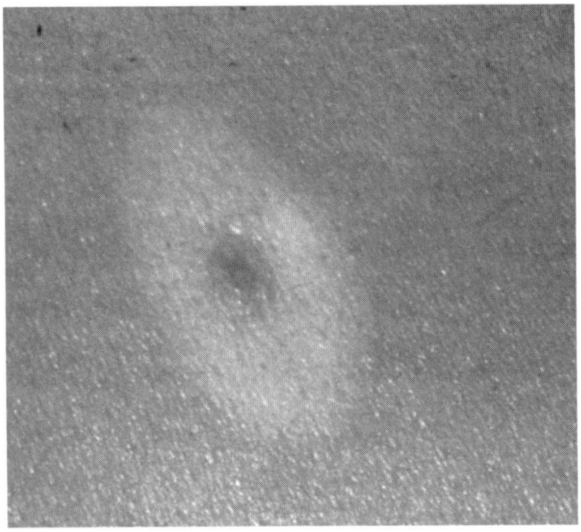

Fig. 30.1 Halo naevus. There is a sharply outlined ring of depigmentation surrounding an otherwise normal-appearing intradermal naevi. As the lesion progresses, the central naevus begins to disappear.

similar to that of typical naevus cells. Many patients have more than one halo naevus, possibly as many as two or three (Kopf *et al.* 1965). However, the majority of pigmented naevi in an affected individual almost invariably remain normally pigmented.

Halos of depigmentation or leukoderma acquisitum centrifugum may occur around other lesions including neurofibromas (Kopf *et al.* 1965; Smith & Moseley 1976), blue naevus (Kopf *et al.* 1965), Spitz naevus (Kopf *et al.* 1965; Larsson & Liden 1980), congenital naevus (Albert *et al.* 1992) and in the choroid of the ocular fundus. The common feature of these other lesions is that almost all are neoplasms of pigment cells or derivatives of the neural crest. In these conditions, the naevus usually does not regress, although there are exceptions (Tokura *et al.* 1994). There is usually no discernible precipitating factor. There is an association between halo naevus and vitiligo or melanoma. Halo naevi are not genetically determined, although occasional familial cases can occur (Kopf *et al.* 1965; Larsson & Liden 1980). Leukoderma centrifigum acquisitum has also been rarely observed around lesions not of neural crest origin such as seborrheic keratoses, angiomas, skin tags and other similar benign lesions. The significance is not known.

Histology

The histological findings depend on the stage of evolution at which the biopsy is taken. The most characteristic findings are naevus cells, a dense lymphocytic infiltrate within the naevus, and loss of melanocytes and melanin in the halo. There is a sharp transition between the depigmented halo and the normal adjacent epidermis. In the completely depigmented halo, epidermal melanocytes are absent and there is an increased number of Langerhan's cells in the basal cell layer (Mishima *et al.* 1972). The central naevus is usually a compound naevus (Wayte *et al.* 1968; Akasu *et al.* 1994), though it may be entirely dermal or junctional (Wayte *et al.* 1968). There is usually no discernible atypia of naevus cells or of melanocytes in early lesions (Kopf *et al.* 1965; Wayte *et al.* 1968). As the regression progresses, mild atypia of naevus cells may become apparent, probably as a result of the inflammatory infiltrate.

Resolution of the central naevus is characterized by a dense lymphocytic infiltrate which initially appears as a band in the deepest portion of the naevi and proceeds toward the surface (Stegmaier 1959). The infiltrate is composed of lymphocytes, plasma cells, and histiocytes. While the density of the infiltrate changes as regression evolves, its composition remains constant (Akasu *et al.* 1994). Approximately 80% of the cells are T cells. Of these, a relatively high proportion are CD8+ cells (Bergman *et al.* 1985); and approximately 25% are CD4+ (Akasu *et al.* 1994). In fully regressed lesions, the histology resembles that of vitiligo with total absence of naevus cells and melanocytes, few or no inflammatory cells (Jacobs *et al.* 1975), and some fibrosis.

Relation between halo naevus and vitiligo

Halo naevi and vitiligo share a common terminal event—the destruction of normal melanocytes—and both appear to be associated with anti-pigment cell immune responses, although these responses may be different. Between 1% and 48% of patients with halo naevus are reported to have vitiligo (Kopf *et al.* 1965; Wayte *et al.* 1968, 1973; Gauthier *et al.* 1975). This large variation reflects the small number of patients in each study. At times it might be difficult to distinguish a regressed halo naevus from vitiligo. Conversely, the incidence of halo naevi in vitiligo also appears to be elevated. It ranged from 0.5 to 14% (average of 5.9%) in five large studies involving at least 100 patients each (Barona *et al.* 1995; Bystryn & Xie 1998); an incidence approximately five-fold greater than that in a normal population.

Several observations argue that the trigger for the two conditions is different. Halo naevi always begins around a naevus while vitiligo rarely does so. A lymphocytic infiltrate is always present in the naevocellular cells of an active halo naevus but is exceptional in lesions of vitiligo. Pigmented naevi can be present within lesions of vitiligo, an unexpected event if the cause of the two diseases is similar. Thus different immune mechanisms may appear to be responsible for destruction of melanocytes in the halo and within lesions of vitiligo. In any event, the persistence of pigmented naevi within lesions of vitiligo argues for there being antigenic differences between melanocytes and naevus cells; and for the immune reactions in vitiligo and halo naevi to be targeting the unique antigens associated with each type of cell.

Association between halo naevi and melanoma

Individual case reports associate halo naevi with melanoma (Kopf *et al.* 1965). How often this occurs is unclear. There are few studies of the incidence of halo naevi in large populations of melanoma patients. The halo naevi may appear together with, or following, the removal of the melanoma.

Management

Management of halo naevi is controversial, for the reason that a few observers have suggested but not proven that halo naevi results from naevus cells that are atypical or undergoing malignant transformation. Most observers consider the lesions to be harmless and requiring no therapy but recommend careful follow-up and excision of lesions with features suggestive of melanoma, such as if the halo is asymmetric or if the lesion is of concern to the patient.

Leukoderma with melanoma

Three different types of depigmentation are associated with melanoma:

1 leukoderma within the tumour;
2 leukoderma acquisitum centrifugum around the tumour;
3 vitiligo-like depigmentation at distal sites (Kopf *et al.* 1979).

Leukoderma and regression within melanoma

Partial depigmentation of the tumour is a common manifestation of primary melanoma (see Fig. 30.2). It results from the local regression of the melanoma. White colour within a pigmented lesion is a feature used to diagnose primary melanoma. Histologically it is characterized by destruction of melanoma cells and a dense lymphohistiocytic infiltrate (McGovern & Murad 1985). The destruction of melanoma cells is very selective. It usually does not involve normal melanocytes in adjacent normal skin. The leukoderma may involve any part of the tumour, may halt at any time, or may progress to eventual disappearance of the melanoma. Histological evidence of partial melanoma regression is seen in 10% to 50% of primary melanoma (Bystryn & Xie 1998).

Approximately 3–15% of patients that present with metastatic melanoma have no detectable primary lesions (McGovern & Murad 1985; Bystryn & Xie 1998). It is believed that the primary melanoma has spontaneously and completely regressed in these patients. This is supported by the presence in some of these patients of small white macules in the area drained by the node involved with metastases that are clinically and histo-

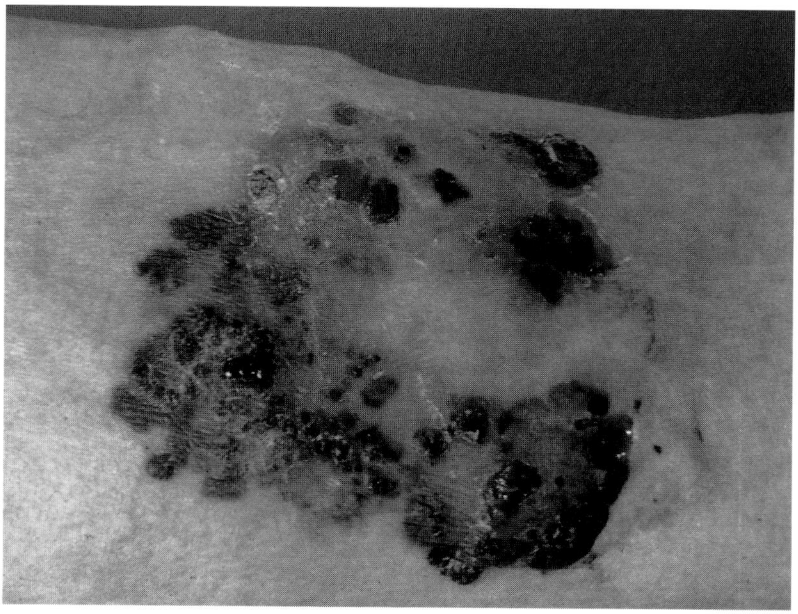

Fig. 30.2 Depigmentation within a melanoma. There is an irregular area of partial and complete loss of pigmentation within the tumour. This represents areas of melanoma cell regression. In some cases the regression can progress to result in complete disappearance of the melanoma.

logically typical of end stage halo naevi (Avril *et al.* 1992; Shai *et al.* 1994), and which can be documented to result from the regression of a primary melanoma in some cases (Avril *et al.* 1992).

It is suspected that partial regression is the result of an immune attack on a single clone of melanoma cells (McGovern & Murad 1985), which differs antigenically from other clones within the same tumour. This possibility is supported by evidence that the antigenic properties of melanoma are heterogeneous, and that antigenically different clones of melanoma cells are present within the same tumour.

Leukoderma acquisitum centrifugum around melanoma

Partial or complete rings of depigmentation can also occur in the normal skin surrounding primary or metastatic lesions of melanoma. This can occur independently of regression within the melanoma. It results from the destruction of melanocytes in normal skin adjacent to the tumour. It is clinically and histologically similar to the halo of a halo naevus. Unlike a halo naevus, the perilesional pigment loss usually appears only along a part of the perimeter of the melanoma rather than being completely circumferential. The incidence of leukoderma acquisitum centrifugum around melanoma is not clear. It was reported in 3% of 1130 patients with American Joint Commission for Cancer (AJCC) stage I or II melanoma (Bystryn *et al.* 1987). As described below, leukoderma acquisitum centrifugum is associated with an improved prognosis.

Vitiligo-like depigmentation distal from the tumour

Sharply outlined macules of depigmentation that resemble vitiligo, and for which no explanation can be found, can appear at sites distant from the tumour in patients with melanoma. Histologically these lesions resemble those of vitiligo with absent or abnormal melanocytes and absence of inflammatory cell infiltrate (Takahashi *et al.* 1979). Some consider these macules to be of classic vitiligo as their clinical appearance and histology is similar to vitiligo. However, as the mechanism of pigment loss and its relation to that of vitiligo remains unknown it is best to refer to it as vitiligo-like leukoderma until the relation is clarified (see Chapter 1).

Vitiligo-like leukoderma has been reported in 5–20% of patients, all of whom had stage III metastatic melanoma (Nordlund *et al.* 1983; Merinsky *et al.* 1994). In our experience it is rarer, at least in those individuals with earlier melanomas. It was found in only 15 (1.3%) of 1130 unselected melanoma patients with mostly AJCC stage I and II disease followed by the NYU Melanoma Cooperative Group (Bystryn *et al.* 1987). It is possible, though no data are available to reach a conclusion, that vitiligo-like depigmentation becomes more common as melanoma progresses. It may precede or follow the development of melanoma (Nordlund *et al.* 1983). The relation between this type of leukoderma, and that in vitiligo, halo naevi or leukoderma acquisitum centrifugum, remains unknown. These different leukodermas may have different pathogenesis.

Prognostic implication of leukoderma associated with melanoma

As the suspected manifestation of anti-melanoma immune responses, one would expect that leukoderma appearing in patients with melanoma carries a favourable prognosis. The available data suggest that the prognostic impact depends on the nature of the leukoderma. When depigmentation and regression occur within a melanoma, the prognostic significance is uncertain. Most studies describe it as of no prognostic value (McGovern & Murad 1985; Bystryn & Xie 1998), and some investigators suggest it is associated with an increased risk of metastasis (Paladugu & Yonemoto 1983; Shai *et al.* 1994). One explanation for these unexpected results is that the true thickness of a regressed melanoma is difficult to ascertain and is probably underestimated. At the time it is measured it is likely to be falsely thin as the depth of the regressed elements cannot be measured. This technical problem is likely to result in misclassification of the melanoma into a better prognostic group, resulting in an actual outcome worse than predicted and to the false conclusion that regression is associated with a poorer prognosis. The prognosis of primary melanoma that has completely regressed but becomes metastatic is poor (Avril *et al.* 1992), but no different from that of similar patients with a known primary (Wong *et al.* 1987).

By contrast, leukoderma acquisitum centrifugum around, or vitiligo-like depigmentation distal from, melanoma is associated with an improved prognosis. The effects of leukoderma on prognosis was examined by Bystryn *et al.* (1987) in a prospective study of 1130 patients with melanoma. A prognostic index developed by Rigel *et al.* (1985) was used to control for the multiple risk factors that affect the prognosis of melanoma. The 5 years survival of patients with leukoderma either around or distal from the tumour was significantly better than predicted (86.3% vs. 74.8%, respectively, $P = 0.03\%$). When patients with leukoderma acquisitum centrifugum around the melanoma, as opposed to those with distal, vitiligo-like leukoderma, were analysed separately, the actual survival of each subgroup (83.4% and 93.1%, respectively) was again significantly better than predicted (70.3% and 77.2%, respectively, $P = 0.04$ and 0.01%). There was no difference in survival between patients with depigmentation around, as opposed to away from, the tumour. Similar results were obtained by Koh *et al.* (1983) and Nordlund *et al.* (1983) in smaller studies.

Pathogenesis of leukodermas associated with neoplasia

Two possibilities can be entertained for the pathogenesis of leukodermas associated with neoplasms. One is that they result from toxic factors released by or near neoplasms of pigment cells. The other is that they result from abnormal immune responses to pigment cells. The latter possibility is supported by:

1 the possible presence of humoral and/or cellular immune responses to pigment cells in these patients (Wayte *et al.* 1968). These data must be interpreted cautiously as they are based on a small number of patients, often using techniques no longer considered reliable and that lack appropriate controls;

2 the clinical links between melanoma and vitiligo-like leukoderma;

3 the evidence that vitiligo is mediated by autoimmune responses to pigment cells.

It is unclear whether a common or different mechanisms are involved in all forms of leukodermas associated with pigmented tumours. The second possibility is more likely as discussed below. The relation between these leukodermas and classical vitiligo is also unknown.

Immune responses to pigment cells in halo naevi and leukoderma associated with melanoma

The report that had the most profound impact on our thinking about the pathogenesis of halo naevi is that of Copeman *et al.* (1973) (Lewis & Copeman 1972) who reported that patients with halo naevi or with melanoma both had similar antibodies to cytoplasmic melanoma antigens, and argued that halo naevi represented an accelerated and successful rejection of a naevus developing malignant changes. However, the indirect immunofluorescence assay used is not reliable for the detection of antimelanoma antibodies. Subsequent studies are too small or poorly controlled to confirm this observation (Bystryn & Xie 1998).

Cellular immune mechanisms might play a role in the pathogenesis of halo naevi and of some other leukodermas associated with neoplasia, based on the presence of dense lymphocytic infiltrates in regressing halo naevi and melanomas. In addition, there are reports that lymphocytes of patients with halo naevi, but not those of patients with vitiligo or normal individuals, can kill cultured human melanoma cells *in vitro*. The significance of these reports is questionable as they are based on a small number of patients, usually without controls, and using outdated assays no longer considered reliable. The expression of class I HLA-A, B and C antigens is up-regulated in naevus cells adjacent to inflammatory infiltrates. These molecules are necessary both for the induction of cytolytic CD8+ T-cells and for the recognition and killing of target cells by CD8+ lymphocytes. However, they appear late in the disease process, suggesting that their role, if any, is to amplify rather than induce anti-pigment cell immune responses.

Links between leukoderma and melanoma

A number of observations link leukoderma with melanoma (see Table 30.2)

Table 30.2 Observations linking vitiligo and melanoma.

Clinical observations
Vitiligo-like leukoderma associated with melanoma
Horses and pigs with melanoma regularly develop vitiligo
Vitiligo-like leukoderma improves the prognosis of melanoma in humans and animals
Immunization of animals to melanoma cells can induce vitiligo
Laboratory observations
Swine born with melanoma develop antimelanoma antibodies that react with melanocytes. The frequency and level of these antibodies correlates with the appearance of vitiligo-like leukoderma and the regression of melanoma
Most patients with melanoma or vitiligo develop antibodies to similar pigment cell antigens, which are expressed by both melanocytes and melanoma cells

and suggest that the link results from immune responses to common pigment cell antigens.

1 Vitiligo-like leukoderma is associated with melanoma in humans and in some animals (Berkelhammer *et al.* 1982; Lerner & Cage 1973).

2 The appearance of vitiligo-like leukoderma improves the prognosis of melanoma in both humans and animals (Oxenhandler *et al.* 1982; Bystryn *et al.* 1987).

3 Immunization of animals to melanoma cells can induce depigmentation (Hornung & Krementz 1974).

4 Swine born with melanoma spontaneously develop antimelanoma antibodies that also react with melanocytes, and the frequency and level of these antibodies correlates with the appearance of vitiligo and the regression of melanoma (Cui *et al.* 1995). The antibody appearance can precede melanoma regression, so that they do not appear to be secondary to tumour cell destruction.

5 Patients with melanoma or vitiligo both develop antibodies to similar pigment cell antigens which are expressed by both melanocytes and melanoma cells (Cui & Bystryn 1995).

Taken together, these observations suggest that loss of pigmentation in, and regression or slow progression of, melanoma in humans and some animals results from the destruction of melanocytes and of melanoma cells by immune responses to common antigens shared by these two types of cells. By extension, it implies that similar mechanisms may cause vitiligo-like leukoderma (see Chapter 1).

References

Akasu, R., From, L. & Kahn, H.J. (1994) Characterization of the mononuclear infiltrate involved in regression of halo nevi. *Journal of Cutaneous Pathology* **21**, 302–311.

Albert, V.A., Barnhill, R. & Sober, A.J. (1992) Leukoderma in association with giant congenital nevi: Report of two cases. *Dermatology* **185**, 140–142.

Avril, M.F., Charpentier, P., Margulis, A. & Guillame, C. (1992) Regression of primary melanoma with metastases. *Cancer* **69**, 1377–1381.

Barona, M.I., Arrunategui, A., Falabella, R. & Alzate, A. (1995) An epidemiologic case-control study in a population with vitiligo. *Journal of the American Academy of Dermatology* **33**, 621–625.

Bergman, W., Willemze, R., Graaff-Reitsma, C. & Ruiter, D.J. (1985) Analysis of major histocompatibility antigens and the mononuclear cell infiltrate in halo nevi. *Journal of Investigative Dermatology* **85**, 25–29.

Berkelhammer, J., Ensign, B.M., Hook, R.R., Hecker, C.J. & Smith, G.D. (1982) Growth and spontaneous regression of swine melanoma: Relationship of *in vitro* leukocyte reactivity. *Journal of the National Cancer Institute* **68**, 461–468.

Bystryn, J.-C. & Xie, Z. (1998) Neoplastic hypomelanoses. In: *The Pigmentary System: Physiology and Pathophysiology* (eds J.J.Nordlund, R.E.Boissy, V.J.Hearing, R.A.King & J.P.Ortonne), pp. 647–662, Oxford University Press, New York.

Bystryn, J.-C., Rigel, D., Friedman, R.J. & Kopf, A. (1987) Prognostic significance of hypopigmentation in malignant melanoma. *Archives of Dermatology* **123**, 1053–1055.

Copeman, P.W.M., Lewis, M.G., Phillips, T.M. & Elliott, P.G. (1973) Immunological associations of the halo nevus with cutaneous malignant melanoma. *British Journal of Dermatology* **88**, 127–137.

Cui, J. & Bystryn, J.-C. (1995) Melanoma and vitiligo are associated with antibody responses to similar antigens on pigment cells. *Archives of Dermatology* **131**, 314–318.

Cui, J., Chen, D., Misfeldt, M., Swinfard, R.W. & Bystryn, J.C. (1995) Antimelanoma antibodies in swine with spontaneously regressing melanoma. *Pigment Cell Research* **8**, 60–63.

Gauthier, Y., Surleve-Bazeille, J.E., Gauthier, O. & Texier, L. (1975) Ultrastructure of halo nevi. *Journal of Cutaneous Pathology* **2**, 71–81.

Hornung, M.O. & Krementz, E.X.T. (1974) Specific tissue and tumor responses of chimpanzees following immunization against human melanoma. *Surgery* **75**, 477.

Jacobs, J.B., Edelstein, L.M., Snyder, L.M. & Fortier, N. (1975) Ultrastructural evidence for destruction in the halo nevus. *Cancer Research* **35**, 352–357.

Koh, H.K., Sober, A.J., Nakagawa, H., Albert, D.M., Mihm, M.C. & Fitzpatrick, T.B. (1983) Malignant melanoma and vitiligo-like leukoderma: an electron microscopic study. *Journal of the American Academy of Dermatology* **9**, 696–708.

Kopf, A.W., Morrill, S.D. & Silberberg, I. (1965) Broad spectrum of leukoderma acquisitum centrifugum. *Archives of Dermatology* **92**, 14–35.

Kopf, A.W., Bart, R.S., Rodrigues-Sains, R.S. & Ackerman, A.B., eds. (1979) *Malignant Melanoma*, pp. 162–165. Masson, New York.

Larsson, P.-A. & Liden, S. (1980) Prevalence of skin disease among adolescents 12–16 yr of age. *Acta Dermato-Venereologica (Stockholm)* **60**, 415–423.

Lerner, A.B. & Cage, G.W. (1973) Melanomas in horses. *Yale Journal of Biology and Medicine* **46**, 646–649.

Lewis, M.G. & Copeman, P.W.M. (1972) Halo nevus: a frustrated malignant melanoma. *British Medical Journal* **2**, 47–48.

McGovern, V.J. & Murad, T.M. (1985) Pathology of melanoma: An overview. In: *Cutaneous Melanoma: Clinical Management and Treatment Results Worldwide* (eds C.Balch & G.W.Milton), pp. 29–53, J.B. Lippincott, Philadelphia.

Merinsky, O., Shoenfeld, Y., Yecheskel, G., Chaitchik, S., Azizi, E. & Fishman, P. (1994) Vitiligo- and melanoma-associated hypopigmentation: a similar appearance but a different mechanism. *Cancer Immunology Immunotherapy* **38**, 411–416.

Mishima, Y., Kawasaki, H. & Pinkus, H. (1972) Dendritic cell dynamics in progressive depigmentations. *Archives of Dermatological Research* **243**, 67–87.

Mosher, D.B., Fitzpatrick, T.B., Hori, Y. & Ortonne, J.-P. (1993) Disorders of pigmentation. In: *Dermatology in General Medicine,* 4th edn, Vol. 1 (eds T.B.Fitzpatrick, A.Z.Eisen, K.Wolff, I.M.Freedberg & K.F.Austen), p. 957. McGraw-Hill, New York.

Nordlund, J.J., Kirkwood, J.M., Forget, B.M., Milton, G. & Lerner, A.B. (1983) Vitiligo in patients with metastatic melanoma: a good prognostic sign. *Journal of the American Academy of Dermatology* **9**, 689–696.

Ortonne, J.-P., Mosher, D.B. & Fitzpatrick, T.B., eds. (1983) Leukoderma acquisitum centrifugum: Halo nevus and other hypomelanoses associated with neoplasms. In: *Vitiligo and Other Hypomelanoses of Hair and Skin*, pp. 567–611. Plenum, New York and London.

Oxenhandler, R.W., Berkelhammer, J., Smith, G.D. & Hook, R.R. Jr (1982) Growth and regression of cutaneous melanomas in Sinclair miniature swine. *American Journal of Pathology* **109**, 259–269.

Paladugu, R.R. & Yonemoto, R.H. (1983) Biologic behavior of thin malignant melanomas with regressive changes. *Archives of Surgery* **118**, 41–44.

Rigel, D.S., Rogers, G.S. & Friedman, R.J. (1985) Prognosis in malignant melanoma. *Dermatologic Clinics* **3**, 309–314.

Shai, A., Avinoach, I. & Sagi, A. (1994) Metastatic malignant melanoma with spontaneous and complete regression of the primary lesion. *Journal of Dermatologic Surgery and Oncology* **20**, 342–345.

Smith, W.E. & Moseley, J.C. (1976) Multiple halo neurofibromas. *Archives of Dermatology* **112**, 987–990.

Stegmaier, O.C. (1959) Natural regression of the melanocytes nevus. *Journal of Investigative Dermatology* **32**, 413–421.

Takahashi, M., Sober, A.J., Mosher, D.B., Fitzpatrick, T.B. & Farinelli, W.A. (1979) Vitiligo-like leukoderma in patients with metastatic malignant melanoma. In: *Proceedings of the 10th International Pigment Cell Conference, in*, Vol. 4, *Biologic Basis of Pigmentation. Cambridge, Mass, 1977*; S Karger, Basel, New York.

Tokura, Y., Yamanaka, K., Wakita, H., Kurokawa, S., Horiguchi, D., Usui, A., Sayama, S. & Takigawa, M. (1994) Halo congenital nevus undergoing spontaneous regression. *Archives of Dermatology* **130**, 1036–1041.

Wayte, D.M., Major, R.A.M.C. & Helwig, E.B. (1968) Halo nevi. *Cancer* **22**, 69–90.

Wong, J.H., Cagle, L.A. & Morton, D.L. (1987) Surgical treatment of lymph nodes with metastatic melanoma from unknown primary sites. *Archives of Surgery* **122**, 1380–1383.

31: Physiological Alterations in the Depigmented Skin of Patients with Vitiligo

SUNGBIN IM AND JAMES J. NORDLUND

Introduction

The epidermis is composed mainly of three types of cells, keratinocytes comprising 90% of the cells of the epidermis, Langerhans cells (5%) and melanocytes (5%). In addition there are smaller populations of other cells such as the Merkel cells that are thought to be neurotransducer cells. Vitiligo is a disorder that causes destruction or disappearance of melanocytes from the epidermis (Chapter 5) (Nordlund & Ortonne 1998) as well as the Merkel cells (Bose 1994a, b, c). Clinically the manifestation is leukoderma or depigmentation. Histologically the epidermis has only two cell types rather than the normal four types of cells.

The concept of the epidermal melanin unit was first proposed in the 1960s. The concept suggested that a melanocyte worked as a unit with about 30 surrounding keratinocytes. This insight was most significant and helped explain how the cells of the epidermis worked together. At that time, the Langerhans cells were considered effete or dying melanocytes and could not be included in the unit. Of course that concept is no longer accepted. However the Langerhans cells still are considered unrelated to the other cells of the epidermis. Yet it is very clear that many cytokines that affect the function of Langerhans cells also alter the function of melanocytes (for review see Nordlund & Ortonne 1998; Nordlund *et al.* 1998; Norris *et al.* 1998). In like fashion, melanogenic factors like MSH that augment pigment formation also alter the function of the Langerhans cells and the inflammatory response (for review see Nordlund & Ortonne 1992; Nordlund & Ortonne 1998; Nordlund *et al.* 1998 and see also Cannon *et al.* 1986; Lipton *et al.* 1991; Lyson & McCann 1993; Catania & Lipton 1993, 1994; Ceriani *et al.* 1994; Nordlund & Majumder 1997). Thus we have suggested that the Langerhans cell be incorporated into the epidermal melanin unit and the three cells functioning as a unit be called the KLM unit (keratinocytes, Langerhans cells and melanocytes) (Nordlund & Boissy 1999).

That this concept is correct is supported by the numerous data indicating that depigmented skin in patients with vitiligo has an altered physiology in response to a variety of stimuli as outlined below. Without a unit composed of at least the three major cell types, i.e. the KLM unit, it is difficult to understand and to explain the alteration in the function of epidermis that is devoid of melanocytes and Merkel cells as observed in vitiligo. On the other hand, it is equally feasible that these physiological aberrations are the cause of rather than the effect of the morphological abnormalities found in the depigmented and depigmenting skin of patients with vitiligo. If we can learn how these physiological aberrations are related to the loss of melanocytes, we will have a much greater understanding of the individual cells, the epidermis and the skin.

Contact dermatitis

It has been observed that the depigmented skin of vitiligo has an altered or muted response to contact allergens and to various irritants (Uehara *et al.* 1984; Hatchome *et al.* 1987; van der Kerkhof & Fokkink 1989; Westerhof *et al.* 1989). Several investigators sensitized the pigmented skin of patients with vitiligo using contact allergens and found that only the pigmented skin but not the white skin responded to a challenge application of allergen (Uehara *et al.* 1984; Hatchome *et al.* 1987). One investigator reversed the experiment and, using other antigens, sensitized individuals with vitiligo on the white skin. He challenged both the white and pigmented skin and found that only the pigmented skin responded to a challenge dose (Hatchome *et al.* 1987). This latter finding suggests that the afferent limb of the skin-associated immune system sensitization is normal in both the white and pigmented skin and is able to induce an allergic response. In contrast, the efferent limb of the immune reaction in the pigmented skin is normal but in the depigmented skin is incapable of producing a reaction to a second exposure of an antigen. That is, the efferent limb is anomalous within the depigmented, vitiligo skin.

The response of the depigmented epidermis to contact allergens was markedly abrogated in these studies. However, the dermal response to immunogens like *Candida* seemed normal in both pigmented and depigmented skin (Uehara *et al.* 1984). This observation suggests that the impairment of the inflammatory/immune response was limited to the epidermis and was not a generalized phenomenon in the body of those with vitiligo. Thus the white epidermis of vitiligo skin seems exclusively affected and is deficient in some manner so that it cannot produce a response to an allergen. One explanation for the deficiency is the absence of the melanocytes and/or the Merkel cells that might be involved in some way with the cutaneous inflammatory response.

Very similar results have been observed in mice homozygous for the mi^{vit}/mi^{vit} gene (Rheins *et al.* 1986). These animals have a pigmentary syndrome that resembles human vitiligo but probably does not have the same pathophysiology. The depigmentation is clearly related to mutations in the *mi* gene for which the animals are homozygous. The mice develop depigmentation of the fur and epidermis starting around 6 weeks after birth (Lerner *et al.* 1986; Rheins *et al.* 1986; Boissy *et al.* 1987; Palkowski *et al.* 1987; Amornsiripanitch *et al.* 1988; Lamoreux *et al.* 1992; Nordlund *et al.* 1995; Smith *et al.* 1995). The mice respond poorly to sensitization with potent contact allergens. They respond normally to dermal-injected antigens. In general their immune system and lymphocytes seem to be normal. The only abnormality found in these mice to explain the inability of these animals to respond to contact allergens is low expression of ICAM-1 (Nordlund *et al.* 1995), a molecule that is essential for normal immune responses in the skin (Norris 1990; Norris *et al.* 1998). One hypothesis to explain these observations is that the melanocytes produce an essential cytokine, or other factors involved in a critical way in the afferent/efferent limbs of the epidermal immune response to allergens and irritants.

Applications of monobenzone to the skin of patients with extensive vitiligo showed similar results, a marked inflammatory reaction to the chemical limited to the pigmented skin but absent from the depigmented skin (Figs 31.1, 31.2). Histological examinations of the skin showed the inflammatory infiltrated locally, specifically to the pigmented, normal-appearing skin (Figs 31.3, 31.4) (Nordlund *et al.* 1985). Others have applied irritants like dithranol to the pigmented and depigmented skin of patients with vitiligo (van der Kerkhof & Fokkink 1989; Westerhof *et al.* 1989). They observed that the type of inflammatory infiltrate in the pigmented skin was mainly mononuclear whereas that in the depigmented skin was

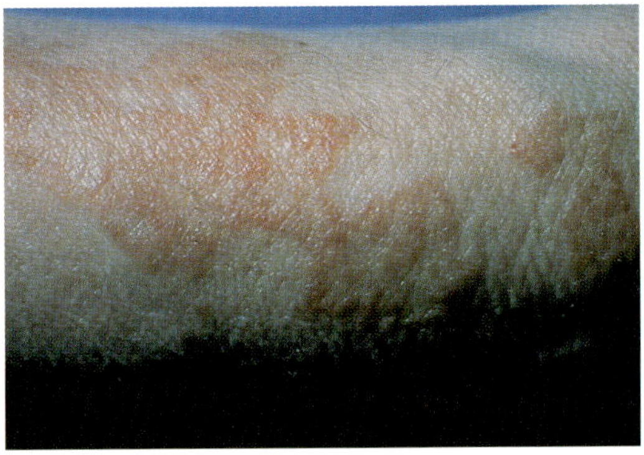

Fig. 31.1 The skin of patient 1 inflamed following the application of monobenzone. The inflammation is restricted exclusively to the pigmented skin.

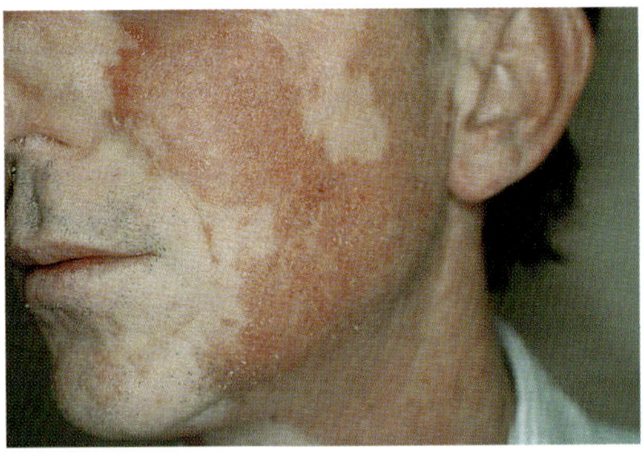

Fig. 31.2 The skin of a young man who was applying monobenzone to which he was very sensitive. Note the inflammation has a bizarre distribution that corresponds exclusively to his pigmented skin.

neutrophilic. The investigators noted that the erythema was more pronounced in the white skin than in the pigmented skin (Westerhof *et al.* 1989). These observations support the idea that the inflammatory response in depigmented skin lacking melanocytes (and Merkel cells) is unlike that of pigmented skin.

The easiest explanation for the altered response to allergens and inflammatory stimuli is that vitiliginous skin is depleted of Langerhans cells or that they are physiologically abnormal. However, results of many studies show that the population density of Langerhans cells in both humans and mice with depigmentation are normal or increased (Birbeck *et al.* 1961; Brown *et al.* 1967; Claudy & Rouchouse 1984; Kano *et al.* 1984; Uehara *et al.* 1984; Rheins *et al.* 1986; Westerhof *et al.* 1986; Hatchome *et al.* 1987; Palkowski *et al.* 1987; Le Poole *et al.* 1996). A few studies have found a decreased population of Langerhans cells (Kao & Yu 1990). Because of the results of the histological studies, some investigators have suggested that the Langerhans cells in vitiligo skin are functionally altered (Hatchome *et al.* 1987). In the mi^{vit}/mi^{vit} mice, Langerhans cells function normally in all standard assays (Nordlund *et al.* 1995).

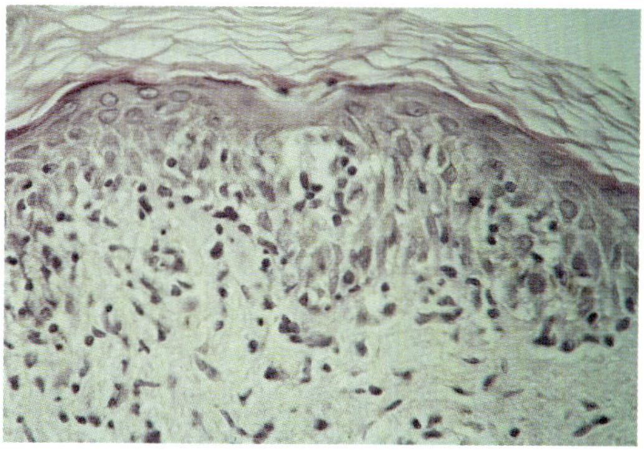

Fig. 31.3 The histological appearance of the inflamed skin of patient 1 (Fig. 31.1) showing a microvesicular dermatitis (H & E).

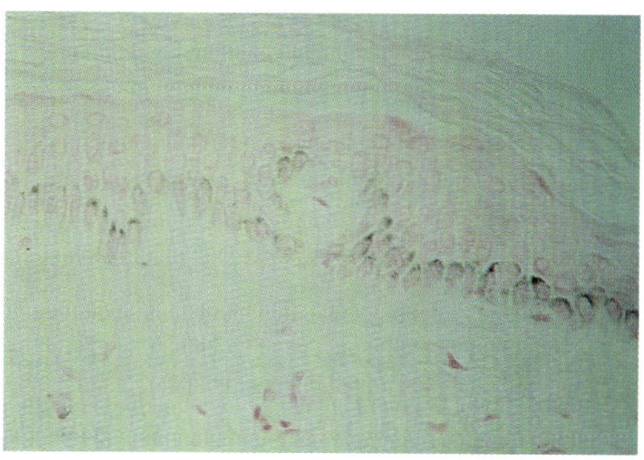

Fig. 31.4 Histology of skin from the border of vitiligo and normal skin. The biopsy was stained with Fontana-Masson to show melanin. Note the microvesicle in the centre and a positive melanin stain to one side.

Other investigators injected γ-IFN into the pigmented and depigmented skin of those with vitiligo. This cytokine should induce a marked shift of Langerhans cells from the epidermis into the dermis. In the depigmented skin of those with vitiligo, this shift is not observed (Gilhar *et al.* 1993). This observation again suggests a functional defect in depigmented skin. Others have observed in the depigmenting mi^{vit}/mi^{vit} an abnormally low production of ICAM-1 in response to injections of γ-IFN (Nordlund *et al.* 1995). Other investigators noted abnormal expression of ICAM-1 in perilesional skin (al Badri *et al.* 1993; Gilhar *et al.* 1993; Ahn *et al.* 1994). The important conclusion is that molecules that are critical for a normal inflammatory or immune response (Norris 1990) are altered in depigmented or depigmenting skin. These results all support that epidermis devoid of melanocytes (and possibly Merkel cells) has an altered immune/inflammatory response. What is still unclear is whether the absence of melanocytes is the cause or the result of these immune/inflammatory alterations.

Merkel cells

Melanocytes are not the only cells missing in depigmented skin. It has been observed by electron microscopy that there are holes along the basal lamina of depigmented skin (Bose & Ortonne 1994). Subsequent studies have shown that these holes are due to absence of Merkel cells from vitiliginous skin (Bose 1994a, b, c). Whether the absence of Merkel cells is responsible for abrogating the inflammatory response of depigmented skin, or is related to other physiological changes in the skin, remains to be determined.

Vitiligo and other inflammatory dermatoses

There are a large number of inflammatory disorders that affect the skin. Some of these can occur by chance alone in association with vitiligo (Table 31.1). Psoriasis is a common cutaneous disorder that affects about 4% of the population of the US and Europe. Vitiligo affects about 0.5% of the population. In these countries alone millions of individuals with psoriasis would be expected by chance alone to have vitiligo. Regardless, sometimes psoriasis is confined exclusively to the depigmented skin of an individual with vitiligo and at other times seems specifically to spare these same areas (Moragas & Winkelmann 1970; Chapman 1973; Howsden *et al.* 1973; Koransky & Roenigk 1982; Mancuso & Gasponi 1983; Powell & Dicken 1983; Iakovleva & Sen'kin 1984; Roberts 1984; Enhamre *et al.* 1986; Duvic *et al.* 1987; Menter *et al.* 1989). Lichen planus and vitiligo have been reported to occur together and, in some reports, lichen planus has been noted to spare depigmented skin (Babanov & Schieferstein 1970; Tan 1974a, 1974b; Brenner *et al.* 1979; Saha *et al.* 1979; Anstey & Marks 1993; Porter *et al.* 1994; Rubisz-Brzezinska *et al.* 1996). Another association is vitiligo with dermatitis herpetiformis (Humbert *et al.* 1989; Allende & Reed 1964; Ortonne *et al.* 1976; Olholm-Larsen & Kavli 1980; Hogan & Lane 1986; Hazelrigg

Table 31.1 Dermatoses coexisting with vitiligo.

Acne conglobata
Alopecia areata
Anetoderma
Ataxia telangiectasia
Atopic and eczematous dermatitis
Cicatricial pemphigoid
Cutaneous Crohn's disease
Dermatitis herpetiformis
Erythema dyschromicum perstans
Hailey-Hailey disease
Ichthyosis vulgaris
Lichen planus
Lichen sclerosis et atrophicus
Morphea
Mucocutaneous candidiasis
Parapsoriasis (small-plaque)
Pityriasis rubra pilaris
Porokeratosis of Mibelli
Porphyria cutanea tarda
Psoriasis
Sutton's naevus

1987). The list of disorders occurring at least several times with vitiligo is given in Table 31.1. It is hard to draw any definitive conclusion about the associations (see Chapter 12). If vitiligo affects 0.5% of the population, then as many as 20 000 000 individuals worldwide have this disorder. Clearly some of the reported associations are chance events. Others might have great biological implications. Currently we cannot distinguish which associations, or which disorders affecting depigmented skin or involving only pigmented skin, are in the former (meaningful) or the latter (unimportant) category.

Alterations in sweating, temperature and blood flow through depigmented skin

Patients with vitiligo almost never complain of symptoms referable to the depigmentation itself. They, at times, report mild itching or sensitivity to sunburn but the depigmented macules cause no other complaints. Sensory exteroceptors such as touch, temperature and pain receptors seem to be normal in depigmented skin.

The eccrine glands of the skin are innervated by the sympathetic nerves that release acetylcholine rather than norepinephrine. Many years ago, one group of workers observed that sweating in depigmented skin was increased (Chanco-Turner & Lerner 1965). The investigators also observed that the surface temperature of the depigmented skin was warmer than the surrounding pigmented skin and that the bleeding time was prolonged (Chanco-Turner & Lerner 1965). From these and other findings they proposed that dysfunction of the sympathetic nerves in the depigmented skin was responsible for these findings (Chanco-Turner & Lerner 1965; Lerner *et al.* 1966).

Others have not noted abnormalities in sweating in depigmented skin (Sharquie & Assaf 1985). More recent reports suggest that cholinergic activity is deficient in depigmented skin of vitiligo (Elwary *et al.* 1997). If so then one might expect decreased, not increased sweating. Consistent with this latter conclusion are the findings of Gokhale *et al.* who noted there were degenerative changes in the sweat glands and ducts, dermal nerves and nerve endings in depigmented skin (Gokhale *et al.* 1977). Other investigators have not noted these findings in their studies on vitiligo-affected skin (Morohashi *et al.* 1977; Kumakiri *et al.* 1982; Moellmann *et al.* 1982).

Epidermal keratinocytes have the capacity to synthesize acetylcholine (Grando *et al.* 1993) as well as adrenergic agonists (Iyengar & Misra 1988a, 1988b; Morrone *et al.* 1992; Schallreuter *et al.* 1993, 1995). The precise and specific functions of these neurotransmitters produced by keratinocytes and melanocytes are not known but they are autocrine/paracrine agonists that must be involved in regulation of the various epidermal cells. These agonists might have effects on both sweating as well as blood flow and thus skin temperature.

Besides these neurotransmitters, there are other factors produced within the skin that might have effects on sweating, blood flow and therefore skin temperature. It is well known that interleukins such as IL-1, IL-6 and other peptides like α-MSH affect the hypothalamus and regulate, in part, body temperature (for review see Nordlund & Ortonne 1998; Nordlund *et al.* 1998; Norris *et al.* 1998; Nordlund & Boissy 1999). It also is possible that some of these cytokines could have effects on the melanocytes, Merkel cells and other components of the epidermis (Norris 1990; Plettenberg *et al.* 1995).

Bleeding times also have been measured in depigmented and normal-appearing skin of individuals with vitiligo. It is prolonged in depigmented skin (Chanco-Turner & Lerner 1965). Bleeding time is a complex assay that involves blood flow, clotting factors, platelets, capillary integrity, and contractility of capillaries. It is possible that the bleeding time is a manifestation of anomalous autonomic innervation, either decreased sympathetic activity or increased cholinergic activity. It is also possible that some other entirely different factor is involved. It would be worth repeating these studies with more modern technology to determine their accuracy and to improve our understanding of their mechanism.

Vitiligo and skin cancers

The pigment system is popularly thought to be the most important protection against development of skin cancers. Indeed, melanin has a sun protective factor (SPF) of about 2–5, depending on the depth of colour of the skin. Even an SPF of 2 indicates that 50% of the incident sunlight is absorbed and blocked from striking the basilar keratinocytes. Thus melanin does contribute to prevention of squamous and basal cell carcinomas. Many observers have reported that there is a notable paucity of cancers observed or reported in depigmented skin of patients with vitiligo. Biologically, melanomas cannot occur in depigmented skin devoid of melanocytes.

This depigmented skin has no pigment whatsoever and should be as sensitive or more sensitive to formation of cancers as the skin of individuals with albinism. This is especially true since vitiligo is treated with PUVA which is known to cause squamous and basal cell carcinomas in those with psoriasis (Gupta & Anderson 1987). Yet there are very few reports of cancers (for review see Nordlund & Ortonne 1998). One observer noted actinic and lichenoid keratoses in those treated with PUVA but no cancers (Harrist *et al.* 1984). Others have observed little less evidence of sun damage in the white skin than in the pigmented skin (Cohen *et al.* 1984; Calanchini-Postizzi & Frenk 1987; Abdullah & Keczkes 1989; Wildfang *et al.* 1992; Halder *et al.* 1995; Park *et al.* 1996). Some of the patients in these studies were treated with PUVA, others exhibited only the damage from ambient sunlight. In contrast there are numerous reports of squamous and basal cell carcinomas developing in albino skin, especially type OCA-2 found most commonly in Africa, where the tumours affect about 25% of albinos and cause the death of some. Actinic keratoses and actinic damage to the skin is universal in the exposed skin of albinos living in equatorial Africa, even in infants only 6 months of age. Yet patients with long-standing vitiligo, i.e. 5–20 years, have no evidence of epidermal actinic damage although their skin manifests marked solar elastosis (personal observations).

The explanation for the paucity of cancers or sun damage is not known. It seems likely that for those living in the western, affluent countries, the availability of sunscreens and indoor occupations would lessen the probability of skin cancers. Yet vitiligo typically affects the face and hands and the skin in these areas might be expected to form at least a few cancers. The enigma is more difficult from observations in east African nations that are located on or near the equator. Many people live at high altitude. Yet even these individuals fail to exhibit manifestations of sun damage. There are no sunscreens available in East African nations and the number of indoor jobs is very few. It is possible that the paucity of skin cancers in vitiligo skin has a trivial explanation. The observation might hold some important secrets but at this time its significance remains unknown.

There have been many reports of melanoma being associated with depigmentation (Chapter 30). As many as 20% of those with metastatic melanoma develop depigmentation (Burdick & Hawk 1964; Friederich 1967; Goldman *et al.* 1967; Balabanov *et al.* 1969; Frenk 1969; Milton *et al.* 1971; Donaldson *et al.* 1974; Fodor & Bodrogi 1975; Gregor 1976; Perrot *et al.*

1976; Pantoja *et al.* 1977; Albert *et al.* 1978; Ortonne & Perrot 1978; Sober & Haynes 1978; Cohen *et al.* 1979; Hamm & Fiedler 1979; Forrest & Forrest 1980; Moroc *et al.* 1980; Albert *et al.* 1982; Agdal *et al.* 1983; Koh *et al.* 1983; Nordlund *et al.* 1983; Chang *et al.* 1986; Gross *et al.* 1990; Kossard & Commens 1990; Alabi *et al.* 1991; Duhra & Ilchyshyn 1991; Schallreuter *et al.* 1991; Harris *et al.* 1994; Merimsky *et al.* 1994; Cavallari *et al.* 1996). It is very controversial whether the depigmentation is vitiligo vulgaris or some other disorder that results in destruction of melanocytes that resembles vitiligo (Chapter 1). A distinction is made between vitiligo and depigmentation with melanoma because the clinical presentations of these two types of depigmentation are very different. It is the opinion of these writers that the depigmentation associated with melanoma is not the same as vitiligo. The significance is discussed in Chapter 30.

There have been many other types of cancer associated with vitiligo (Table 32.2). However these malignancies might have occurred by chance alone. Until the cause of vitiligo is known, the significance of these associations remains unclear.

Table 31.2 Malignancies coexisting with vitiligo.

Skin cancers, premalignancies and neoplasms
Melanoma
Actinic keratosis
Extramammary Paget's disease
Squamous cell carcinoma
Keratoacanthoma
Basal cell carcinoma
Kaposi's sarcoma
Sezary syndrome
Sarcoma cutis
Internal malignancies
Lymphatic malignancies
Dysgammaglobulinaemia
Hodgkin's disease
Multiple myeloma
Mycosis fungoides
Sezary syndrome
Thymomas
Gastrointestinal malignancies
Adenocarcinoma of colon
Abdominal carcinomatosis
Hepatoma
Others
Breast tumour
Bronchogenic carcinoma
Intracranial tumour
Squamous cell carcinoma of the bladder
Thyroid carcinoma
Uterine tumour

Conclusions

It is popular to consider the pigmentary system as an atavism with little importance. Yet the entire animal kingdom has invested enormous energies into developing and preserving a pigmentary system that has, it seems, many functions, one of which is to provide protection against the deleterious effects of excessive and intense sunlight (for an extensive review see Nordlund & Ortonne 1998). That the behaviour of skin changes in so many ways when the pigment cells are lost suggests that the melanocyte has functions other than merely protecting us against sunlight, which itself is not evil. Sunlight also is responsible for beneficial effects such as production of vitamin D. The pigment system is activated during every inflammatory disorder of the skin manifested as postinflammatory hyperpigmentation or hypopigmentation, which strongly suggests that the melanocyte is involved in the inflammatory process in some way. And the oddities noted about cancers suggest that the mechanisms that protect us from sun-induced malignancies are more complex and interesting than currently believed.

References

Abdullah, A.N. & Keczkes, K. (1989) Cutaneous and ocular side-effects of PUVA photochemotherapy—a 10-year follow-up study. *Clinical and Experimental Dermatology* **14**, 421–424.

Agdal, N., Christensen, J.D. & Roed, J. (1983) Malignant melanoma with secondary vitiligo. *Ugeskrift for Laeger* **145**, 3659–3660.

Ahn, S.K., Choi, E.H., Lee, S.H., Won, J.H., Hann, S.K. & Park, Y.K. (1994) Immunohistochemical studies from vitiligo—comparison between active and inactive lesions. *Yonsei Medical Journal* **35**, 404–410.

al Badri, A.M., Foulis, A.K., Todd, P.M., Gariouch, J.J., Gudgeon, J.E., Stewart, D.G., Gracie, J.A. & Goudie, R.B. (1993) Abnormal expression of MHC class II and ICAM-1 by melanocytes in vitiligo. *Journal of Pathology* **169**, 203–206.

Alabi, G.O., Falope, Z.F. & Lekwauwa, U.G. (1991) Coexisting malignant melanoma and vitiligo in a Nigerian. *West African Journal of Medicine* **10**, 443–446.

Albert, D.M., Sober, A.J. & Fitzpatrick, T.B. (1978) Iritis in patients with cutaneous melanoma and vitiligo. *Archives of Ophthalmology* **96**, 2081–2084.

Albert, D.M., Todes-Taylor, N., Wagoner, M., Nordlund, J.J. & Lerner, A.B. (1982) Vitiligo or halo nevi occurring in two patients with choroidal melanoma. *Archives of Dermatology* **118**, 34–36.

Allende, M.F. & Reed, E. (1964) Dermatitis herpetiformis and vitiligo. *Archives of Dermatology* **89**, 156–158.

Amornsiripanitch, S., Barnes, L.M., Nordlund, J.J., Trinkle, L.S. & Rheins, L.A. (1988) Immune studies in the depigmenting C57BL/Ler-vit/vit mice. An apparent isolated loss of contact hypersensitivity. *Journal of Immunology* **140**, 3438–3445.

Anstey, A. & Marks, R. (1993) Colocalization of lichen planus and vitiligo (letter). *British Journal of Dermatology* **128**, 103–104.

Babanov, G.P. & Schieferstein, G. (1970) Case of circumscribed and progressive scleroderma with lichen planus. *Hautarzt* **21**, 225–228.

Balabanov, K., Andreev, V.C. & Tchernozemski, I. (1969) Malignant melanoma and vitiligo. *Dermatologica* **139**, 211–219.

Birbeck, M.S., Breathnach, A.S. & Everall, J.D. (1961) An electron microscope study of basal melanocytes and high-level clears cells (Langerhans cells) in vitiligo. *Journal of Investigative Dermatology* **37**, 51–64.

Boissy, R.E., Moellmann, G.E. & Lerner, A.B. (1987) Morphology of melanocytes in hair bulbs and eyes of vitiligo mice. *American Journal of Pathology* **127**, 380–388.

Bose, S.K. (1994a) Absence of Merkel cells in lesional skin. *International Journal of Dermatology* **33**, 481–483.

Bose, S.K. (1994b) Absence of Merkel cells in lesional skin of vitiligo [corrected] [published erratum appears in *International Journal of Dermatology* 34: 66, 1995]. *International Journal of Dermatology* **33**, 481–483.

Bose, S.K. (1994c) Probable mechanisms of loss of Merkel cells in completely depigmented skin of stable vitiligo. *Journal of Dermatology* **21**, 725–728.

Bose, S.K. & Ortonne, J.P. (1994) Focal gaps in the basement membrane of involved and uninvolved skin of vitiligo: are they normal? *Journal of Dermatology* **21**, 152–159.

Brenner, W., Diem, E. & Gschnait, F. (1979) Coincidence of vitiligo, alopecia areata, onychodystrophy, localized scleroderma and lichen planus. *Dermatologica* **159**, 356–360.

Brown, J., Winklemann, R.K. & Wolff, K. (1967) Langerhans cells in vitiligo: a qualitative study. *Journal of Investigative Dermatology* **49**, 386–390.

Burdick, K.H. & Hawk, W.A. (1964) Vitiligo in a case of vaccinia virus treated melanoma. *Cancer* **19**, 708–712.

Calanchini-Postizzi, E. & Frenk, E. (1987) Long-term actinic damage in sun-exposed vitiligo and normally pigmented skin. *Dermatologica* **174**, 266–271.

Cannon, J.G., Tatro, J.B., Reichlin, S. & Dinarello, C.A. (1986) Alpha melanocyte stimulating hormone inhibits immunostimulatory and inflammatory actions of interleukin 1. *Journal of Immunology* **137**, 2232–2236.

Catania, A. & Lipton, J.M. (1993) Alpha-melanocyte stimulating hormone in the modulation of host reactions. *Endocrine Reviews* **14**, 564–576.

Catania, A. & Lipton, J.M. (1994) The neuropeptide α-MSH: a key component of neuroimmunomodulation. *Neuroimmunomodulation* **1**, 93–99.

Cavallari, V., Cannavo, S.P., Ussia, A.F., Moretti, G. & Albanese, A. (1996) Vitiligo associated with metastatic malignant melanoma. *International Journal of Dermatology* **35**, 738–740.

Ceriani, G., Macaluso, A., Catania, A. & Lipton, J.M. (1994) Central neurogenic anti-inflammatory action of alpha-MSH: modulation of peripheral inflammation induced by cytokines and other mediators of inflammation. *Neuroendocrinology* **59**, 138–143.

Chanco-Turner, M.L. & Lerner, A.B. (1965) Physiologic changes in vitiligo. *Archives of Dermatology* **91**, 390–396.

Chang, M.A., Fournier, G., Koh, H.K., Sober, A.J., Nakagawa, H., Fitzpatrick, T.B. & Albert, D.M. (1986) Ocular abnormalities associated with cutaneous melanoma and vitiligo like leukoderma. *Graefes Archive for Clinical and Experimental Ophthalmology* **224**, 529–535.

Chapman, R.S. (1973) Coincident vitiligo and psoriasis in the same individual. *Archives of Dermatology* **107**, 776.

Claudy, A.L. & Rouchouse, B. (1984) Langerhans' cell and vitiligo: quantitative study of T6 and HLA-DR antigen-expressing cells. *Acta Dermato-Venereologica (Stockholm)* **64**, 334–336.

Cohen, L.E., Tanner, D.J., Schaefer, H.G. & Levis, W.R. (1984) Common and uncommon cutaneous findings in patients with ataxia-telangiectasia. *Journal of the American Academy of Dermatology* **10**, 431–438.

Cohen, Y., Haim, S., Bartal, A. & Robinson, E. (1979) Vitiligo associated with BCG-methanol extraction residue in malignant melanoma. Report of a case. *Dermatologica* **158**, 8–12.

Donaldson, R.C., Canaan, S.A. Jr, McLean, R.B. & Ackerman, L.V. (1974) Uveitis and vitiligo associated with BCG treatment for malignant melanoma. *Surgery* **76**, 771–778.

Duhra, P. & Ilchyshyn, A. (1991) Prolonged survival in metastatic malignant melanoma associated with vitiligo. *Clinical and Experimental Dermatology* **16**, 303–305.

Duvic, M., Rapini, R., Hoots, W.K. & Mansell, P.W. (1987) Human immunodeficiency virus-associated vitiligo: expression of autoimmunity with immunodeficiency? *Journal of the American Academy of Dermatology* **17**, 656–662.

Elwary, S.M., Headley, K. & Schallreuter, K.U. (1997) Calcium homeostasis influences epidermal sweating in patients with vitiligo. *British Journal of Dermatology* **137**, 81–85.

Enhamre, A., Ros, A.M. & Nordlind, K. (1986) Co-existing vitiligo and small-plaque parapsoriasis [letter]. *Dermatologica* **173**, 103–104.

Fodor, J. & Bodrogi, I. (1975) Vitiligo and malignant melanoma. *Neoplasia* **22**, 445–448.

Forrest, J.B. & Forrest, H.J. (1980) Case report: malignant melanoma arising during drug therapy for vitiligo. *Journal of Surgical Oncology* **13**, 337–340.

Frenk, E. (1969) Depigmentations vitiligineuses chez des patients atteints de melanommes malins. *Dermatologica* **139**, 84–91.

Friederich, H.C. (1967) Vitiligo as an undesired side-effect in the management of melanoma. A contribution to experimental vitiligo research. *Archiv für Klinische und Experimentelle Dermatologie* **229**, 223–230.

Gilhar, A., Aizen, E., Ohana, N. & Etzioni, A. (1993) Vitiliginous vs. pigmented skin response to intradermal administration of interferon gamma. *Archives of Dermatology* **129**, 600–604.

Gokhale, B.B., Mehta, L.N. & Damle, P.S. (1977) Skin resistance to electric current and its correlation with sweat gland histology in vitiligo. *Indian Journal of Medical Research* **66**, 859–864.

Goldman, L., Wilson, R.G., Glasgow, R. & Richfield, R. (1967) Perilesional leucoderma in metastatic melanoma. The use of the Wood's light for early detection of this rare reaction. *Acta Dermato-Venereologica (Stockholm)* **47**, 369–372.

Grando, S.A., Kist, D.A., Qi, M. & Dahl, M.V. (1993) Human keratinocytes synthesize, secrete and degrade acetylcholine. *Journal of Investigative Dermatology* **101**, 32–36.

Gregor, R.T. (1976) Vitiligo and malignant melanoma: a significant association? *South African Medical Journal* **50**, 1447–1449.

Gross, D.J., Singer, P.G. & Schosser, R.H. (1990) Adult-onset leukoderma and malignant melanoma (letter). *Archives of Dermatology* **126**, 1240–1241.

Gupta, A.K. & Anderson, T.F. (1987) Psoralen photochemotherapy. *Journal of the American Academy of Dermatology* **17**, 703–734.

Halder, R.M., Battle, E.F. & Smith, E.M. (1995) Cutaneous malignancies in patients treated with psoralen photochemotherapy (PUVA) for vitiligo. *Archives of Dermatology* **131**, 734–735.

Hamm, G. & Fiedler, H. (1979) Vitiligo and malignant melanoma (author's translation). *Dermatologische Monatsschrift* **165**, 838–842.

Harris, J., Bines, S. & Das Gupta, T. (1994) Therapy of disseminated malignant melanoma with recombinant alpha 2b-interferon and piroxicam: clinical results with a report of an unusual response-associated feature (vitiligo) and unusual toxicity (diffuse pulmonary interstitial fibrosis). *Medical and Pediatric Oncology* **22**, 103–106.

Harrist, T.J., Pathak, M.A., Mosher, D.B. & Fitzpatrick, T.B. (1984) Chronic cutaneous effects of long-term psoralen and ultraviolet radiation therapy in patients with vitiligo. *National Cancer Institute Monographs* **66**, 191–196.

Hatchome, N., Aiba, S., Kato, T., Torinuki, W. & Tagami, H. (1987) Possible functional impairment of Langerhans' cells in vitiliginous skin. Reduced ability to elicit dinitrochlorobenzene contact sensitivity reaction and decreased stimulatory effect in the allogeneic mixed skin cell lymphocyte culture reaction. *Archives of Dermatology* **123**, 51–54.

Hazelrigg, D.E. (1987) Dermatitis herpetiformis and vitiligo (letter). *Cutis* **39**, 232.

Hogan, D.J. & Lane, P.R. (1986) Dermatitis herpetiformis and vitiligo. *Cutis* **38**, 195–197.

Howsden, S.M., Herndon, J.H. Jr & Freeman, R.G. (1973) Vogt-Koyanagi–Harada syndrome and psoriasis. *Archives of Dermatology*, 108, 395–398.

Humbert, P., Dupond, J.L., Vuitton, D. & Agache, P. (1989) Dermatological autoimmune diseases and the multiple autoimmune syndromes. *Acta Dermato-Venereologica (Stockholm). Supplementum* **148**, 1–8.

Iakovleva, N.I. & Sen'kin, V.I. (1984) Case of alopecia associated with vitiligo and psoriasis. *Vestnik Dermatologii I Venerologii* **10**, 70–71.

Iyengar, B. & Misra, R.S. (1988a) Neural differentiation of melanocytes in vitiliginous skin. *Acta Anatomica* **133**, 62–65.

Iyengar, B. & Misra, R.S. (1988b) Reaction of dendritic melanocytes in vitiligo to the substrates of tyrosine metabolism. *Acta Anatomica* **129**, 203–205.

Kano, Y., Shiohara, T. & Nagashima, M. (1984) Epidermal Langerhans cells in various skin diseases (2) Langerhans cells in vitiligo. *Journal of Dermatology* **11**, 103–110.

Kao, C.H. & Yu, H.S. (1990) Depletion and repopulation of Langerhans cells in nonsegmental type vitiligo. *Journal of Dermatology* **17**, 287–296.

Koh, H.K., Sober, A.J., Nakagawa, H., Albert, D.M., Mihm, M.C. & Fitzpatrick, T.B. (1983) Malignant melanoma and vitiligo-like leukoderma: an electron microscopic study. *Journal of the American Academy of Dermatology* **9**, 696–708.

Koransky, J.S. & Roenigk, H.H. Jr (1982) Vitiligo and psoriasis. *Journal of the American Academy of Dermatology* **7**, 183–189.

Kossard, S. & Commens, C. (1990) Hypopigmented malignant melanoma simulating vitiligo. *Journal of the American Academy of Dermatology* **22**, 840–842.

Kumakiri, M., Kimura, T., Miura, Y. & Tagawa, Y. (1982) Vitiligo with an inflammatory erythema in Vogt-Koyanagi-Harada disease: demonstration of filamentous masses and amyloid deposits. *Journal of Cutaneous Pathology* **9**, 258–266.

Lamoreux, M.L., Boissy, R.E., Womack, J.E. & Nordlund, J.J. (1992) The vit gene maps to the mi (microphthalmia) locus of the laboratory mouse. *Journal of Heredity* **83**, 435–439.

Le Poole, I.C., van den Wijngaard, R.M., Westerhof, W. & Das, P.K. (1996) Presence of T cells and macrophages in inflammatory vitiligo skin parallels melanocyte disappearance. *American Journal of Pathology* **148**, 1219–1228.

Lerner, A.B., Snell, R.S., Chanco-Turner, M.L. & McGuire, J.S. (1966) Vitiligo and sympathectomy. The effect of sympathectomy and alpha-melanocyte stimulating hormone. *Archives of Dermatology* **94**, 269–278.

Lerner, A.B., Shiohara, T., Boissy, R.E., Jacobson, K.A., Lamoreux, M.L. & Moellmann, G.E. (1986) A mouse model for vitiligo. *Journal of Investigative Dermatology* **87**, 299–304.

Lipton, J.M., Macaluso, A., Hiltz, M.E. & Catania, A. (1991) Central administration of the peptide alpha-MSH inhibits inflammation in the skin. *Peptides* **12**, 795–798.

Lyson, K. & McCann, S.M. (1993) Alpha-melanocyte-stimulating hormone abolishes IL-1 and IL-6-induced corticotropin-releasing factor release from the hypothalamus *in vitro*. *Neuroendocrinology* **58**, 191–195.

Mancuso, G. & Gasponi, A. (1983) The vitiligo-psoriasis combination. Genetic and immunologic study. *Giornale Italiano Di Dermatologia E Venereologia* **118**, 369–372.

Menter, A., Boyd, A.S. & Silverman, A.K. (1989) Guttate psoriasis and vitiligo: anatomic cohabitation. *Journal of the American Academy of Dermatology* **20**, 698–700.

Merimsky, O., Shoenfeld, Y., Yecheskel, G., Chaitchik, S., Azizi, E. & Fishman, P. (1994) Vitiligo- and melanoma-associated hypopigmentation: a similar appearance but a different mechanism. *Cancer Immunology Immunotherapy* **38**, 411–416.

Milton, G.W., McCarthy, W.H. & Carlon, A. (1971) Malignant melanoma and vitiligo. *Australian Journal of Dermatology* **12**, 131–142.

Moellmann, G., Klein-Angerer, S., Scollay, D.A., Nordlund, J.J. & Lerner, A.B. (1982) Extracellular granular material and degeneration of keratinocytes in the normally pigmented epidermis of patients with vitiligo. *Journal of Investigative Dermatology* **79**, 321–330.

Moragas, J.M. & Winkelmann, R.K. (1970) Psoriasis and vitiligo. *Archives of Dermatology* **101**, 235–237.

Moroc, A., Kral, V., Duchkova, H. & Richter, J. (1980) Vitiligo and malignant melanoma. *Ceskoslovenska Dermatologie* **55**, 284–285.

Morohashi, M., Hashimoto, K., Goodman, T.F. Jr, Newton, D.E. & Rist, T. (1977) Ultrastructural studies of vitiligo, Vogt–Koyanagi syndrome, and incontinentia pigmenti achromians. *Archives of Dermatology* **113**, 755–766.

Morrone, A., de Picardo, M., Luca, C., Terminali, O., Passi, S. & Ippolito, F. (1992) Catecholamines and vitiligo. *Pigment Cell Research* **5**, 65–69.

Nordlund, J.J. & Boissy, R.E. (1999) The biology of the melanocyte. In: *Basic Science Review for Dermatology Residents* (eds D.Woodley & R.Frankel) Chicago.

Nordlund, J.J. & Majumder, P.P. (1997) Recent investigations on vitiligo vulgaris [review]. *Dermatologic Clinics* **15**, 69–78.

Nordlund, J.J. & Ortonne, J.P. (1992) Vitiligo and depigmentation. *Current Problems in Dermatology* **4**, 3–30.

Nordlund, J.J. & Ortonne, J.P. (1998) Vitiligo vulgaris. In: *The Pigmentary System: Physiology and Pathophysiology* (eds J.J.Nordlund, R.E.Boissy, V.J.Hearing, R.A.King & J.-P.Ortonne), pp. 513–551. Oxford University Press, New York.

Nordlund, J.J., Kirkwood, J.M., Forget, B.M., Milton, G., Albert, D.M. & Lerner, A.B. (1983) Vitiligo in patients with metastatic melanoma: a good prognostic sign. *Journal of the American Academy of Dermatology* **9**, 689–696.

Nordlund, J.J., Forget, B., Kirkwood, J. & Lerner, A.B. (1985) Dermatitis produced by applications of monobenzone in patients with active vitiligo. *Archives of Dermatology* **121**, 1141–1144.

Nordlund, J.J., Csato, M., Babcock, G. & Takei, F. (1995) Low ICAM-1 expression in the epidermis of depigmenting C57BL/6J-mi^{vit}/mi^{vit} mice: a possible cause of muted contact sensitization. *Experimental Dermatology* **4**, 20–29.

Nordlund, J.J., Boissy, R.E., Hearing, V.J., King, R.A. & Ortonne, J.-P., eds. (1998) *The Pigmentary System: Physiology and Pathophysiology*. Oxford University Press, New York.

Norris, D.A. (1990) Cytokine modulation of adhesion molecules in the regulation of immunologic cytotoxicity of epidermal targets. *Journal of Investigative Dermatology* **95**, 111S–120S.

Norris, D.A., Morelli, J.G. & Fujita, M. (1998) Melanocyte interactions in the skin. In: *The Pigmentary System: Physiology and Pathophysiology* (eds J.J.Nordlund, R.E.Boissy, V.J.Hearing, R.A.King & J.-P.Ortonne), pp. 123–133. Oxford University Press, New York.

Olholm-Larsen, P. & Kavli, G. (1980) Dermatitis herpetiformis and vitiligo. *Dermatologica* **160**, 41–44.

Ortonne, J.P. & Perrot, H. (1978) Giant melanin granules in vitiliginous achromia with malignant melanoma. *Acta Dermato-Venereologica (Stockholm)* **58**, 475–480.

Ortonne, J.P., Perrot, H. & Thivolet, J. (1976) Clinical and statistical study of 100 patients with vitiligo. II. Associated lesions. *Semaine Des Hopitaux* **52**, 679–686.

Palkowski, M.R., Nordlund, M.L., Rheins, L.A. & Nordlund, J.J. (1987) Langerhan's cells in hair follicles of the depigmenting C57BL/Ler-vit/vit mouse. A model for human vitiligo. *Archives of Dermatology* **123**, 1022–1028.

Pantoja, E., Wendth, A.J. & Beecher, T.S. (1977) Perilesional vitiligo in melanoma. *Cutis* **19**, 51–53.

Park, S.H., Hann, S.K. & Park, Y.K. (1996) Ten-year experience of phototherapy in Yonsei Medical Center. *Yonsei Medical Journal* **37**, 392–396.

Perrot, H., Schmidt, D. & Ortonne, J.P. (1976) Vitiliginous achromia in malignant melanoma. Ultrastructural study of achromic and normal skin. *Journal of Cutaneous Pathology* **3**, 140.

Plettenberg, A., Ballaun, C., Pammer, J., Mildner, M., Strunk, D., Weninger, W. & Tschachler, E. (1995) Human melanocytes and melanoma cells constitutively express the Bcl-2 proto-oncogene in situ and in cell culture. *American Journal of Pathology* **146**, 651–659.

Porter, S.R., Scully, C. & Eveson, J.W. (1994) Coexistence of lichen planus and vitiligo is coincidental [letter]. *Clinical and Experimental Dermatology* **19**, 366.

Powell, F.C. & Dicken, C.H. (1983) Psoriasis and vitiligo. *Acta Dermato-Venereologica (Stockholm)* **63**, 246–249.

Rheins, L.A., Palkowski, M.R. & Nordlund, J.J. (1986) Alterations in cutaneous immune reactivity to dinitrofluorobenzene in graying C57BL/vi.vi mice. *Journal of Investigative Dermatology* **86**, 539–542.

Roberts, D.L. (1984) Irritancy of anthralin in patients with psoriasis and widespread vitiligo [letter]. *British Journal of Dermatology* **110**, 247–248.

Rubisz-Brzezinska, J., Buchner, S.A. & Itin, P. (1996) Vitiligo associated with lichen planus. Is there a pathogenetic relationship? *Dermatology* **192**, 176–178.

Saha, K.C., Arya, M. & Saha, A.K. (1979) Neurohistological studies in lichen planus and vitiligo. *Indian Journal of Dermatology* **24**, 51–55.

Schallreuter, K.U., Levenig, C. & Berger, J. (1991) Vitiligo and cutaneous melanoma. A case study. *Dermatologica* **183**, 239–245.

Schallreuter, K.U., Wood, J.M., Pittelkow, M.R., Swanson, N.N. & Steinkraus, V. (1993) Increased *in vitro* expression of beta 2-adrenoceptors in differentiating lesional keratinocytes of vitiligo patients. *Archives of Dermatological Research* **285**, 216–220.

Schallreuter, K.U., Lemke, K.R., Pittelkow, M.R., Wood, J.M., Korner, C. & Malik, R. (1995) Catecholamines in human keratinocyte differentiation. *Journal of Investigative Dermatology* **104**, 953–957.

Sharquie, K.E. & Assaf, F. (1985) Sweating in vitiligo in relation to electrical skin resistance (letter). *Clinical and Experimental Dermatology* **10**, 598–599.

Smith, S.B., Bora, N., McCool, D., Kutty, G., Wong, P., Kutty, R.K. & Wiggert, B. (1995) Photoreceptor cells in the vitiligo mouse die by apoptosis. TRPM-2/clusterin expression is increased in the neural retina and in the retinal pigment epithelium. *Investigative Ophthalmology and Visual Science* **36**, 2193–2201.

Sober, A.J. & Haynes, H.A. (1978) Uveitis, poliosis, hypomelanosis, and alopecia in a patient with malignant melanoma. *Archives of Dermatology* **114**, 439–441.

Tan, R.S. (1974a) Ulcerative colitis, myasthenia gravis, atypical lichen planus, alopecia areata, vitiligo. *Proceedings of the Royal Society of Medicine* **67**, 195–196.

Tan, R.S.-H. (1974b) Thymoma, acquired hypogammaglobulinaemia, lichen planus, alope. *Proceedings of the Royal Society of Medicine* **67**, 196–198.

Uehara, M., Miyauchi, H. & Tanaka, S. (1984) Diminished contact sensitivity response in vitiliginous skin. *Archives of Dermatology* **120**, 195–198.

van der Kerkhof, P.C. & Fokkink, H.J. (1989) Irritancy of dithranol in normally pigmented and depigmented skin of patients with vitiligo. *Acta Dermato-Venereologica (Stockholm)* **69**, 236–238.

Westerhof, W., Groot, I., Krieg, S.R., Bos, J.D. & Cormane, R.H. (1986) Langerhans' cell population studies with OKT6 and HLA-DR monoclonal antibodies in vitiligo patients treated with oral phenylalanine loading and UVA irradiation. *Acta Dermato-Venereologica (Stockholm)* **66**, 259–262.

Westerhof, W., Buehre, Y., Pavel, S., Bos, J.D., Das, P.K., Krieg, S.R. & Siddiqui, A.H. (1989) Increased anthralin irritation response in vitiliginous skin. *Archives of Dermatological Research* **281**, 52–56.

Wildfang, I.L., Jacobsen, F.K. & Thestrup-Pedersen, K. (1992) PUVA treatment of vitiligo: a retrospective study of 59 patients. *Acta Dermato-Venereologica (Stockholm)* **72**, 305–306.

32: Chemical Leukoderma

LEIGH MIYAMOTO AND JAMES S. TAYLOR

Introduction

Chemical leukoderma is a form of cutaneous pigment loss resembling vitiligo that is caused by exposure to a variety of chemicals which selectively destroy epidermal melanocytes. Most cases result from direct contact of the chemical with the skin but ingestion or inhalation of chemicals may also be routes of exposure. Chemical leukoderma has been referred to as occupational vitiligo, but nonoccupational cases have also been reported.

A number of chemicals have been implicated as causing leukoderma from the results obtained from both human and animal *in vivo* studies, and also by experimental *in vitro* work (Table 32.1). The largest and best studied group of chemicals are derivatives of phenol and catechols (Fig. 32.1). Hydroxylation of the 4-(para)-position and substitution of a nonpolar alkyl side group in the 1-position has been observed to increase the melanotoxicity of the compound (Riley 1969). Alkyl phenols are commonly used in the industrial setting as antioxidants or rust inhibitors. In commercial products they may be found in deodorants, disinfectants, germicides, insecticides, motor oils, oil additives, de-emulsifiers, paints, photographic chemicals, printing inks, varnishes, lacquers, plasticizers, adhesives, resins and rubber (Calnan 1973; Gellin & Maibach 1983).

Monobenzyl ether of hydroquinone (MBEH)

In 1939 and 1940, Oliver, Schwartz, and Warren from the US Public Health Service were the first investigators to document an outbreak of occupational leukoderma in tannery workers wearing rubber gloves (Oliver *et al.* 1939; Schwartz *et al.* 1940). Depigmentation was caused by the rubber antioxidant monobenzyl ether of hydroquinone (MBEH), also known as 'Agerite Alba'. Twenty-five (52%) of 48 exposed workers who wore acid-cured rubber gloves containing 0.2% MBEH were affected. In some the leukoderma occurred on the hands and half way up the forearms with a uniform, sharp cut-off line corresponding to areas covered by the gloves. In others there was a patchy, guttate, confetti-like pigment loss at sites distant to obvious exposure. The face and trunk were also involved in some workers, possibly from direct contact with the gloves.

Patch testing with various chemicals in the gloves confirmed that MBEH

Table 32.1 Selected chemicals associated with chemical leukoderma. From Gellin and Maibach (1985), Ortonne *et al.* (1983) and Taylor *et al.* (1993).

Phenol/Catechol Derivatives
Monobenzyl ether of hydroquinone (MBEH)
Monomethyl ether of hydroquinone (MMEH) (p-methoxyphenol; p-hydroxyanisole)
Monoethyl ether of hydroquinone (MEEH) (p-ethoxyphenol)
Hydroquinone (HQ) (1,4-dihydroxybenzene; 1,4-benzenediol; quinol; p-hydroxyphenol)
p-tert-butylcatechol (PTBC)
p-tert-butylphenol (PTBP)
p-tert-amylphenol (PTAP)
p-phenylphenol
p-octylphenol
p-nonylphenol
p-isopropylcatechol
p-methylcatechol
Butylated hydroxytoluene (BHT)*
Butylated hydroxyanisole (BHA)*
Pyrocatechol (1,2-benzenediol)
p-cresol
Sulphydryls
β-mercaptoethylamine hydrochloride (MEA) (cysteamine)
N-(2-mercaptoethyl)-dimethylamine hydrochloride (MEDA)
Sulphanolic acid
Cysteamine dihydrochloride
3-mercaptopropylamine hydrochloride
Miscellaneous
Mercurials
Arsenic
Cinnamic aldehyde
p-phenylenediamine (PPDA)
Benzyl alcohol
Azaleic acid*
Corticosteroids
Optic Preparations
Eserine (physostigmine)
Diisopropyl fluorophosphate
Thio-tepa (N, N′, N″-triethylenethiophosphoramide)
Guanonitrofuracin
Systemic Medications
Chloroquine
Fluphenazine (Prolixin)

* Depigmentation weak or not known.

was the cause of the pigment loss. Leukoderma occurred at most positive patch test sites within 14 days to several months. There was no direct correlation between intensity of patch test reactions and subsequent leukoderma. Hydroquinone was present as an impurity at less than one percent

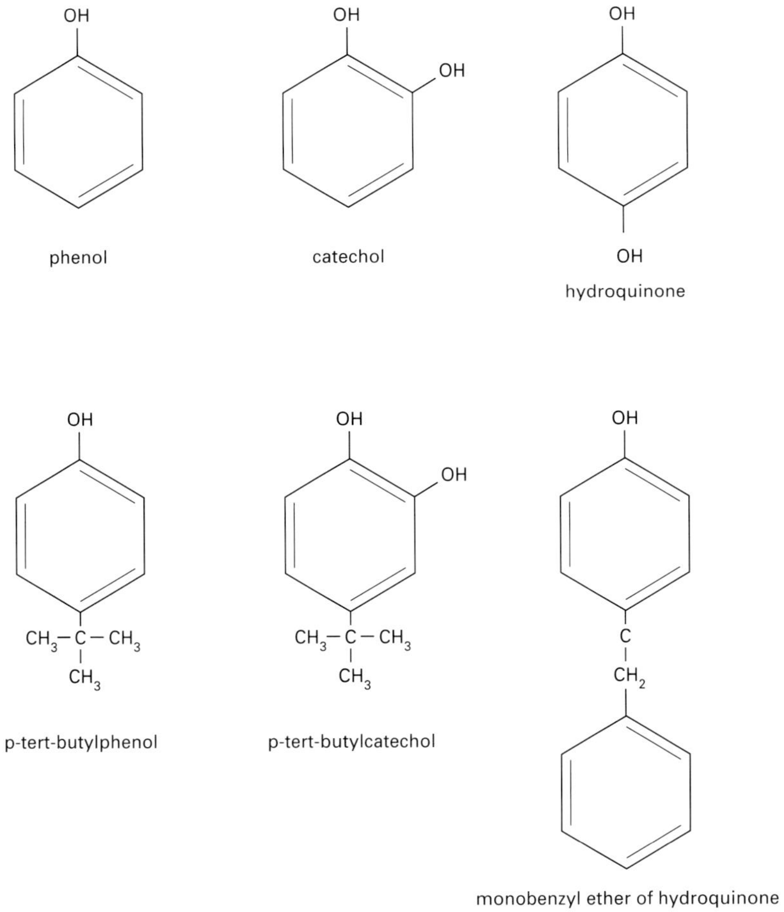

Fig. 32.1 Chemical structures of selected phenol and catechol derivatives.

concentration and was not considered a significant factor in the leukoderma. Several months after workers discontinued wearing the gloves, the onset of perifollicular repigmentation was noted.

Around the same time, McNally reported similar cases of depigmentation, initially involving the hands and arms, in 34 tannery workers. The leukoderma was associated with the use of a new brand of rubber gauntlet gloves which were found to contain the same antioxidant, MBEH, as well as unchanged hydroquinone (McNally 1939).

Leukoderma from MBEH has been reported from a number of other rubber devices including tape, diaphragms, condoms, finger cots, clothing, aprons, dolls, and shoes (Ortonne *et al.* 1983; Fisher 1995). It has also been identified in synthetic neoprene rubber (Ortonne *et al.* 1983). The US rubber industry has not used MBEH as an antioxidant for many years (Taylor 1986). In 1959, Botvinick reported dermatitis and secondary leukoderma from a fabric-lined household glove containing MBEH, and reproduced the dermatitis and leukoderma with patch testing (Botvinick 1951). In 1992

Bajaj, Gupta, and Chatterjee identified a patient in India with depigmentation at the site of a hearing aide which was found by high pressure liquid chromatography analysis to contain MBEH (Bajaj *et al.* 1992). Bajaj also described cases of depigmentation of the breast corresponding to the site of contact with a synthetic leather wallet and 19 cases of depigmentation of the feet corresponding to contact with footwear material (bathroom slip-ons, rain shoes). All incriminated objects were confirmed, on analysis, to contain MBEH (Bajaj *et al.* 1991, 1996).

Monomethyl ether of hydroquinone (MMEH)

Monomethyl ether of hydroquinone (MMEH) has also been shown to cause depigmentation. Riley performed *in vitro* studies in black guinea pigs and demonstrated that MMEH caused depigmentation (Riley 1969). Chivers described two cases of depigmentation out of eight workers exposed to MMEH in a vinylidene chloride plant (Chivers 1972).

Hydroquinone and pyrocatechol

Hydroquinone (HQ), at concentrations of up to 4%, is present in bleaching creams which are used to lighten hyperpigmented skin such as in melasma. HQ is a weak lightening agent at 1% concentration, but is a stronger lightening agent at higher concentrations and with different vehicles. Prolonged use of HQ followed by sun exposure may lead to exogenous ochronosis with colloid milium production (Elder 1986).

Fisher reported four patients who developed leukoderma following the use of bleaching creams containing 2% HQ. Markey described confetti-like depigmentation in the beard area of a dark skinned man after application of a HQ-containing cream (Fisher 1982; Markey *et al.* 1989). Three other, separate anecdotal reports of depigmentation due to HQ present in photographic developer, in concentrations ranging from 0.06% to 7%, have also been reported (Frenk & Loi-Zedda 1980; Kersey & Stevenson 1981; Das & Tandon 1988). Cummings and Nordlund argue that pure HQ is not a melanocytotoxin and that the case reports of HQ chemical leukoderma are anecdotal and unproven. They do agree that 'pure HQ is a weak whitening agent' (Cummings & Nordlund 1995). *In vivo* black guinea pig studies identified that hydroquinone may be a weak depigmenting agent through a mild toxic effect on melanocytes (Bleehen *et al.* 1968; Jimbow *et al.* 1974). Animals ingesting hydroquinone in their food grow white hair. However the fur of animals regains its normal colour when feeding of hydroquinone is discontinued. This observation suggests that the HQ might inhibit the production of melanin rather than destroy the melanocytes as occurs in those with MBEH-induced leukoderma.

Kligman proposed a combination of retinoic acid, hydroquinone and steroids as a lightening agent. He clinically depigmented the skin of several African-Americans. However, on histological examination, he found the number of melanocytes in the depigmented skin greater than in control skin, although the melanocytes were inhibited from producing melanin.

Pyrocatechol has a toxicological profile similar to that of HQ and is structurally similar to HQ. Pyrocatechol did not depigment rabbit skin at 1% concentration but did so at 3%. The most frequent use of HQ and pyrocatechol is in rinse off type hair dyes and colours in which the use concentration is 1% or less (Elder 1986).

Para tertiary butylphenol (PTBP) and para tertiary amylphenol (PTAP)

Cases of occupational leukoderma occurring in Russian, Japanese, and Dutch factories producing PTBP were summarized by Malten (Malten *et al.* 1971). PTBP and PTAP are both used as phenolic germicides. PTAP was more widely used as a commercial germicide then PTBP, and PTAP was much more toxic to epidermal and bacterial cells than was PTBP (Kahn 1970). Kahn reported 12 hospital workers who developed depigmentation of the hands and forearms following exposure to the phenolic detergent germicides. Leukoderma developed in spite of the fact that some employees wore gloves, and patch testing confirmed that PTBP and PTAP were able to produce depigmentation at the test sites (Kahn 1970).

James reported leukoderma in 54 of 198 exposed workers at a PTBP manufacturing factory. The occurrence of depigmentation was related to duration of PTBP exposure and even more so to intensity of exposure, which included vapour inhalation and dust contact (James *et al.* 1977).

PTBP had been known to cause contact dermatitis in shoe manufacturers and wearers, and in automobile assemblymen (Kahn 1970). PTBP formaldehyde resin (PTBPFR) is also a contact sensitizer present in neoprene adhesives used in the manufacture of car seats, roof linings, and car interiors. Depigmentation on the hands and forearms was observed in 11 of 99 British automobile factory workers who were exposed to a PTBPFR glue without wearing protective gloves (Calnan & Cooke 1974). Malten attributed the leukoderma to excess PTBP in the glue (Malten 1984).

Malten also reported depigmentation as a consequence of contact with a PTBPFR glue in a wrist watch strap (Malten 1975). He believed that depigmentation from consumer products containing PTBPFR was infrequent because PTBP is rarely added in excess. However one hundred cases of depigmentation caused by PTBP present at a concentration of 80% in an adhesive used to apply *bindi*, the circular red mark worn on the forehead of married Indian women, has been documented (Bajaj *et al.* 1990). A recent report from Italy described allergic contact dermatitis and depigmentation of the lip margins from a PTBP-containing lip liner. The PTBP patch test site depigmented and the presence of PTBP was confirmed by gas chromatography and mass spectroscopy (Angelini *et al.* 1993).

Para tertiary butylcatechol (PTBC) and 4-isopropyl catechol (4-IPC)

Gellin documented occupational leukoderma in 4 out of 75 tappet assembly workers who were exposed to PTBC present in an assembly oil (Gellin *et al.* 1970). Each had preceding dermatitis, and patch tests demonstrated allergic contact reaction to PTBC, tested at 0.1% concentration in acetone in three of four cases. Depigmentation at distant sites was present in three of the cases, with one showing extensive (75%) involvement. One of the workers who had a strong allergic contact reaction developed depigmentation at the patch test site. Horio reported one case of chemical leukoderma to PTBC in a worker in a polyester resin plant (Horio 1977). Testing revealed an allergic contact reaction to 0.5% PTBC with depigmentation at this site after 2 weeks. Cross reactivity to 0.05% PTBP was also observed, but without depigmentation.

In a comprehensive review, Bleehen tested the depigmenting capacity of 33 compounds on black guinea pigs and found that 4-IPC was the most potent (Bleehen *et al.* 1968). Animal studies with black guinea pigs confirmed that PTBC and even PTBP induced depigmentation that was reversible two months after chemical application ceased (Gellin *et al.* 1970). The reversibility suggests that the compound might have induced the leukoderma by blocking melanin formation rather than the complete destruction of melanocytes, a condition that might be permanent.

Other phenolic derivatives

Data supporting butylated hydroxyanisole (BHA) and butylated hydroxytoluene (BHT) as depigmenters are inconclusive. Riley found that low concentrations of BHA were toxic to cultured guinea pig melanocytes, but Gellin *et al.* could not produce depigmentation when they applied BHA to guinea pigs or to black mice (Riley 1971; Gellin *et al.* 1979). Maibach was unable to reproduce depigmentation from 60 day occlusive application of BHT to darkly pigmented men (Maibach *et al.* 1975). Bentley-Phillips also did not observe pigment loss in patch testing 0.5% and 3% BHT on 50 African volunteers (Bentley-Phillips & Bayles 1974). The Cosmetic Ingredient Review panel considers 'BHA is safe as a cosmetic ingredient in the present practices of use' (Elder 1984).

Mercaptoamines

The depigmenting potential of β-mercaptoethylamine hydrochloride (MEA) and N-(2-mercaptoethyl)-dimethylamine hydrochloride (MEDA) was first demonstrated in black goldfish by Chavin and Schlesinger and later in a mammalian model of the black guinea pig (Pathak *et al.* 1966; Bleehen *et al.* 1968; Frenk & Loi-Zedda 1980). MEDA was shown to have greater depigmenting potency than MEA. Sulphanolic acid, cysteamine dihydrochloride, and 3-mercaptopropylamine hydrochloride were also shown to weakly depigment skin of black guinea pigs (Bleehen *et al.* 1968).

Miscellaneous

Mathias and colleagues reported perioral leukoderma simulating vitiligo in a patient who used cinnamic-aldehyde-containing toothpaste. The patch test site of cinnamic aldehyde depigmented (Mathias *et al.* 1980).

We reported three cases of circumferential contact leukoderma of the scalp associated with the application of permanent and semipermanent hair colours. Depigmentation developed at the sites of patch testing or re-challenge with paraphenylenediamine (PPDA) and/or the hair colour, but not at sites of positive patch test reactions to other chemicals. We observed no obvious clinical evidence of vitiligo in these patients. We also reported a similar patient with partial scalp depigmentation following the use of a benzyl-alcohol-containing hair colour; there was no pigment loss at the site of the positive patch test reaction (Taylor *et al.* 1993). Brancaccio and Cohen reported a case of leukoderma of the upper lip following exposure to PPDA in moustache colouring solution. However, patch tests were negative for both allergic contact dermatitis and depigmentation (Brancaccio & Cohen 1995).

P-cresol, the active chemical in laundry-ink, has been shown to cause depigmentation in agouti and black mice (Shelley 1974).

Several cases of periocular leukoderma associated with the use of various mitotic ophthalmic preparations such as eserine and diisopropyl fluorophosphate have been described (Jacklin 1965; Koldys & Frye 1973). In addition, use of thiotepa following pterygium surgery and guanonitrofuracin for treatment of conjunctivitis and blepharitis has also been reported to cause eyelid depigmentation (Harben *et al.* 1979; Ortonne *et al.* 1983).

Clinical features

Chemical leukoderma occurs in individuals with all skin types and colours. The appearance of chemical leukoderma may be identical to vitiligo including the anatomical distribution. Depigmentation usually begins from small confetti-like round to oval grouped macules. The pattern of spread may be a helpful clue in differentiating chemical leukoderma from vitiligo; 'a history of gradual coalescence of small discrete macules, rather than development of large macules with perifollicular sparing suggests chemical leukoderma' (Ortonne *et al.* 1983).

Chemical leukoderma, especially in the occupational setting, initially often involves the hands and forearms, presumably where there is contact with the inciting agent (Schwartz *et al.* 1940; Gellin *et al.* 1970; Kahn 1970; Malten *et al.* 1971; Horio 1977). Some individuals with chemical leukoderma develop depigmentation at distant sites which is usually symmetrical and may, at times, become extensive (Schwartz *et al.* 1940; Kahn 1970; Malten *et al.* 1971; Calnan & Cooke 1974). The mechanism for spread may involve either the transfer of the chemical by the hands to other parts of the body or absorption of the chemical through inhalation or ingestion (Malten *et al.* 1971). Scalp hair is rarely involved in chemical leukoderma except for the case reports of scalp depigmentation and poliosis attributed to PPDA (Taylor *et al.* 1993).

The period of chemical exposure required for depigmentation to appear ranges from 2 weeks to up to 4–6 months (Kahn 1970; Malten *et al.* 1971). Depigmentation appears after the reservoir of pre-existing melanin has been metabolized, a process which may take weeks to months (Schwartz *et al.* 1940).

Most cases of chemical leukoderma are preceded by inflammation of the affected skin (Gellin *et al.* 1970; Horio 1977; Taylor *et al.* 1993). The development of allergic contact dermatitis, as demonstrated by patch testing, although frequent, is not a prerequisite (Malten *et al.* 1971; James *et al.* 1977). Depigmentation at patch test sites in reported cases of chemical leukoderma has not been consistently demonstrated (Gellin *et al.* 1970; Malten *et al.* 1971; Horio 1977).

In most studies, there was some degree of spontaneous follicular-based repigmentation after avoidance of the chemical presumed responsible. However, depigmentation at times is permanent (Kahn 1970; Malten *et al.* 1971; Horio 1977). Malten found that the more limited the extent of chemical leukoderma and the shorter its duration before avoidance, the earlier that spontaneous repigmentation was apt to occur (Malten *et al.* 1971).

Differential diagnosis

Other causes of depigmentation should also be considered and excluded before attributing the cause to chemicals. The main differential diagnoses are postinflammatory pigment loss and idiopathic vitiligo. Postinflammatory pigment changes usually consist of off-white patches corresponding to the site of preceding inflammation. The opposite is also true, namely, that the absence of preceding dermatitis at all areas of pigment loss excludes postinflammatory leukoderma (Mosher *et al.* 1993).

Vitiligo may be indistinguishable from chemical leukoderma. Histopathological examination is not usually helpful in differentiating the two entities because both have decreased to absent numbers of melanocytes (Fisher 1995). Additionally, the differential diagnosis also includes pigment loss from physical agents such as burns or trauma; discoid lupus erythematosus, or pityriasis alba; genetic disorders such as albinism and Waardenburg syndrome; endocrine disorders such as hypopituitarism, Addison's disease, and hyperthyroidism.

Pathology

Histopathology does not reliably distinguish between chemical leukoderma and vitiligo. On light microscopy, both chemical leukoderma and vitiligo demonstrate reduced numbers of melanocytes. There may be a decreased number of dopa positive melanocytes as well as tyrosinase activity. In this study the remaining melanocytes were abnormal in shape and had lost their dendrites (Bleehen *et al.* 1968).

Some electron microscopic studies have shown that there is a decreased to absent number of melanocytes in chemically induced depigmentation and those remaining possess structural abnormalities, such as vacuolization and swollen mitochondria (Malten *et al.* 1971). In a case of adhesive-tape-induced depigmentation described by Frenk and Kocsis, 'electron microscopy revealed numerous indeterminate clear cells but no melanocytes in between the basal keratinocytes' (Frenk *et al.* 1974).

Diagnosis/evaluation

Diagnosis of chemical leukoderma is more easily made when a number of cases are clustered, typically in a factory, and there is exposure to known depigmenting agents; when pigment loss follows contact dermatitis; or when the person affected is an adult with no personal or family history of vitiligo or its associated diseases (Gellin & Maibach 1985). A detailed history is especially important in isolated cases and in cases involving litigation to exclude other causes such as medications, trauma, and burns. A history of exposure to known depigmenters, either through direct contact or through systemic absorption should be established.

The role of patch testing is important in documenting cases of suspected chemical leukoderma. Patch testing should be performed carefully, especially in darker skinned individuals, so as to minimize potential for depigmentation in cosmetically important anatomical sites (Taylor *et al.* 1993). Peripheral and distant spread of pigment loss is possible. The material or chemical in question should be tested using a nonirritating concentration derived from standard dilution techniques. The patch test sites should be evaluated for dermatitis after 2 days and again after 4–7 days and for pigment loss after 4–6 weeks and, in some cases, after 4–6 months. A delayed reading at 4–6 weeks is necessary when testing for chemical leukoderma since the reservoir of preformed melanin must be first shed by the epidermis prior to detecting depigmentation (Fisher 1994).

Treatment

In the workplace it is important to prevent and minimize exposure to known depigmenting agents through environmental engineering and industrial hygiene measures. These include good work practices, local exhaust ventilation, chemical substitution and, as a last resort, the use of personal protective equipment. Prevention is especially important for those with chemical leukoderma.

Spontaneous repigmentation has been reported in cases following avoidance of the causative agent (Kahn 1970; Malten *et al.* 1971; Horio 1977). Repigmentation is perifollicular, gradual in onset and has been noted variably over a period of weeks to months.

Photochemotherapy with psoralen and ultraviolet light A (PUVA) has had limited success. Ehrnfeld's case of depigmentation from a phenolic detergent germicide responded to PUVA at weekly intervals for two months with follicular repigmentation occurring after six treatments (Ehrenfeld 1971). Limited therapy with systemic PUVA resulted in partial follicular repigmentation in one of our patients with leukoderma from hair dye (Taylor *et al.* 1993). Almost total repigmentation from PUVA occurred in an unreported patient of ours with chemical leukoderma of the hands from rubber gloves.

References

Angelini, E., Marinaro, C., Carrozzo, A., Bianchi, L., Delogu, A., Giannello, G. & Nini, G. (1993) Allergic contact dermatitis of the lip margins from para-tertiary-butylphenol in a lip liner. *Contact Dermatitis* **28**, 146–148.

Bajaj, A.K., Gupta, S.C. & Chatterjee, A.K. (1990) Contact depigmentation from free para-tertiary-butylphenol in bindi adhesive. *Contact Dermatitis* **22**, 99–102.

Bajaj, A.K., Gupta, S.C. & Chatterjee, A.K. (1991) Contact depigmentation of the breast [published errata appear in Contact Dermatitis 1991 October; 25 (4) 272 and 1992 May **26** (5), 360]. *Contact Dermatitis* 24, 58.

Bajaj, A.K., Gupta, S.C. & Chatterjee, A.K. (1992) Hearing aid depigmentation. *Contact Dermatitis* **27**, 126–127.

Bajaj, A., Gupta, S. & Chatterjee, A. (1996) Footwear depigmentation. *Contact Dermatitis* **35**, 117–118.

Bentley-Phillips, B. & Bayles, M. (1974) Butylated hydroxytoluene as a skin lightener. *Archives of Dermatology* **109**, 216–217.

Bleehen, S.S., Pathak, M.A., Hori, Y. & Fitzpatrick, T.B. (1968) Depigmentation of skin with 4-isopropylcatechol, mercaptoamines and other compounds. *Journal of Investigative Dermatology* **50**, 103–117.

Botvinick, I. (1951) Dermatitis and secondary leukoderma due to fabric-lined rubber gloves. *Archives of Dermatology and Syphilology* **63**, 334–335.

Brancaccio, R. & Cohen, D. (1995) Contact leukoderma secondary to paraphenylenediamine. *Contact Dermatitis* **32**, 313.

Calnan, C.D. (1973) Occupational leukoderma from alkyl phenols. *Proceedings of the Royal Society of Medicine* **66**, 258–260.

Calnan, C.D. & Cooke, M.A. (1974) Leucoderma in industry. *Journal of Sociology and Occupational Medicine* **24**, 59–61.

Chivers, C. (1972) Two cases of occupational leucoderma following contact with hydroquinone monomethyl ether. *British Journal of Industrial Medicine* **29**, 105–107.

Cummings, M.P. & Nordlund, J.J. (1995) Chemical leukoderma: fact or fancy. *American Journal of Contact Dermatitis* **6**, 122–127.

Das, M. & Tandon, A. (1988) Occupational vitiligo. *Contact Dermatitis* **19**, 184–185.

Ehrenfeld, I. (1971) Depigmentation due to phenolic detergent germicide. Treated with methoxsalen and blacklite. *Archives of Dermatology* **104**, 216–217.

Elder, R. (1984) Final report on the safety assessment of butylated hydroxyanisole. *Journal of the American College of Toxicology* **3**, 83–146.
Elder, R. (1986) Final report on the safety assessment of hydroquinone and pyrocatechol. *Journal of the American College of Toxicology* **15**, 123–165.
Fisher, A. (1982) Leukoderma from bleaching creams containing 2% hydroquinone. *Contact Dermatitis* **8**, 272–273.
Fisher, A.A. (1994) Differential diagnosis of idiopathic vitiligo. Part III: Occupational leukoderma [news]. *Cutis* **53**, 278–280.
Fisher, A. (1995) Contact leukoderma (vitiligo) hyperpigmentation and discolorations from contactants. In: *Fisher's Contact Dermatitis* (eds R.Rietschel & J.J.Fowler), 4th edn, pp. 765–777. Williams & Wilkins, Baltimore.
Frenk, E. & Loi-Zedda, P. (1980) Occupational depigmentation due to a hydroquinone-containing photographic developer. *Contact Dermatitis* **6**, 238–239.
Frenk, M.E. & Kocsis, M. (1974) Depigmentation due to adhesive tape: ultra-structural comparison with vitiligo and vitiliginous depigmentation associated with a melanoma. *Dermatologica* **148**, 276–284.
Gellin, G. & Maibach, H. (1983) Detection of environmental depigmenting chemicals. In: *Dermatotoxicology* (eds F.Marzulli & H.Maibach), 2nd edn, pp. 443–459. Hemisphere, Washington, DC.
Gellin, G. & Maibach, H. (1985) Chemically induced depigmentation. In: *Models in Dermatology* (eds H.Maibach & N.Lowe), pp. 282. Karger, Basel.
Gellin, G., Possick, P. & Davis, I. (1970) Occupational depigmentation due to 4-tertiarybutyl catechol (TBC). *Journal of Occupational Medicine* **12**, 386–389.
Gellin, G.A., Maibach, H.I. & Misiaszek, M.H. (1979) Detection of environmental depigmenting substances. *Contact Dermatitis* **5**, 201–213.
Harben, D., Cooper, P. & Rodman, O. (1979) Thiotepa-induced leukoderma. *Archives of Dermatology* **115**, 973–974.
Horio, T. (1977) Depigmentation due to para tertiary butyl catechol. *International Archives of Occupational and Environmental Health* **39**, 127–133.
Jacklin, H. (1965) Depigmentation of the eyelids in eserine allergy. *American Journal of Ophthalmology* **59**, 89–92.
James, O., Mayes, R.W. & Stevenson, C.J. (1977) Occupational vitiligo induced by *p-tert*-butylphenol: a systemic disease? *Lancet* **2**, 1217–1219.
Jimbow, K., Obata, H., Pathak, M.A. & Fitzpatrick, T.B. (1974) Mechanism of depigmentation by hydroquinone. *Journal of Investigative Dermatology* **62**, 436–449.
Kahn, G. (1970) Depigmentation caused by phenolic detergent germicides. *Archives of Dermatology* **102**, 177–187.
Kersey, P. & Stevenson, C.J. (1981) Vitiligo and occupational exposure to hydroquinone from servicing self-photographing machines. *Contact Dermatitis* **7**, 285–287.
Koldys, K. & Frye, L. (1973) A perplexing pigmentary problem. *Cutis* **12**, 420–423.
Maibach, H., Gellin, G. & Ring, M. (1975) Is the antioxidant butylated hydroxytoluene a depigmenting agent in man? *Contact Dermatitis* **1**, 295–296.
Malten, K. (1975) Paratertiary butylphenol depigmentation in a 'consumer'. *Contact Dermatitis* **1**, 181–182.
Malten, K.E. (1984) Dermatological problems with synthetic resins and plastics in glues. Part I. *Dermatosen in Beruf und Umwelt. Occupational and Environmental Dermatoses* **32**, 81–86.
Malten, K.E., Seutter, E., Hara, I. & Nakajima, T. (1971) Occupational vitiligo due to paratertiary butylphenol and homologues. *Transactions of the St. Johns Hospital Dermatological Society* **57**, 115–134.
Markey, A.C., Black, A.K. & Rycroft, R.J. (1989) Confetti-like depigmentation from hydroquinone. *Contact Dermatitis* **20**, 148–149.
Mathias, C.G., Maibach, H.I. & Conant, M.A. (1980) Perional leukoderma simulating vitiligo from use of a toothpaste containing cinnamic aldehyde. *Archives of Dermatology* **116**, 1172–1173.

McNally, W.D. (1939) A depigmentation of the skin by rubber gloves. *Industrial Medicine* **8**, 405–410.

Mosher, D., Fitzpatrick, T., Hori, H. & Ortonne, J.-P. (1993) Disorders of pigmentation. In: *Dermatology in General Medicine* (eds T.Fitzpatrick, A.Eisen, K.Wolff, I.Freedberg & K.Austen), 4th edn, pp. 903–995. McGraw-Hill, New York.

Oliver, E.A., Schwartz, L. & Warren, L.H. (1939) Occupational leukoderma. *JAMA* **113**, 927–928.

Ortonne, J., Mosher, D. & Fitzpatrick, T. (1983) Chemical hypomelanosis. In: *Vitiligo and Other Hypomelanosis of Hair and Skin* (eds J.Ortonne, D.B.Mosher & T.B.Fitzpatrick), pp. 479–508. Plenum Medical Book Company, New York.

Pathak, M.A., Frenk, E., Szabo, G. & Fitzpatrick, T.B. (1966) Cutaneous depigmentation. *Clinical Research* **14**, 272.

Riley, P.A. (1969) Hydroxyanisole depigmentation: *in vivo* studies. *Journal of Pathology* **97**, 185–191.

Riley, P. (1971) Acquired hypomelanosis. *British Journal of Dermatology* **84**, 290–293.

Schwartz, L., Oliver, E. & Warren, L. (1940) Occupational leukoderma. *Public Health Reports* **55**, 1111–1130.

Shelley, W. (1974) Cause of ink-induced hair depigmentation in mice. *British Journal of Dermatology* **90**, 169–174.

Taylor, J. (1986) Rubber. In: *Contact Dermatitis* (ed. A.Fisher), 3rd edn, pp. 603–643. Lea & Febiger, Philadelphia.

Taylor, J.S., Maibach, H.I., Fisher, A.A. & Bergfeld, W.F. (1993) Contact leukoderma associated with the use of hair colors. *Cutis* **52**, 273–280.

33: Animal Models

LYNN LAMOREUX AND RAYMOND E. BOISSY

Introduction

Vitiligo vulgaris of man is an acquired, progressive disorder characterized by the destruction of melanocytes in the skin and other organs (Nordlund *et al.* 1998). Causative factors responsible for the selective elimination of melanocytes in vitiligo may include environmental insult (Cummings & Nordlund 1995), autoimmune response (Fishman *et al.* 1997), and/or an inherited predisposition (see below). It therefore appears that the aetiology of vitiligo is multiple (Lamoreux *et al.* 1987; Boissy & Lamoreux 1988; Le Poole *et al.* 1993; Norris *et al.* 1994).

Animal models may be used in a number of ways to evaluate the pathology of human disorders which are inherited or environmentally caused. If a human disorder is a simple, one locus, inherited disease, then identification of the homologous gene locus in an animal model makes available an abundant source of information about the gene function, biochemical processes affected, aetiology and pathogenesis. Because gene functions are generally conserved across species lines, even if the disorder is expressed differently in the animal, the animal model can be used to study the disorder at all levels from the molecular to the organismal to determine the function of the gene and develop practical approaches to treat the symptoms or attempt to replace the defective gene product.

Vitiligo, however, is not a simple, one-locus disease, and inheritance is not its only cause (see Chapter 4). Therefore, in the case of vitiligo, animal models must be used with the knowledge that the disorder observed in the genetically defective animal will not be homologous with the disorder of the average human vitiligo patient. Vitiligo has multiple causes and, probably, it is often true that multiple insults are necessary to initiate vitiligo in any one individual. Thus, the study of one animal model, especially if the defect is caused by one gene locus in the model, can make only a small contribution to our understanding of human vitiligo. However, one should not abandon these valuable models simply because they provide only one portion of the overall answer. When we have a complex question to answer, we need multiple sources of information, each of which is simple enough to elucidate one or a few parameters in the dynamic web of interacting factors which regulate normal melanocyte survival.

Available animal models

The Smyth chicken

In the early 1970s, Dr J.Robert Smyth, Jr. identified a Brown line female chicken which, as an adult, developed complete feather amelanosis and which subsequently developed blindness (Smyth *et al.* 1981). This hen was mated to phenotypically normal birds and her descendants were selected by Dr Smyth for expression of the aberrant traits. The birds were originally named DAM, or delayed amelanotic chickens (Smyth *et al.* 1981) but have been renamed the Smyth chickens (Smyth 1989).

The Smyth chicken expresses the major features of human vitiligo, the delayed development of cutaneous amelanosis, most commonly appearing during adolescence or at young adulthood, and variable in occurrence, location and extent (Fig. 33.1). Birds of the Smyth line express many of the associated disorders presented by patients with vitiligo. These include ocular depigmentation and uveitis, alopecia-areata-like trait, autoimmune thyroiditis and a low incidence of spontaneous repigmentation. The blindness that frequently develops in Smyth chickens results from degeneration of retinal pigment epithelium, the neural retina and optic nerve fibres, abnormalities occurring after extensive uveitis (Boissy *et al.* 1983; Fite *et al.* 1983, 1985). Autoimmune thyroiditis occurs in several chicken models, with or without vitiligo, and is itself thought to result from the convergence of multiple genetic and environmental factors, including MHC genes (Rose 1994).

Much of the variability of phenotypic expression of vitiligo in humans and probably in the chickens results from the fact that neither is inbred. Sublines of the Smyth chicken have been developed which express high incidence of some of these traits, an observation suggesting that the syndrome is influenced at several genetic loci. Thus the Smyth chicken is an excellent model for the human condition in that (i) the birds are not inbred, the phenotype exhibits variable expression, and (ii) the underlying pathophysiol-

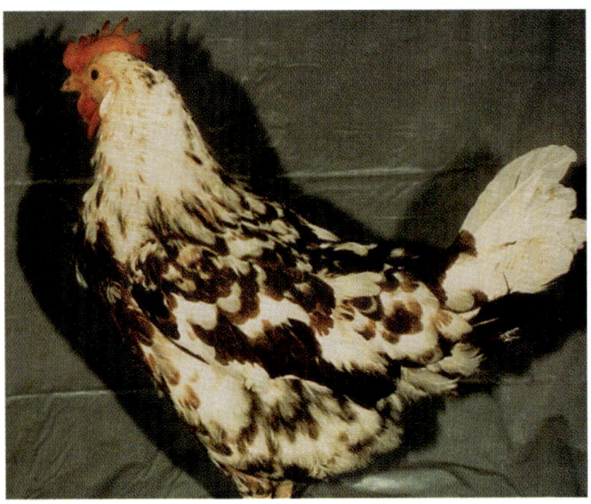

Fig. 33.1 Mature Smyth line chicken exhibiting partial feather amelanosis.

ogy is clearly polyfactorial and has a genetic component. That the trait can be selected by inbreeding argues for a modest number of genetic loci contributing to its expression and their availability for analyses.

The aetiology of vitiligo in the Smyth chicken appears to include an inherent defect in the melanocyte and an associated autoimmune response (Smyth 1989). However, the molecular interactions between these two components have yet to be resolved. Melanocytes isolated in culture from neural tubes of Smyth line embryos develop melanosomal abnormalities and large autophagosomes that accumulate with time (Boissy *et al.* 1986). Similarly, histological and ultrastructural evaluations of feather and ocular tissue prior to the expression of amelanosis reveal cytological abnormalities within the melanocytes prior to the appearance of cells of the immune/inflammatory system (Boissy *et al.* 1983, 1984, 1988b). The appearance of abnormally structured melanosomes, large autophagocytic-like bodies in the cytoplasm, and fragmentation of the melanocytes suggest that melanocytes undergo premature cell death in the Smyth chicken. Thus several lines of evidence suggest that an inherent melanocyte defect exists in the Smyth line chicken. However, these morphological abnormalities have been observed also in bursectomized Smyth line chickens which remained normally pigmented (Boissy *et al.* 1984), an observation suggesting active depigmentation involves a response of the immune system to an inherent melanocyte abnormality.

The involvement of the immune system in the aetiology of vitiligo in Smyth chickens is further indicated by an influx of immunocytes which is commonly observed in the dermal pulp and occasionally in the epidermal layer of the feather during development of amelanosis (Boissy *et al.* 1983). In addition, lymphocytes and macrophages become abundant in the uveal tract in concert with ocular melanocyte damage (Smyth *et al.* 1981; Boissy *et al.* 1983; Fite *et al.* 1983). Corticosteroid therapy of young preamelanotic Smyth line chicks significantly decreases the incidence of feather amelanosis (Boyle *et al.* 1987). This suggests that the immune system plays an active role in melanocyte destruction and/or removal in the Smyth line chicken.

The role of antibody-producing B cells in the Smyth chicken was initially assessed by surgical removal of the bursa. Elimination of the humoral immune system in the Smyth chicken by neonatal bursectomy resulted in a significant decrease in the expression and severity of the feather amelanosis (Lamont & Smyth 1981). It has subsequently been demonstrated that serum autoantibodies, specific for melanocytes, develop immediately prior to or at the time of feather amelanosis (Austin *et al.* 1992; Searle *et al.* 1993). Also, when Smyth line chickens spontaneously develop complete repigmentation, these serum autoantibodies are no longer detectable (Austin *et al.* 1992). The predominant serum autoantibody detected in vitiliginous Smyth chickens recognizes tyrosinase-related protein-1 (TRP-1), a protein homologous with that produced at the *brown* ($Tyrp1^b$) locus of the mouse (Austin & Boissy 1995).

The cellular component of the immune system also appears to be involved in the aetiology of vitiligo in Smyth line chickens. Cyclosporin-A, a potent inhibitor of interleukin-1 and 2 release which influences helper/inducer T lymphocyte functions, effectively reduces the incidence and severity of feather amelanosis and ocular pathology (Fite *et al.* 1986; Pardue *et al.* 1987). Concurrent with the development of the amelanosis, mononuclear cell infiltration and altered T cell profiles are observed in the pulp of developing feathers (Erf *et al.* 1995) and altered leucocyte profiles exist in the blood (Erf & Smyth 1995) of Smyth chickens. In addition, the expression of amelanosis in chickens of the Smyth line can be influenced by loci of the major histocompatability complex (Auclair *et al.* 1984).

In general, Smyth line chickens seem to have a hyperactive immune system. Affected Smyth birds can produce higher serum antibody titres after administration of exogenous antigen than can their normally pigmented siblings (Lamont *et al.* 1982). In fact, the extent of this elevated antibody response correlates positively with the severity of the amelanosis and visual defect, an indication that the development of amelanosis is associated with the immune competency of the animal (Lamont & Smyth 1984).

Thus, it is clear that there is an autoimmune component to the development of depigmentation in the Smyth chicken, and that one gene locus which may participate antigenically in this autoimmune syndrome is the Tyrp1 locus. It is also clear that Smyth chicken vitiligo is polyfactorial. However, it is not clear which genes, other than the one encoding TRP-1, cause which defects and in what combinations.

The Smyth chicken is an excellent model for the study of human vitiligo in that it parallels the human condition in variability, complexity, mode of expression and polyfactorial aetiology. Disadvantages of this model include the fact that such a complex system is difficult to analyse without isolating the interacting factors and developing separate normal controls for each aberrant trait. Quantitative trait linkage (QTL) analysis of the Smyth line chicken is underway (Sreekuman *et al.* 1997) in an attempt to map the loci which are interacting inappropriately to cause progressive loss of melanocytes. Using this method, specific contributing loci can be identified, whether or not they individually cause leukoderma, and analysed separately from the syndrome as a whole. When this is accomplished, the Smyth chicken may well be our most productive vitiligo model. However, it is not the only model and does not incorporate all the genetic and environmental factors which may or do cause vitiligo in humans.

Other birds

Two additional avian vitiligo models have been proposed, each of which is a single locus phenotype rather than a polyfactorial population model. These are the White Leghorn and the Barred Plymouth Rock (Bowers *et al.* 1992). The White Leghorn chicken is a mutant that has an abnormality at the *I* locus; the Barred Rock chicken is mutant with an anomaly at the sex-linked avian *B* locus (Smyth 1990) (the avian *B* locus is not homologous with the murine *B* locus).

The White Leghorn (*I*/–) chicken expresses congenital amelanosis resulting from premature cell death of melanocytes in the collar of the developing feather follicle, which occurs during each feather growth cycle, prior to the successful transfer of melanosomes to the keratinocytes (Jimbow *et al.* 1974). The Barred Plymouth Rock (*B*/–) chicken exhibits an alternating black and white banding pattern along the length of the feathers. This pattern appears to result from premature autophagic degeneration of melanocytes at the proximal edge of the black band, resulting in a white band devoid of melanocytes (Bowers 1988). Transplantation studies have demonstrated that the pigment defect in both cases is autonomous to the mutant melanocyte (Willier & Rawles 1940). In addition, neither the White Leghorn chicken nor the Barred Plymouth Rock chicken expresses an immune response during the development of feather amelanosis. Therefore, these mutant conditions represent separate defects of melanocytes which result in the inability of melanocytes to survive and function normally in the feather follicle. It is therefore surprising that melanocytes mutant at either locus are able to function normally in culture conditions (Bowers *et al.* 1992). Bowers and co-authors suggest that a toxic substance in the avascular feather epithelium is responsible for inducing cell death of sensitive melanocytes.

Single locus mutations are much more available for evaluation at the cellular and molecular level than are polyfactorial traits. Therefore, while the Smyth chicken may be a more closely parallel model of the human condition, the single locus mutants provide an opportunity to study the relationship between the melanocyte and its tissue environment. To take full advantage of this opportunity, single-locus traits should be evaluated against one or preferably more than one inbred background.

The Sinclair pig

The Sinclair miniature pig was developed by selection as a model for melanoma which is similar to human melanoma. Sinclair swine exhibit a high incidence of congenital malignant melanoma which spontaneously regresses in 85% to 90% of the affected pigs. Tumour regression appears to be mediated by an immune response (Cui *et al.* 1995; Morgan *et al.* 1996), and is sometimes associated with the development of depigmentation that closely resembles human vitiligo, and which may progress over most of the body of the pig (Morgan *et al.* 1996) (Fig. 33.2). Therefore, the development of depigmentation may be secondary to the immune processes involved in regression of the melanoma (Misfeldt & Grimm 1994).

Using classic cytogenetic techniques, Pathak and Amoss (1997) identified chromosomes 2, 3, 6, 7, 12 and 17 as causative in the regression of the melanoma. Using complex segregation analysis, Blangero *et al.* (1996) developed a two locus model involving an unknown major locus and a

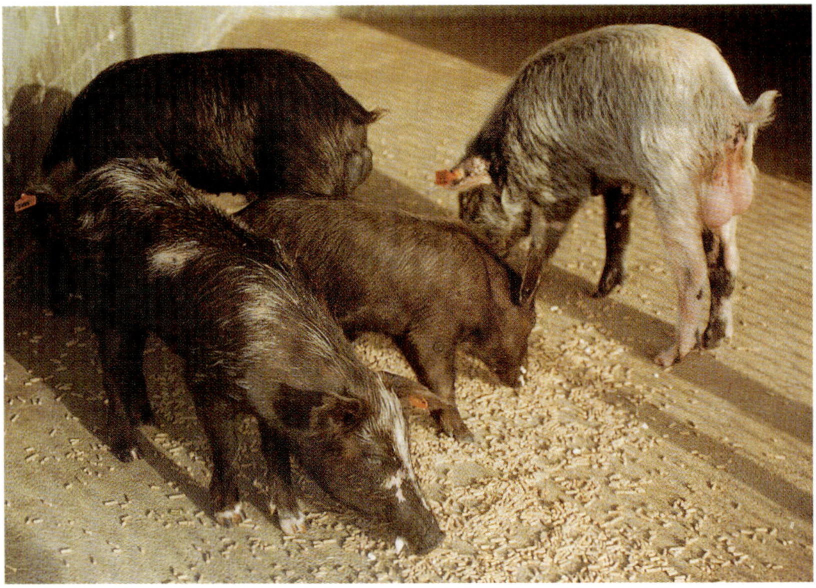

Fig. 33.2 The Sinclair pig.

second locus that lies within or close to the swine leucocytic antigen (SLA) complex. These loci also account for approximately 20% of the phenotypic variation in quantitative tumour burden, further supporting the hypothesis that the regression of the melanoma tumour and associated development of leukoderma both result from immune response to the original melanoma.

An observation that needs further study is the relationship between pheomelanin and melanoma/depigmentation in the Sinclair swine. Sinclair pigs that are pheomelanic rarely develop melanoma and, when they do, the tumour never progresses (Amoss, personal communication). In addition, leukoderma does not develop in these rare tumour-bearing pheomelanic pigs. Selection among black pigs for melanoma resistance resulted in an increase of yellow offspring (Amoss, personal communication). Production of pheomelanin in mammals is mediated by the *extension* and *agouti* loci, and the yellow allele at the *extension* locus is recessive. Taken together, these observations suggest that:

1 a tumour and leukoderma resistance gene might be located at or near the *extension* locus, or

2 tumour and leukoderma resistance are biochemically influenced by pheomelanogenesis.

While melanoma-associated depigmentation accounts for only a subset of human depigmentation, the Sinclair miniature pig is an excellent model for this type of pigment loss. The fact that the depigmentation is apparently secondary to the melanoma might be considered a disadvantage. However, depigmentation in humans apparently develops sometimes as a secondary response to melanoma (Koh *et al.* 1983; Nordlund *et al.* 1983; Bystryn *et al.* 1987; Merinsky *et al.* 1994), and it has been demonstrated that patients with metastatic melanoma who are being treated for the disease with immunotherapy frequently develop depigmentation (Rosenberg & White 1996; Kawakami & Rosenberg 1997). These observations, plus consideration of the Smyth chicken may clarify cause and effect relationships between the genetic defect, the immune response, and some types of depigmentation including vitiligo. The immune response is clearly a factor in the aetiology of human vitiligo, though it may not be the primary genetic defect. Thus, the study of melanoma-associated depigmentation in the pig should lead to insights that are applicable to all or at least many depigmentations such as vitiligo.

Another advantage of the pig model is that the depigmentation is clearly expressed in the skin in a way more similar to man than is true in most other models, which may depigment feathers or hair but not skin. Further, while inbred strains are not now available, the pig model has recently developed increased potential for genetic analyses. The linkage map, including microsatellite markers, of the pig is becoming available for use in mapping studies (Marklund *et al.* 1996), and embryo manipulation including the creation of transgenic pigs is now possible (Shim *et al.* 1997; Piedrahita *et al.* 1998).

With current technology and development of this model, the Sinclair pig now represents a wealth of information regarding survival needs of melanocytes *in vivo*, and evaluation of the immune responses involved in vitiligo, and the relationship between melanoma-cell survival and melanocyte survival.

The disadvantage of the Sinclair pig model is primarily the expense of maintaining pigs, especially in the numbers required for mapping and embryo manipulation.

Water buffalo and elephants

Water buffalo (Cerundolo *et al.* 1993) and elephants also have depigmentation that affects skin melanocytes. Because they are both domestic animals, the potential exists for their study. Histological evaluation of melanocytes at the border of the depigmented lesion in the water buffalo demonstrates profiles of dilated rough endoplasmic reticulum (Cerundolo *et al.* 1993) similar to melanocytes from patients with vitiligo (Boissy *et al.* 1991) and those from the mi^{vit}/mi^{vit} mouse (Boissy *et al.* 1991). The disadvantages of attempting genetic studies in animals of this size are obvious.

The grey horse

Grey horses always exhibit progressive loss of hair and skin pigment over their lives (Lerner & Cage 1973), but only rarely develop defined patches of depigmentation similar to symmetrical or asymmetrical vitiligo of man (Lamoreux, personal observation). Differences have not been studied between the consistent, progressive, overall greying of the horse and the occasional appearance of discrete depigmented patches. Some statements appear in the literature regarding congenital white spotting of the face and feet. Many horses have congenital white spotting, including many grey horses, but this is not a pleiotropic effect of the gene which causes greying in horses, nor is it vitiligo.

The dominant grey (*G*) gene is responsible for the grey horse phenotype, and is common in most purebred and mixed breed populations. Homozygous (*G/G*) horses are relatively rare. Their depigmentation proceeds more rapidly and thoroughly than that of the *G/g* animals. Immunological differences between grey (*G/–*) horses and non-grey (*g/g*) horses have been reported (Naughton *et al*. 1986).

Melanoma-like tumours are very common in aged grey horses. One investigator suggested these tumours are neurocristal haematomas. It is not known if the neoplasm arises secondarily to the depigmentation (which would apparently be the reverse of the Sinclair swine model) or if the tumour is a direct result of the mutant gene function. Certainly there is no evidence of a neoplasm prior to onset of depigmentation, which becomes obvious in the foal at first moult.

The primary advantage of the grey horse is the opportunity to study relationships among melanoma, depigmentation and the immune system in a model in which the three seem again to be interrelated, but are expressed in an apparently different causative sequence than in other models. *In vitro* study of melanocytes and melanoma cells from the grey horse might help illuminate the reasons for these differences.

The disadvantages of this model are obviously its size, appetite, and long generation time.

The vitiligo mouse

The vitiligo (mi^{vit}/mi^{vit}) mutant mouse was identified by Dr E. S. Russell at the Jackson Laboratory, on the inbred C57BL/6J background and has subsequently been mapped to the *mitf* locus (Lamoreux *et al*. 1992; Sidman & Neumann 1988), which encodes a basic-helix-loop-helix-zipper transcription factor (Hodgkinson *et al*. 1993). The vitiligo ($mitf^{mi*vit}$) mutant allele contains an Asp 222 to Asn substitution in helix 1 of the gene product. Numerous other alleles at this locus result in a range of phenotypes from a completely white, microphthalmic mouse with skeletal abnormalities to a phenotypically apparently normal animal (Moore 1995). Most alleles, in homozygous condition, result in mice that do not express depigmentation, but several of the heterozygous combinations produce depigmentation that is more pronounced than that seen in the 'vitiligo' mouse (Lamoreux, personal observation).

The $mitf^{mi*vit}/mitf^{mi*vit}$ mouse is born dark grey, rather than black, and is characterized by white spotting (or piebaldism, defined as congenital absence of pigment cells) that is somewhat variable in extent, as well as vitiligo (defined as progressive loss of pigment cells) (Fig. 33.3). The vitiligo

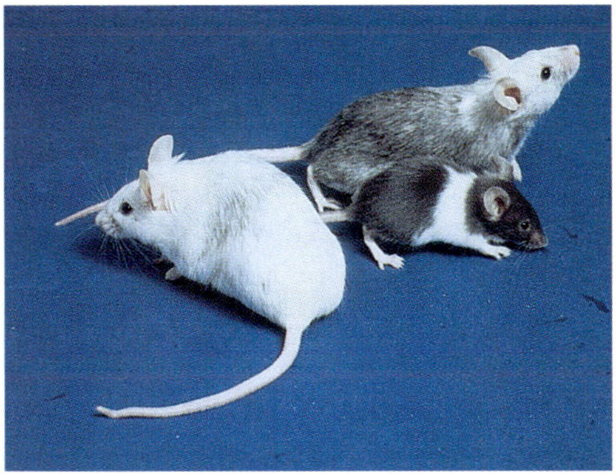

Fig. 33.3 Vitiligo (*mi*^{vit}/*mi*^{vit}) mice: a three week old mouse (centre) demonstrating grey pigmented pelage and congenital white spotting on the upper trunk, abdomen and legs, a six month old mouse (background) demonstrating partial pelage depigmentation, and a one year old mouse (left) demonstrating complete pelage depigmentation.

is expressed with each new hair coat as the animal becomes progressively less pigmented until in old age when pigmentation is much reduced over the entire body (Lerner *et al.* 1986; Boissy *et al.* 1987). Accompanying the development of cutaneous amelanosis is the loss of ocular pigment cells and retinal degeneration (Boissy *et al.* 1987; Smith *et al.* 1994; Smith & Defoe 1995). Prior to the loss of pigment cells, melanocytes in the anagen hair express autophagocytic vesicles and cellular fragmentation (Boissy *et al.* 1987). When isolated in culture, *mitf*^{mi*vit}/*mitf*^{mi*vit} melanocytes derived from neonatal skins demonstrate dilated rough endoplasmic reticulum and premature cell death (Boissy *et al.* 1991).

No immune component is obvious in the process of melanocyte destruction in *mitf*^{mi*vit}/*mitf*^{mi*vit} mice. Immunocytes are rarely apparent in either the hair or ocular tissue concurrent with the expression of aberrant melanocytes (Boissy *et al.* 1987), and the administration of immunosuppressive agents like cyclosporin-A does not influence the expression of the trait (Boissy, personal observation). Skin transplantation studies demonstrate that the development of hair depigmentation is autonomous to the mutant skin and not influenced by surrounding normal tissues (Lerner *et al.* 1986). However, the mice are unable to mount a normal inflammatory response to applied contact allergens (Nordlund *et al.* 1995).

The retinal degeneration of the vitiligo mouse has been described in detail (Smirnakis *et al.* 1991; Smith & Hamasaki 1994; Smith & Defoe 1995; Smith & Wiggert 1995; Kosaras & Sidman 1996; Smith *et al.* 1994, 1995, 1997, 1998). Ultrastructural evidence of retinal degeneration has been demonstrated in animals as early as 12 days of age (Nir *et al.* 1995; Tang *et al.* 1996). It seems clear that pigment cells in the retinal pigmented epithelium (RPE) are necessary for normal optic development (Raymond & Jackson 1995) and maintenance (Kosaras & Sidman 1996; Sidman *et al.* 1996). Thus the retinal degeneration of the vitiligo mouse may be secondary to the pigment-cell defect noted in these mice as early as embryonic day 18, when twice as many RPE cells are present in *mitf^mi*vit^/mitf^mi*vit^* mice compared with controls (Tang *et al.* 1997).

Because this mouse is inbred, and the mutant is coisogenic with its controls, we can be confident that the various defects observed in the vitiligo mutant mouse result from the *mitf^mi*vit^* mutation itself, and because the gene has been identified and sequenced we are in a position to evaluate the relationship between the specific DNA lesion and the progressive loss of melanocytes.

Mouse models in general are powerful in that they have available all the advantages of sophisticated modern technological and genetic methodologies. A specific gene can be evaluated against multiple and contrasting inbred strains; mapping is advanced; either polymorphic or individual loci can be located; and embryos can be manipulated. All these advances allow mutagenesis by design, by adding, subtracting, or by mutating defined genes to facilitate experimental investigation. Thus, the genetic defect which causes vitiligo is available for analysis at almost any level and will inform us regarding the factors which are necessary for development and maintenance of normal pigmentation.

The mouse model has a few disadvantages. It is not polyfactorial and therefore does not parallel the human condition as closely as do the Sinclair pig or the Smyth chicken. Furthermore, unlike humans and pigs, mice have little interfollicular epidermal pigmentation. The vitiligo of mice resembles the early greying that is always seen in grey horses and sometimes seen in humans, rather than the discretely outlined epidermal depigmented patches that are usually defined as vitiligo in humans and only occasionally occurs in grey horses.

Other mouse models

All of the mouse models might better be described as models for the early greying type of depigmentation. *London Grey* (Steel 1981) mice are born with hairs that are rather uniformly brownish grey and progress with age to hairs that are more extensively depigmented at their bases and an increasing number of hairs that are fully white. *Faded* (Oh *et al.* 1986; Oh & Tomita 1987), when crossed from the original multiple mutant stock onto C57BL/6J, expresses a phenotype similar to that of C57BL/6J-*London Grey*, but with a somewhat more uniform shade of slate grey, rather than brownish grey. *Faded* is known to be linked with *mitf*. Neither *Faded* nor *London Grey* has been studied as a vitiligo model, but both are available.

Other mouse genes which cause depigmentation that progresses with the age of the mouse, and throughout the growth cycles of the individual hairs, include *silver* (Dunn & Thigpen 1930) and the *B-light* allele at the *Tyrp1* locus (Quevedo & Chase 1958), and reportedly the slaty-light allele at the *Tyrp2* locus (Jackson *et al.* 1992). These three loci, *silver*, *Tyrp1* and *Tyrp2* encode proteins that are structurally similar to each other and to tyrosinase, the enzyme that is essential for initiation of melanogenesis. Further, the protein products of these loci are major components of a melanogenic complex embedded in the melanosomal membranes in eumelanic mice (Orlow *et al.* 1994). Some of the components of this complex are absent from pheomelanic melanosomes, because TRP-1, TRP-2 and silver proteins are not produced in pheomelanosomes (Lamoreux *et al.* 1995). Likewise pheomelanic mice which are homozygous for the *B-light* and/or *silver* mutant alleles do not exhibit the melanocyte destruction characteristic of similar mice that are eumelanic. Neither has melanocyte destruction been observed in pheomelanic *slaty-light* mice (Lamoreux, personal observation). Taken together, these facts suggest that progressive destruction of melanocytes in these mice may result from disruption of the melanogenic complex by the aberrant structures of its member proteins, while absence of these proteins does not result in melanocyte destruction.

Silver, *B-light* and *slaty-light* were identified on strain backgrounds that differ from C57BL/6J. When backcrossed onto C57BL/6J, the phenotypes of these mice differ from the literature reports. Inbred C57BL/6J mice of these mutant genotypes have much less of the early greying phenotype than they exhibit on their strains of origin (Lamoreux, personal observation). Thus, one or more loci in the background genomes must influence expression of these mutant phenotypes.

With the advent of modern technology, new avenues are opening for the study of vitiligo in mice. Bcl-2-deficient knockout mice turn grey at first moult as a result of melanocyte loss (Veis *et al.* 1993; Nakayama *et al.* 1994; Yamamura *et al.* 1996). TRP-1 proteins, altered to enhance their antigenicity, were used to immunize mice against melanoma and also resulted in a patchy depigmentation of their coats (Hara *et al.* 1995; Naftzger *et al.* 1996), mirroring similar efforts in humans (Rosenberg & White 1996; Wang *et al.* 1996).

The most obvious advantage of the mouse models is that the murine system is the most sophisticated animal model resource, especially for traits in which there is a genetic component. The most obvious disadvantage of mouse models is that all of them appear to represent early greying pigmentary changes rather than the discrete patches often seen in human vitiligo patients. It is possible that this difference between the human and the model results from the relative absence of melanocytes in the interfollicular epidermis of mice. It is also possible that, if some of these murine 'greying' factors were combined in the same mice, we would be able to create a polyfactorial vitiligo model that expresses vitiligo more similar to that seen in humans.

Summary

Among the animal models reviewed above, the most obvious cause of vitiligo is the abnormal function of the immune system, observed in different manifestations in the Smyth chicken and the Sinclair pig. Other components of vitiligo include genetically determined autodestruction of melanocytes, which is the probable cause of melanocyte loss in most of the single locus mutants including the mouse models and the chicken models other than the Smyth chicken. A self destructive mechanism of the melanocyte, of course, does not preclude subsequent autoimmune reactions.

Because we have considerable knowledge about the functions of the *silver*, *B-light* and *slaty-light* gene products, we are able to speculate about the nature of the cell-autonomous death of their melanocytes (and tyrosinase falls into the same category and has been implicated as an antigen in some human studies) (Song *et al.* 1994). Similarly we can speculate about the reasons why pheomelanic mice and pigs are not subject to some kinds of depigmentation (but yellow mice which are homozygous for the $mitf^{mi*vit}$ gene do show loss of pigmentation similarly to non-yellow *vitiligo* mice) (Lamoreux, personal observation).

A viral sensitivity in some strains of B10 H-2 congenic mice is implicated in their greying with age (Morse *et al.* 1985) and a viral contribution to the chicken syndrome has been suggested (Sreekumar *et al.* 1997).

The swine model suggests that vitiligo results from the presence of melanoma; the horse model does not, though depigmentation and melanoma are associated in both cases.

Thus our animal models confirm the human observations, which suggest that human vitiligo is a complex, multifactorial syndrome which will require a complex, multifaceted approach to its solution. Each animal model has its own information to contribute. The appropriate animal models will be chosen in light of several considerations:

1 how closely does the model approximate the human condition?

2 how powerful is the model species—that is, how many types of biological analysis are possible using the species?

3 in the case of genetic models, what types of questions are amenable to evaluation given the nature of the genetic lesion?

The overall question is twofold: what kills melanocytes *in vivo*, and what do melanocytes require for survival? The primary agents of melanocyte death appear to be environmental and genetic.

To study the environmental contribution to melanocyte death, and the resulting physiological responses, one need only find an animal which responds appropriately to the application of suitable stimuli. Even in a straightforward stimulus/response study, however, the availability of genetic controls in the chosen animal model is desirable. In order to evaluate the genetic component to susceptibility, it is useful to know whether the research animals are genetically uniform or not. Because the human population is not genetically uniform, it is desirable to use a nonuniform animal model for some purposes. However, it is also desirable to test the stimulus/response against various inbred backgrounds as another way to approximate the variable human condition, but with the advantage that any genes which influence sensitivity can be more readily identified.

To evaluate the genetic contribution to a polyfactorial disease, one should identify more than one animal model, including:

1 those which have occurred naturally,
2 those which have been created by selective breeding or mutagenesis, and
3 those which occurred or can be created in an inbred animal.

In addition, one would want to use, or design by embryo manipulation, models with which to study expression of suspect genes or evaluate the expression of known genes on differing genetic backgrounds in order to identify interacting factors which may not cause vitiligo individually, but which do influence its expression or severity.

For example, consider the power of the mouse model, used in conjunction with the excellent polyfactorial chicken (or pig) model. As genes are mapped and identified in the chicken model, or the pig model, the homologous genes could be identified or created in the mouse model, where they could be caused to function together or separately in any desired set of combinations against manageable genetic backgrounds. Similarly, factors identified *in vitro* could be tested *in vivo*. Thus, a carefully designed collaborative effort would apply the special strengths of each of the vitiligo models to compensate for the weaknesses of other models, and would test in the mouse room the biological applicability of work done in the laboratory.

References

Auclair, B.W., Smith, J.R. Jr, Lamont, S.J. & Briles, W.E. (1984) Effects of the major histocompatibility complex on delayed amelanosis and associated retinal dystrophy in the DAM chicken. *Poultry Science* **63**, 102.

Austin, L.M. & Boissy, R.E. (1995) Mammalian tyrosinase-related-protein-1 is recognized by autoantibodies from vitiliginous Smyth chickens. An avian model for human vitiligo. *American Journal of Pathology* **146**, 1529–1541.

Austin, L.M., Boissy, R.E., Jacobson, B.S. & Smyth, J.R. Jr (1992) The detection of melanocyte autoantibodies in the Smyth chicken model for vitiligo. *Clinical Immunology and Immunopathology* **64**, 112–120.

Blangero, J., Tissot, R.G., Beattie, C.W. & Amoss, M.S. (1996) Genetic determinants of cutaneous malignant melanoma in Sinclair swine. *British Journal of Cancer* **73**, 667–671.

Boissy, R.E. & Lamoreux, M.L. (1988) Animal models of an acquired pigmentary disorder—vitiligo. *Progress in Clinical & Biological Research* **256**, 207–218.

Boissy, R.E., Smyth, J.R. Jr & Fite, K.V. (1983) Progressive cytological changes during the development of delayed feather amelanosis and associated choroidal defects in the DAM chicken line—a vitiligo model. *American Journal of Pathology* **111**, 197–202.

Boissy, R.E., Lamont, S.J. & Smyth, J.R. Jr (1984) Persistence of abnormal melanocytes in immunosuppressed chickens of the autoimmune 'DAM' line. *Cell and Tissue Research* **235**, 663–668.

Boissy, R.E., Moellmann, G.E., Trainer, A.T., Smyth, J.R. Jr & Lerner, A.B. (1986) Delayed-amelanotic (DAM or Smyth) chicken: Melanocyte dysfunction *in vivo* and *in vitro*. *Journal of Investigative Dermatology* **86**, 149–156.

Boissy, R.E., Moellmann, G.E. & Lerner, A.B. (1987) Morphology of melanocytes in hair bulbs and eyes of vitiligo mice. *American Journal of Pathology* **127**, 380–388.

Boissy, R.E., Gecks, S., Smyth, J.R. Jr & Nordlund, J.J. (1988) Ocular pathology in the minimally depigmented subline of the vitiliginous Smyth chicken. *Pigment Cell Research* **1**, 303–314.

Boissy, R.E., Liu, Y.Y., Medrano, E.E. & Nordlund, J.J. (1991) Structural aberration of the rough endoplasmic reticulum and melanosome compartmentalization in long-term cultures of melanocytes from vitiligo patients. *Journal of Investigative Dermatology* **97**, 395–404.

Bowers, R.R. (1988) the melanocyte of the chicken: a review. *Progress in Clinical and Biological Research* **256**, 49–63.

Bowers, R.R., Harmon, J., Prescott, S., Asano, J. & Wynne, S. (1992) Fowl model for vitiligo: genetic regulation on the fate of the melanocytes. *Pigment Cell Research Supplement* **2**, 242–248.

Boyle, M.L., Pardue, S.L. & Smyth, J.R. Jr (1987) Effect of corticosterone on the incidence of amelanosis in Smyth delayed amelanotic line chickens. *Poultry Science* **66**, 363–367.

Bystryn, J.-C., Rigel, D., Friedman, R.J. & Kopf, A. (1987) Prognostic significance of hypopigmentation in malignant melanoma. *Archives of Dermatology* **123**, 1053–1055.

Cerundolo, R., DeCaprariis, D., Esposito, D.L., Maiolino, P., Restucci, B. & Roperto, F. (1993) Vitiligo in two water buffaloes: histological, histochemical, and ultrastructural investigations. *Pigment Cell Research* **6**, 23–28.

Cui, J., Chen, D., Misfeldt, M.L., Swinfard, R.W. & Bystryn, J.-C. (1995) Antimelanoma antibodies in swine with spontaneously regressing melanoma. *Pigment Cell Research* **8**, 60–63.

Cummings, M.P. & Nordlund, J.J. (1995) Chemical leukoderma; fact or fancy. *American Journal of Contact Dermatitis* **6**, 122–127.

Dunn, L.C. & Thigpen, L.W. (1930) The silver mouse, a recessive color variation. *Journal of Heredity* **21**, 495–498.

Erf, G.F. & Smyth, J.R. Jr (1995) Alterations in blood leukocyte populations in Smyth line chickens with autoimmune vitiligo. *Poultry Science* **75**, 351–356.

Erf, G.F., Trejo-Skalli, A.V. & Smyth, J.R. Jr (1995) T cells in regenerating feathers of Smyth line chickens with vitiligo. *Clinical Immunology and Immunopathology* **76**, 120–126.

Fishman, P., Merimski, O., Baharav, E. & Shoenfeld, Y. (1997) Autoantibodies to Tyrosinase; the bridge between melanoma and vitiligo. *American Cancer Society* **79**, 1461–1464.

Fite, K.V., Whitney, T., Montgomery, N. & Smyth, J.R. Jr (1983) Behavioral and central visual correlates of inherited retinal degeneration in the domestic chicken (*Gallus domesticus*). *Experimental Neurology* **79**, 729–745.

Fite, K.V., Bengston, L. & Doran, P. (1985) Retinal pigment epithelial correlates of avian retinal degeneration: Electron microscopic analysis. *Journal of Comparative Neurology* **231**, 310–322.

Fite, K.V., Pardue, S., Bengston, L., Hayden, D. & Smith, J.R. Jr (1986) Effects of cyclosporine in spontaneous, posterior uveitis. *Current Eye Research* **5**, 787–796.

Hara, I., Yoshizumi, T. & Houghton, A.N. (1995) Implicating a role for immune recognition of self in tumor rejection: passive immunization against the brown locus protein. *Journal of Experimental Medicine* **182**, 1609–1614.

Hodgkinson, C.A., Moore, K.J., Nakayama, A., Steingrimsson, E., Copeland, N.G., Jenkins, N.A. & Arnheiter, H. (1993) Mutations at the mouse microphthalmia locus are associated with defects in a gene encoding a novel basic helix-loop-helix-zipper protein. *Cell* **74**, 395–404.

Jackson, I.J., Chambers, D.M., Tsukamoto, K., Copeland, N.J., Gilbert, D.J., Jenkins, N.A. & Hearing, V. (1992) A second tyrosinase-related protein, TRP-2, maps to and is mutated at the mouse slaty locus. *EMBO Journal* **11**, 527–535.

Jimbow, K., Szabo, G. & Fitzpatrick, T.B. (1974) Ultrastructure investigation of autophagocytosis of melanosomes and programmed cell death of melanocytes in White Leghorn feather: a study of morphogenetic events leading to hypomelanosis. *Developmental Biology* **36**, 8–23.

Kawakami, Y. & Rosenberg, S.A. (1997) Immunobiology of human melanoma antigens MART-1 and gp100 and their use for immuno-gene therapy. *International Reviews of Immunology* **14**, 173–192.

Koh, H.K., Sober, A.J., Nakagawa, H., Albert, D.M., Mihm, M.C. & Fitzpatrick, T.B. (1983) Malignant melanoma and vitiligo-like leukoderma: an electron microscopic study. *Journal of the American Academy of Dermatology* **9**, 696–708.

Kosaras, B. & Sidman, R.L. (1996) Phagosome number and distribution in retinal pigment epithelial cells of vitiligo mutant mice. *Experimental Eye Research* **63**, 151–158.

Lamont, S.J. & Smyth, J.R. Jr (1981) Effect of bursectomy on development of a spontaneous postnatal amelanosis. *Clinical Immunology and Immunopathology* **21**, 407–411.

Lamont, S.J. & Smyth, J.R. Jr (1984) Effect of selection for delayed amelanosis on immune response in chickens. 1. Antibody production. *Poultry Science* **63**, 436–439.

Lamont, S.J., Boissy, R.E. & Smyth, J.R. Jr (1982) Humoral immune response and expression of spontaneous postnatal amelanosis in DAM line chickens. *Immunology Communications* **11**, 121–127.

Lamoreux, M.L., Gerrity, L. & Boissy, R.E. (1987) Animal Models of Human Disease: Vitiligo. *Comparative Pathology Bulletin* XIX, **2**, May.

Lamoreux, M.L., Boissy, R.E., Womack, J.E. & Nordlund, J.J. (1992) The vit gene maps to the mi (microphthalmia) locus of the laboratory mouse. *Journal of Heredity* **83**, 435–439.

Lamoreux, M.L., Zhou, B.K., Rosemblat, S. & Orlow, S.J. (1995) The pinkeyed-dilution protein and the eumelanin/pheomelanin switch: in support of a unifying hypothesis. *Pigment Cell Research* **8**, 263–270.

Le Poole, I.C., Das, P.K., van den Wijngaard, R.M., Bos, J.D. & Westerhof, W. (1993) Review of the etiopathomechanism of vitiligo: a convergence theory. *Experimental Dermatology* **2**, 145–153.

Lerner, A.B. & Cage, G.W. (1973) Melanomas in Horses. *Yale Journal of Biology and Medicine* **46**, 646–649.

Lerner, A.B., Shiohara, T., Boissy, R.E., Jacobson, K.A., Lamoreux, M.L. & Moellmann, G.E. (1986) A possible mouse model for vitiligo. *Journal of Investigative Dermatology* **87**, 299–304.

Marklund, L.M., Moller, M.J., Hoyheim, B., Davies, W., Fredholm, M., Juneja, R.K., Mariani, P., Coppieters, W., Ellegren, H. & Andersson, L. (1996) A comprehensive linkage map of the pig based on a wild pig-Large White intercross. *Animal Genetics* **27**, 255–269.

Merinsky, O., Shoenfeld, Y., Yecheskel, G., Chaitchik, S., Azizi, E. & Fishman, P. (1994) Vitiligo and melanoma-associated hypopigmentation: a similar appearance but a different mechanism. *Cancer Immunology Immunotherapy* **38**, 411–416.

Misfeldt, M.L. & Grimm, D.G. (1994) Sinclair miniature swine: an animal model of human melanoma. *Veterinary Immunology and Immunopathology* **43**, 167–175.

Moore, K.J. (1995) Insight into the microphthalmia gene. *Trends in Genetics* **11**, 442–448.

Morgan, C.D., Measel, J.W. Jr, Amoss, M.S. Jr, Rao, A. & Greene, J.F. Jr (1996) Immunophenotypic characterization of tumor infiltrating lymphocytes and peripheral blood lymphocytes isolated from melanomatous and non-melanomatous Sinclair miniature swine. *Veterinary Immunology and Immunopathology* **55**, 189–203.

Morse, H.C. III, Yetter, R.A., Stimpfling, J.H., Pitts, O.M., Fredrickson, T.N. & Hartley, J.W. (1985) Graying with age in mice: relation to expression of murine leukemia viruses. *Cell* **41**, 439–448.

Naftzger, C., Takechi, Y., Kohda, H., Hara, I., Vijayasaradhi, S. & Houghton, A.N. (1996) Immune response to a differentiation antigen induced by altered antigen: a study of tumor rejection and autoimmunity. *Proceedings of the National Academy of Sciences of the United States of America* **93**, 14809–14814.

Nakayama, K., Nakayama, K., Negishi, I., Kuida, K., Sawa, H. & Loh, D.Y. (1994) Targeted disruption of Bcl-2ab in mice: occurrence of gray hair, polycystic kidney disease and lymphocytopenia. *Proceedings of the National Academy of Sciences of the United States of America* **91**, 3700–3704.

Naughton, G.K., Mahaffey, M. & Bystryn, J.-C. (1986) Antibodies to surface antigens of pigmented cells in animals with vitiligo. *Proceedings of the Society for Experimental Biology and Medicine* **181**, 423–426.

Nir, I., Ransom, N. & Smith, S.B. (1995) Ultrastructural features of retinal dystrophy in mutant vitiligo mice. *Experimental Eye Research* **61**, 363–377.

Nordlund, J.J., Kirkwood, J.M., Forget, B.M., Milton, G., Albert, D.M. & Lerner, A.B.

(1983) Vitiligo in patients with metastatic melanoma: a good prognostic sign. *Journal of the American Academy of Dermatology* **9**, 689–696.

Nordlund, J.J., Csato, M., Babcock, G. *et al.* (1995) Low ICAM-1 expression in the epidermis of depigmenting C57GL/6J-mi^{vit}/mi^{vit} mice: a possible cause of muted contact sensitization. *Experimental Dermatology* **4**, 20–29.

Nordlund, J.J., Boissy, R.E., Hearing, V.J., King, R.A. & Ortonne, J.-P., eds. (1998). *The Pigmentary System: Physiology and Pathophysiology*. Oxford University Press, New York.

Norris, D.A., Horikawa, T. & Morell, J.G. (1994) Melanocyte destruction and repopulation in vitiligo. *Pigment Cell Research* **7**, 193–203.

Oh, Y.-S. & Tomita, T. (1987) Linkage of faded gene to chromosome 6 of the mouse. *Experimental Animals* **36**, 73–77.

Oh, Y.-S., Tomita, T. & Kondo, K. (1986) Faded, a mutation in the KSB strain of mouse which shows age-related pigment change. *Experimental Animals* **35**, 131–138.

Orlow, S.J., Zhou, B.-K., Chakraborty, A.K., Drucker, M., Pifko-Hirst, S. & Pawelek, J. (1994) High molecular weight forms of tyrosinase and tyrosinase-related proteins: evidence for a melanogenic complex. *Journal of Investigative Dermatology* **103**, 196–201.

Pardue, S.L., Fite, K.V., Bengston, L., Lamont, S.J., Boyle, M.L. III & Smyth, J.R. Jr (1987) Enhanced integumental and ocular amelanosis following the termination of cyclosporine administration. *Journal of Investigative Dermatology* **88**, 758–761.

Pathak, S. & Amoss, M.S. (1997) Genetic predisposition and specific chromosomal defects associated with Sinclair swine malignant melanoma. *International Journal of Oncology* **11**, 53–57.

Piedrahita, J.A., Moore, K., Oetama, B., Lee, C.-K., Scales, N., Ramsoondar, J., Bazer, F.W. & Ott, T. (1998) Generation of transgenic porcine chimeras using primordial germ cell-derived colonies. *Biology of Reproduction* **58**, 1321–1329.

Quevedo, W.C. Jr & Chase, H.B. (1958) An analysis of the light mutation of coat color in mice. *Journal of Morphology* **102**, 329–346.

Raymond, S.M. & Jackson, I.J. (1995) Requirement for retinal pigmented epithelium in development of the neural retina. *Current Biology* **5**, 1286–1295.

Rose, N.R. (1994) Avian models of autoimmune disease: lessons from the birds. *Poultry Science* **73**, 984–990.

Rosenberg, S.A. & White, D.E. (1996) Vitiligo in patients with melanoma. Normal tissue antigens can be targets for cancer immunotherapy. *Journal of Immunotherapy with Emphasis on Tumor Immunology* **19**, 81–84.

Searle, E.A., Austin, L.M., Boissy, Y.L., Zhao, H., Nordlund, J.J. & Boissy, R.E. (1993) Smyth chicken melanocyte autoantibodies: cross-species recognition, *in vivo* binding, and plasma membrane reactivity of the antiserum. *Pigment Cell Research* **6**, 145–157.

Shim, H., Gutierrez-Adan, A., Chen, L.R., BonDurant, R.H., Behboodi, E. & Anderson, G.B. (1997) Isolation of pluripotent stem cells from cultured porcine primordial germ cells. *Biology of Reproduction* **57**, 1089–1095.

Sidman, R.L. & Neumann, P. (1988) Vitiligo: a new retinal degeneration mutation. *Mouse News Letter* **81**, 60.

Sidman, R.L., Kosaras, B. & Tang, M. (1996) Pigment epithelial and retinal phenotypes in the vitiligo, mi^{vit}, mutant mouse. *Investigative Ophthalmology and Visual Science* **37**, 1097–1115.

Smirnakis, S.M., Tang, M. & Sidman, R.L. (1991) Abnormalities of pigment epithelium precede photoreceptor cell degeneration in vitiligo mutant mice. *Investigative Ophthalmology and Visual Science* **32**, 1056.

Smith, S.B. & Defoe, D.M. (1995) Autoradiographic and biochemical assessment of rod outer segment renewal in the vitiligo (C57BL/6- mi^{vit}/mi^{vit}) mouse model of retinal degeneration. *Experimental Eye Research* **60**, 91–96.

Smith, S.B. & Hamasaki, D.I. (1994) Electroretinographic study of the C57BL/6- mi^{vit}/mi^{vit} mouse model of retinal degeneration. *Investigative Ophthalmology and Visual Science* **35**, 3119–3123.

Smith, S.B. & Wiggert, B.N. (1995) Morphological and biochemical studies of the retinal degeneration in the vitiligo mouse. A model with perturbed retinoid metabolism. In:

Degenerative Diseases of the Retina (ed. R.E.Anderson *et al.*), pp. 155–162, Plenum Press, New York.
Smith, S.B., Zhou, B.K. & Orlow, S.J. (1988) Expression of tyrosinase and the tyrosinase related proteins in the Mitf^{vit} (vitiligo) mouse eye—implications for the function of the microphthalmia transcription factor (Mitf). *Experimental Eye Research* **66**, 403–410.
Smith, S.B., Cope, B.K., McCoy, J.R., McCool, D.J. & Defoe, D.M. (1994) Reduction of phagosomes in the vitiligo (C57BL/6- *mi^{vit}/mi^{vit}*) mouse model of retinal degeneration. *Investigative Ophthalmology and Visual Science* **35**, 3625–3632.
Smith, S.B., Bora, N., McCool, D., Kutty, G., Wong, P., Kutty, R.K. & Wiggert, B. (1995) Photoreceptor cells in the vitiligo mouse die by apoptosis. TRPM-2/Clusterin expression is increased in the neural retina and in the retinal pigment epithelium. *Investigative Ophthalmology and Visual Science* **36**, 2193–2201.
Smith, S.B., Brodjian, S., Desai, S. & Sarthy, V. (1997) Glial fibrillary acidic protein (GFAP) is synthesized in the early stages of the photoreceptor cell degeneration of the *mi^{vit}/mi^{vit}* (vitiligo) mouse. *Experimental Eye Research* **64**, 645–650.
Smith, S.B., McClung, J., Wiggert, B.N. & Nir, I. (1998) Delayed rhodopsin regeneration and altered distribution of interphotoreceptor retinoid binding protein (IRBP) in the *mi^{vit}/mi^{vit}* (vitiligo) mouse. *Journal of Neurocytology* **26**, 605–613.
Smyth, J.R. Jr (1989) the Smyth chicken: model of autoimmune amelanosis. *Critical Reviews in Poultry Science* **2**, 1–9.
Smyth, J.R. Jr (1990) Genetics of plumage, skin and eye pigmentation in chickens. In: *Poultry Breeding and Genetics* (ed. R.D.Crawford), pp. 109–167, Elsevier, Amsterdam.
Smyth, J.R. Jr, Boissy, R.E. & Fite, K.V. (1981) the DAM chicken: a model for spontaneous postnatal cutaneous and ocular amelanosis. *Journal of Heredity* **72**, 150–156.
Song, Y., Connor, E., Li, Y., Zorovich, B., Balducci, P. & Maclaren, N. (1994) The role of tyrosinase in autoimmune vitiligo. *Lancet* **344**, 1049–1052.
Sreekuman, G.P., Smyth, J.R. Jr, Bhogle, A.S., Lakshmanan, M. & Ponce de Leon, F.A. (1995) Incidence of avian leukosis in the Smyth line model for autoimmune vitiligo. *Poultry Science* **74** (Suppl. 2), 25.
Sreekuman, G.P., Smyth, J.R. Jr & Ponce de Leon, F.A. (1997) Genetic and molecular linkage analysis of the Smyth line chicken model for autoimmune human vitiligo. *Pigment Cell Research* **10**, 116.
Steel, K.P. (1981) *Mouse News Letter* **64** (76), 1981.
Tang, M., Ruiz, M., Kosaras, B. & Sidman, R.L. (1996) Increased cell genesis in retinal pigment epithelium of perinatal Vitiligo mutant mice. *Investigative Ophthalmology and Visual Science* **37**, 1116–1124.
Tang, M., Pawlyk, B.S., Kosaras, B., Berson, E.L. & Sidman, R.L. (1997) ERG abnormalities in relation to histopathologic findings in vitiligo mutant mice. *Experimental Eye Research* **65**, 215–222.
Veis, D.J., Sorenson, C.M., Shutter, J.R. & Korsmeyer, S.J. (1993) Bcl-2-deficient mice demonstrate fulminant lymphoid apoptosis, polycystic kidneys and hypopigmented hair. *Cell* **75**, 229–240.
Wang, R.-F., Parkhurst, M.R., Kawakami, Y., Robbins, P.F. & Rosenberg, S.A. (1996) Utilization of an alternative open reading frame of a normal gene in generating a novel human cancer antigen. *Journal of Experimental Medicine* **183**, 1131–1140.
Willier, B.H. & Rawles, M.E. (1940) The control of feather color pattern by melanophores grafted from one embryo to another of a different breed of fowl. *Physiological Zoology* **13**, 177–199.
Yamamura, K., Kamada, S., Ito, S., Nakagawa, K., Ichihashi, M. & Tsujimoto, Y. (1996) Accelerated disappearance of melanocytes in BCL-2-deficient mice. *Cancer Research* **56**, 3546–3550.

Index